Hair Research
for the
Next Millenium

Hair Research
for the
Next Millenium

Proceedings of the First Tricontinental Meeting of Hair Research Societies,
8-10 October 1995, Brussels, Belgium

Editors:

Dominique van Neste

Skin Study Centre
Skinterface sprl
Tournai, Belgium

Valerie A. Randall

Department of Biomedical Sciences
University of Bradford
Bradford , U.K.

Associate Editors:

Howard Baden

Charleston, MA
U.S.A.

Hideoki Ogawa

Tokyo
Japan

Roy Oliver

Dundee
U.K.

1996

ELSEVIER

Amsterdam • Lausanne • New York • Oxford • Shannon • Tokyo

International Congress Series No. 1111
ISBN 0 444 82336 0

This book is printed on acid-free paper.

Published by:
Elsevier Science B.V.
P.O. Box 211
1000 AE Amsterdam
The Netherlands

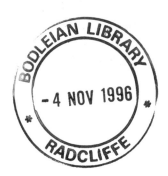

Printed in The Netherlands

Preface

As we go forward into the next millenium interest in hair follicle biology has never been so high. There is growing recognition of the usefulness of the hair follicle as a model system for fundamental research into aspects of cell biology, differentiating systems and/or as a hormone target organ with paradoxically different responses depending on its body site. This is paralleled by the recent recognition that hair regrowth can be stimulated in previously bald scalp in some individuals. Since hair loss, either caused by alopecia areata or male pattern baldness, is both common and distressing to the person concerned, there is obviously a major market for any successful treatment. Market forces have, therefore, contributed to the expansion of interest in both basic hair follicle biology and potential forms of treatment. There is also a growing interest in establishing the pathogenesis of alopecia areata which has been significantly fostered by the efforts of the «National Alopecia Areata Foundation». Nevertheless, the complex nature of the hair follicle, its cycles of growth and rest, mean that less experienced individuals find it difficult to study.

Major aspects of hair research are covered by the extensive range of papers in this book which contains the Proceedings of the First Tricontinental Meeting of Hair Research Societies held in Brussels in October 1995. This exciting milestone conference grew out of a planned, workshop type joint meeting of the «European Hair Research Society» with the «Hair Research Society» of the United States which was predicted to have a maximum of a hundred delegates. During the gestation period Japanese hair scientists formed their own «Society for Hair Science Research» so the meeting became «The Tricontinental». Even so, the organizers were very surprised at the interest the conference generated; 132 abstracts were accepted for presentation and over 300 delegates attended from an even wider area than those covered by the host societies, including Australia and Korea. This is particularly remarkable when almost all the research presented at the two and a half day meeting involved novel studies. The hair science that was to be considered during the meeting also attracted attendees from other remote countries such as Argentina, Brasil, Israel, Mexico, Thailand and Turkey.

Even though, there was no major formal programme for invited speakers reporting their previous work, the Scientific Organizing Committee was able to invite two sponsored plenary lecturers. The «National Alopecia Areata Foundation» sponsored a guest lecture by Dr Catherine Ziller, an embryologist, from the Institute of Cellular and Molecular Embryology, CNRS, Paris, France who updated delegates on highly relevant embryological development, with particular reference to aspects related to the hair follicle. Her paper now starts this book. The second was the «John Ebling Lecture» delivered by Professor W.J. Cunliffe. This lectureship has been awarded each year by the «European Hair Research Society» in honor of the late Professor John Ebling. John Ebling not only made major contributions to our understanding of basic hair follicle and sebaceous gland biology, but also promoted interest in the hair follicle both in Britain and throughout the world. Indeed, the origins of the first joint meeting can arguably be traced back to his influence. At the first meeting of the «European Hair Research Society» organized by Dr Rodney Dawber in 1989, John pointed out that of the forty delegates, over twenty had either worked and/or collaborated with him or he had examined their higher degrees!

The «John Ebling Lectureship» has been sponsored by Unilever Ltd, UK for the last three years in acknowledgement of their longstanding relationship with John Ebling in this field. All the Hair Research Societies and organizers of the Tricontinental meeting are very grateful for this and all the other sponsorship for the meeting, particularly the very generous support provided by L'Oréal, France, Merck & Co Ltd, USA and Procter and Gamble, UK. Without this support it would be almost impossible to organize such conferences or to publish the Proceedings. Obviously, providing the opportunity for hair follicle scientists to come together to present and discuss their science will advance the day when our understanding of the hair follicle increases to the level that good treatments with few side effects can be developed. In this way the sponsorship is beneficial to both parties.

Although we have made great strides recently, there is still much more that we do not know about the complex biology of the hair follicle in health or disease. Hopefully, based on the knowledge in this book we will achieve much greater understanding in the next millenium which will lead to the development of better treatments for hair disorders.

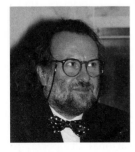

Dominique Van Neste

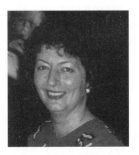

Valerie Anne Randall

Acknowledgements

The publication of this book should not have been possible without the enthusiasm and good will of the many contributors. The following list contains all the sponsors who supported the organization of the meeting:

Barbara Jordan - USA
Bioderma - France
Canfield Scientific - USA
Clairol - USA
Eli-Lilly - USA
Galderma Belgilux - Belgium
Glaxo - USA
Hoyu Co., Ltd. - Japan
Johnson and Johnson - USA
KAO Corporation - Japan
L'Oréal - France
Lundbeck N.V. - Belgium
Merck - USA
NAAF - USA
Neutrogena - USA
Oclassen - USA
Pierre Fabre Cosmétique - France
Pola Laboratories - Japan
Procter & Gamble - UK
Roussel Uclaf - France
Sandoz - USA
Schering - USA
Shiseido - Japan
Taisho Pharmaceutical Co., Ltd. - Japan
The Society of Hair Science Research
Unilever - UK
Upjohn - USA

The processing of all manuscripts, and the preparation of subject index and list of contributing authors would not have been achieved in due time without the expert assistance of Bernadette de Brouwer, Treasurer of the «European Hair Research Society», and the staff members of Skinterface Skin Study Center: Véronique Ronsse who prepared the lay-out, Hannelore Dupont, secretary, and the technicians, Thérèse Leroy, Caroline Tételin and Céline Geveaux.

Their sustained interest in organizing the day-to-day necessary links with the Editors has been much appreciated.

Contents

6

Physical aspects and hair transplantation techniques

8

Structure and function

Alopecia areata

10

Androgens and antiandrogens

12

Sebaceous gland

Paracrine factors in the hair follicle

14

An introduction to morphogenesis

©1996 Elsevier Science B.V. All rights reserved.
Hair research for the next millenium
D.J.J. Van Neste and V.A. Randall (Eds)

Pattern formation in neural crest derivatives

C. Ziller

Institut d'Embryologie Cellulaire et Moléculaire du CNRS et du Collège de France, 49bis, Avenue de la Belle-Gabrielle, 94736 Nogent-sur-Marne cedex, France

Introduction

The neural crest of the vertebrate embryo is a population of cells arising from the lateral ridges of the neural tube at late neurula stage. While the neural tube is closing, the neural crest cells lose their epithelial organization and become mesenchymal. They leave their original position and undergo extensive migrations through the developing embryo, settling in various homing sites where they give rise to a large diversity of different cell types.

The derivatives of the neural crest include most constituents of the peripheral nervous system (PNS), i.e. sensory and autonomic neurons, ganglionic satellite cells and Schwann cells; pigment cells; endocrine and paraendocrine cells; mesectodermal derivatives in the head (bones, cartilage, dermis, connective tissues, meninges).

The migration pathways and phenotypic fates of neural crest cells have been studied with several labeling techniques. The quail-chick labeling system devised by Le Douarin [1] relies on a histological difference between chick and quail cells; in the nucleus of quail cells, a mass of heterochromatin is associated with the nucleolus which thus reacts positively with DNA stains. Embryonic tissues from one species can be grafted into the other at early stages of development and the fate of the implanted cells can be followed in the chimeric embryos. Isotopic transplantations of defined segments of the neural primordium along the neural axis have allowed us to establish precisely the migration pathways and the derivatives of the neural crest. These experiments also show that the neural crest is regionalized; different levels of the neural crest give rise to different sets of derivatives. However, in heterotopic transplantations, when they are translocated from one level of the body axis to another, neural crest cells behave according to the environment in which they are placed experimentally, and not according to their level of origin. In fact, all the levels of the neural crest have the potential to give rise to all types of derivatives (except the cephalic mesenchyme). This demonstrates the pluripotentiality of the neural crest as a population and the important role of the embryonic environment in determining the differentiation of neural crest cells. The neural crest has therefore to be regarded as a pluripotent cell population, whose phenotypic diversification is related to the environments through which neural crest cells travel and into which they become localized. Both while they are en route and when they have reached their sites of arrest, they depend upon cell to cell and cell-matrix interactions, and upon environmental factors required for their survival, proliferation and differentiation.

Heterogeneity of the neural crest

Environmental factors may either select among differently committed precursors or exert an instructive action on pluripotent precursors; an intermediate possibility is that the neural crest is composed of a mixture of pluripotent and more or less restricted progenitors.

The latter hypothesis was confirmed by a number of experiments, carried out mainly *in vitro*, which showed that the neural crest is a heterogeneous population when migration starts. The apparent homogeneity of the early neural crest was challenged both by the finding that several antigenic markers are not uniformly expressed by migrating crest cells [2-5] and by the fact that a subset of neuronal precursors appears to be specified early in development [6].

The state of commitment of neural crest cells was precisely evaluated in cloning experiments, performed *in vivo* and *in vitro,* with avian and mammalian cells [7-9 for reviews and references].

It appeared that in most cases, individual neural crest cells give rise to clones composed of cells which express several different phenotypes, thus revealing the puripotentiality of the founder cell. However, in some clones, all the cells express the same phenotype, for instance neuronal or glial, or pigmented. These monophenotypic colonies derive from apparently committed progenitors. These findings clearly demonstrate the heterogeneity of early neural crest cells, in terms of developmental potentials. Therefore, the differentiation and final fate of neural crest derivatives are the result of an interplay between intrinsic and external influences.

Few cells of early migrating quail cephalic neural crest generate clones that contain representatives of all the main lineages normally arising from the neural crest: neurons, glia, melanocytes and mesenchymal cells (cartilage). These cells can be considered as stem-like cells [10]. Interestingly, this shows that common precursors for mesectodermal, melanocytic and neural derivatives are present in the neural crest at an early migration stage.

The contribution of the neural crest to the head structures

In addition to neural derivatives (peripheral ganglia) and melanocytes, the cephalic neural crest gives rise to mesenchymal structures, the so-called mesectoderm, which includes cartilage, bones, dermis and connective tissue in the head.

By means of the quail-chick marker system, the contribution of the cephalic neural crest to the head has been precisely analyzed [7, 11 for a review and references]. Isotopic and isochronic grafts of precisely defined regions of the quail neural fold into chick embryos were performed prior to the onset of neural crest migration. These experiments showed that the frontal and parietal bones of the skull and the corresponding cephalic dermis are all of neural crest origin. In fact, the neural crest gives rise not only to the facial and hypobranchial skeleton, as had been previously established, but also to the vault of skull. Moreover, the anterior half of the skull basis is also of neural crest origin. In this region, the neural crest contribution to the head structures corresponds to the tip of the notochord. Interestingly, the cephalic mesoderm does not contribute to dermis in any cephalic area except in the occipital region.

These transplantations also allowed the precise localization of the anterior limit of the neural crest in the area of the diencephalon from which the epiphysis arises. Rostrally to this level, the epitheliomesenchymal conversion of the neural epithelium does not occur. The anterior neural fold gives rise to endocrine, neuroepithelial and epithelial structures: the adenohypophysis, the olfactory placodes, the epithelia of the olfactory organ, the roof of the mouth, and the epidermis of the superior lip, nose and frontal area.

At the level of the hindbrain, the patterning of the neural crest has been shown to be controlled by regulatory homeobox-containing genes [8, 9 for reviews]. The expression of *Hox* genes in the rhombencephalon and in the neural crest-derived mesenchyme of the branchial arches was suggestive of a role in generating diversity. This evidence was supported by the result of targeted mutations in the hindbrain of mice: absence of *Hoxa-3* gene product caused a phenocopy of the human Di George syndrome, in which the mesenchymal neural crest derivatives of the hindbrain are essentially missing. Null mutation of the *Hoxa-1* gene mainly induced defects in the neural derivatives of the crest. Other homeobox genes, of the *msh* family, designated as *Msx* 1 and 2, may be involved in patterning cephalic crest-derivatives. Targeted and naturally occurring mutations in these genes cause abnormalities in the cranial bones, in mandibula and maxilla and in tooth, all neural crest-derived skeletal structures.

Control of the development of neural crest-derived melanocytes

In vertebrates, three main cell types migrate extensively before differentiating and depend for their development on the same growth factor encoded by the *Steel* (*Sl*) gene: primordial germ cells, hemopoietic cells, and the melanocyte population, a derivative of the neural crest.

Sl and *Dominant White Spotting* (*W*) mutants have long been known to exhibit the same phenotype characterized by depigmentation, sterility, and anemia [7 for references]. Both mutations are generally lethal in the homozygous condition and exhibit varying degrees of abnormality in heterozygotes, the most prominent of which affect pigmentation, ranging from black-eyed white to white-spotted coat color [12]. The gene products of both the *W* and *Sl* loci have been identified and characterized at the molecular level. The *W* gene corresponds to the proto-oncongene *c-kit* which encodes a tyrosine kinase receptor. The cognate ligand of the *c-kit* receptor is the growth factor encoded by the *Sl* locus called Stem cell growth factor (SCF), Steel factor (SLF), or mast cell growth factor (MCF). The *Sl* cDNA encodes a membrane-bound protein which can be cleaved to produce a soluble form. The soluble recombinant protein encoded by *Sl* is endowed with biological activity, as was shown *in vitro* for primordial germ cells [13] and for melanocyte precursors. Chicken recombinant SCF affects the development of melanocytes from quail neural crest cells in culture [14]: the total number of neural crest cells, of melanocytes and of their precursors is higher in the presence than in the absence of SCF. SCF has a modest and transient mitogenic effect on the neural crest population. It also enhances the differentiation rate of melanocyte precursors, recognized by the «melanocyte early marker» monoclonal antibody [MelEM, 5] and of melanocytes. Finally, SCF increases the survival of the neural crest cell population as a whole. These observations support the notion that SCF has a functional role *in vivo*, by sustaining the survival of the neural crest cell population and stimulating the rate of the melanogenic differentiation process. Moreover, the results of *in vitro* studies and the observations on mutated animals are corroborated by the expression pattern of *c-kit* and *Sl* in the developing skin of mice [15] and avians [16].

Concluding remarks

Recent developments in the field of neural crest ontogeny concern the massive contribution of crest cells to the vertebrate head, their pluripotentiality, and the role of intrinsic (regulatory genes) and extrinsic (growth factors, cell-cell and cell-matrix interactions) factors in their determination. For example, the role of an interplay between a growth factor, SCF and its receptor has been clearly established for the differentiation of pigment cells from pluripotent precursors. Other important growth factors, the neurotrophins, and their receptors, are involved in the development of neural derivatives of the neural crest, as suggested by various effects of neurotrophins, *in vitro* and *in vivo*, and by the analysis of mice with null mutations of the genes encoding neurotrophins and their receptors, which points to a critical role of these molecules in the development of the nervous system.

References

1 Le Douarin NM. The Neural Crest. Cambridge University Press, Cambridge. 1982
2 Barbu M, Ziller C, Rong PM, Le Douarin NM. J Neurosci. 1986; 6: 2215-2225
3 Steel KP, Davidson DC, Jackson IJ. Development. 1992; 115: 1111-1119
4 Kitamura K, Takiguchi-Hayashi K, Sezaki M, Yamamoto H, Takeuchi T. Development. 1992; 114: 367-378
5 Nataf V, Mercier P, Ziller C, Le Douarin NM. Exp Cell Res. 1993; 207: 171-182
6 Ziller C, Dupin E, Brazeau P, Paulin D, Le Douarin NM. Cell. 1983; 32: 627-638
7 Le Douarin NM, Ziller C, Couly, GF. Dev Biol. 1993; 159: 24-49
8 Le Douarin NM, Ziller C. Curr Opin Cell Biol. 1993; 5: 1036-1043
9 Le Douarin NM, Dupin E, Ziller C. Curr Opin Genet Dev. 1994; 4: 685-695
10 Baroffio A, Dupin E, Le Douarin NM. Development. 1991; 112: 301-305
11 Couly GF, Coltey PM, Le Douarin NM. Development. 1993; 117: 409-429
12 Williams DE, de Vries P, Namen AE, Widmer MB, Lyman SD. Dev Biol. 1992; 151: 368-376
13 Godin I, Deed R, Cooke J, Zsebo K, Dexter M, Wylie CC. Nature. 1991; 352: 807-809
14 Lahav R, Ziller C, Lecoin L, Nataf V, Martin FH, Carnahan JF, Langley KE, Boone, TC Le Douarin NM. Differentiation. 1994; 58: 133-139
15 Keshet E, Lyman SD, Williams DE, Anderso DM, Jenkins Na, Copeland NG, Parada LF. EMBO J. 1991; 10: 2425-2435
16 Lecoin L, Lahav R, Martin FH, Teillet MA, Le Douarin NM. Dev Dyn. 1995; 203: 106-118

Clinical conditions:
diagnosis and management

The hair : a diagnostic clue in Menkes syndrome

U. Blume-Peytavi[1], S. Völger[2], J. Föhles[3], K.H. Phan[3], G. Götte[2] and C.E. Orfanos[1]

[1]Department of Dermatology, University Medical Center Benjamin Franklin, Free University of Berlin, Germany
[2]Cristophorus Pediatric Service, Berlin, Germany
[3]German Wool Research Institute, Technic University of Aachen, Germany

Introduction

Menkes steely hair disease, first described by Menkes [1] in 1962, is an x-chromosomal recessive neurodegenerative disorder of copper-metabolism with intracellular accumulation of metallothionein bound copper, decrease of serum copper and decrease in the activity of essential copper-dependent enzymes [2, 3]. Subsequently, an irreversible damage of the nervous and connective tissue originates. Affected male children have growth failure, severe psychomotoric retardation, distinct neurologic defect with myoclonic seizures, typical hair structure anomalies such as pili torti, and mostly die within the first 3 years of life.

Materials and methods

Case report

We report on a 15-months-old boy who was born after an uncomplicated pregnancy as the first child of unrelated parents. Since birth he presented an increased tiredness and failure to thrive, since 5 months of age he developed growth retardation, increasing muscle hypotonia with incapacity of headbearing. At 15 months of age the patient was not able to sit and crawl, he could hold his head only for a few minutes, but had no myoclonic seizures so far. Three of the maternal great-grandmother's sons deceased at 2 years of age, a daughter, our patient's grandmother, developed normally.

Clinical findings

15-months-old boy, height, weight 75th percentile, head circumference 97th percentile, relative normal muscle reflexes, decreased tonus of the muscles. Pasty, pallid skin, white-yellow depigmented, lusterless, stubby hair, no involvement of the eyebrows and eyelashes.

Laboratory findings

Routine laboratory parameters within the normal range, but significant reduction of copper and coeruloplasmin levels in the serum (age-related values), slightly elevated alanine in urine and serum analysis.

X-ray of the hands
Demineralisation of the handroot bones, retardation of development.

Nuclear resonance tomography:
Markedly widened liquor spaces, particularly in the fronto-temporal region, atrophy of the cerebellum with retardation of myelinisation of 3-6 months.

Muscle biopsy
Myopathic pattern with elevated lipid content of the muscular fibres.

Light microscopy
Longitudinal embedding of cut hair showed hair shaft diameter irregularities, pili torti, in several parts trichorrhexis nodosa-like fractures.

Scanning electron microscopy
Hair shaft torsions along the longitudinal axis, with loss of the cuticle in several areas (Fig. 1a), horizontal fissures or fractures (Fig. 1b).

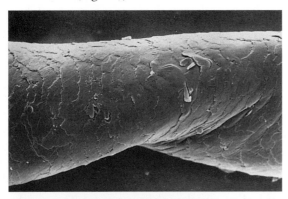

Figure 1a. Scanning electron microscopy with right handed torsion of the hair shaft

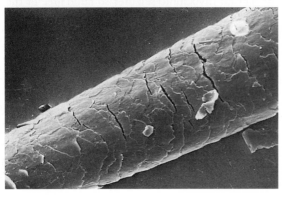

Figure 1b. Deep horizontal fissures of the hair shaft with splitting of the cuticle

Amino acid analysis

Our patient's hair revealed a significant increase of lanthionine in the parietal and occipital region, whereas cysteine was only elevated in the occipital region.

Amino acid	Normal	15-months-old patient with Menkes disease	
	control mmol/g hair	parietal mmol/g hair	occipital mmol/g hair
Cysteine acid	16,2	21,5	12,3
Glutamine acid	877,1	1003,6	1015,3
Lanthionine	0	61,9	75,3
Cysteine	24,0	-	90,0

EDX-analysis (Fig. 2)

The analysis of our patient's hair showed a copper concentration of 3000-5000 ppm. The copper (Cu) content of human hair is about 50-70 ppm; as the detection limit is about 200 ppm for EDX-analysis, normally, copper cannot even be demonstrated in human hair by EDX. However, in our patient distinct copper-peaks could be detected. These different copper peaks are due to the various ionic states of copper leading to different absorption of the Kα- and Kβ-rays used in this technique. Pre-treatment of the hair with gold (Au) before EDX-analysis accounts for the distinct displayed gold (Au) peaks and are thereby solely methodically implied.

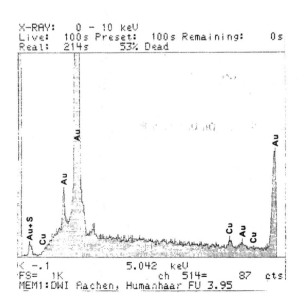

Figure 2. EDX-analysis of the patient's hair revealing distinct copper and gold peaks. The latter are artificially induced by pre-treatment with gold, whereas the copper peaks display significant pathologic copper accumulation in the hair

Discussion

Careful clinical and laboratory examination of our 15-months-old patient with strikingly white-yellow hair revealed pili torti with horizontal fissures, growth failure, psychomotor retardation, muscle hypotonia, progressive cerebral degeneration and decrease of copper and coeruloplasmin in serum. Careful analysis of his hair revealed an important accumulation of copper and an increased level of cysteine and lanthionine in the hair. Thus, in our patient the hair was the diagnostic clue to confirm the clinically suspected diagnosis of Menkes syndrome.

Menkes kinky hair disease, a lethal X-linked recessive trait, is characterized by abnormal copper accumulation in several non-hepatic tissues. It is likely caused by a still unknown defective intracellular copper transportation protein with faultive intracellular copper transport. Various therapeutic attempts with systemic application of copper-histidine complexes have been performed with rather discouraging results. Except when treatment is started before manifestation of neurologic or developmental defects prognosis can be influenced to a certain extent [5, 6].

Recent results support the presumption that the genetic defect is located on the long arm of chromosome 13 (Xq 13.3) [4], however also in 1/3 of all cases there is new mutation. In the case of our patient the family history of the boy's mother confirmed an X-linked recessive inheritance. Careful and correct diagnosis of this lethal proceeding disorder enables an adequate genetic counselling of the parents, and in the next pregnancy a first trimester prenatal diagnosis can be performed [7, 8].

References

1   Menkes JH, Alter M, Steigleder GK, Weakly DR, Sung JH. Pediatrics. 1962; 29: 764-779
2   Leone A. Horiz Biochem Biophys. 1986; 8: 207-256
3   Herd SM, Camakaris J, Christofferson R, Wockey P, Danks DM. Biochem J. 1987; 247: 341-47
4   Horn N, Tonnesen T, Tumer Z. Brain Pathol. 1992; 2: 351-362
5   Tonnesen T, Horn N, Sondergaard F, Jensen OA, Gerdes AM, Girard S, Damsgaard E. Prenat Diagn. 1987; 7: 497-509
6   Tonnesen T, Gerdes AM, Damsgaard E, Miny P, Holzgreve W, Sondergaard F, Horn N. Prenat Diagn. 1989; 9: 159-165
7   Nadal D, Baerlocher K. Eur J Pediatr. 1988; 147: 621-625
8   Kreuder J, Otten A, Fuder H, Tumer Z, Tonnesen T, Horn N, Dralle D. Eur J Pediatr. 1993; 152: 828-832

Trichothiodystrophy associated with urological malformation and primary hypercalciuria

J. Malvehy[1], J. Ferrando[1], A. Tuneu[3], F. Ballesta[2], J. Soler[1] and T. Estrach[1]

[1]Departments of Dermatology and [2]Genetics, Hospital Clinic. Faculty of Medicine. Villarroel 170, 08036 Barcelona, Spain
[3]Department of Dermatology, Hospital Nuestra Senora de Aranzazu, San Sebastian, Spain

Introduction

Trichothiodystrophy (TTD) is a rare hair abnormality with a complex neuroectodermal dysplasia. We report a case of TTD in a patient with congenital ichthyosis, physical and mental retardation, a complex urological malformation and primary hypercalciuria. To our knowledge, this is the first case of trichothiodystrophy associated with urinary malformation.

Materials and methods

Case report

A 20 year-old white male, diagnosed as ectodermal dysplasia, was consulted at the Hospital Clinic of Barcelona for evaluation of a syndrome consisting of congenital ichthyosis, facial dysmorphy and physical and mental retardation.

Clinical background was presided by a complex urologic malformation consisting of right hydronephrosis with a ureteral duplicity and left pyelocalicial ectasia (Fig. 1). Type II hyperabsorptive idiopatic hypercalciuria and hyper IgE (urine) was diagnosed at the age of 18. The patient revealed the following physical and laboratory findings.

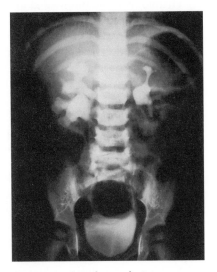

Figure 1. Complex urologic malformation: right hydronephrosis with an ureteral duplicity and left pyelocalicial ectasia

General

Sociable, alert boy with an aged appearance. Weight of 32 kg/height of 148 cm (both below the 3rd percentile). Asymmetric face, hypertelorism and microdolychocephaly, receding chin, dysmorphic and protruding ears with a low implantation. Mental retardation.

Hair

Dark brown, short and sparse (frontal/occipital areas). Breakage and irregular length. Sparse eyebrows with alopecia (external portion). Normal eyelashes and axillary and pubic hairs. Follicular keratosis.

Skin

Ichthyotic brownish scales of 0.5 to 1 cm diameter on the lateral trunk and abdomen (face and folds sparse). Severe hyperkeratosis on palms and soles. Breakable hypoplastic nails with transversal ridging.

Dental

Multiple caries without dysplasic changes.

O.R.L.

Nodules in vocal cords and rough voice.

Laboratory

Histology of the biopsied skin was compatible with lamellar ichthyosis.

Neither haematologic nor biochemic serum alterations were observed. Urinary examination: high levels of calcium (6.22 mg/kg/24h (normal < 4 mg/kg/24h)). Endocrinologic evaluation (thyroid, serum cortisol and growth hormone) was normal.

Chromosome analysis: normal male, 46XY karyotype. Roentgenograms: scoliosis.

Analysis of the hair

Light microscopy: clear transverse fractures through the hair shafts (trichoschisis), with irregular hair surface and diameter. The distal aspect of the broken shaft was of «brush breaks» appearance. The twisting and irregular hairs showed a «trichorrhexis nodosa»-like or a «pili torti» patterns.

Polarizing microscopy: alternance of dark and light bands in a «tiger tail» or «zigzag» pattern.

Scanning electron microscopy: very flattened hairs with severely damaged cuticle, longitudinal grooves and irregular crests with the image of trichoschisis (Figs. 2 and 3).

X-Ray microanalysis: reduction of its sulfur content (25% of normal control).

Phototesting: no photosensitivity to UVA, UVB nor UVC. Increased minimal erythema dose (secondary to ichthyosis). UV studies with cultured fibroblasts were not performed.

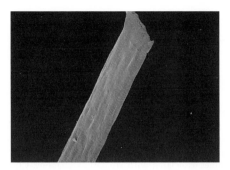 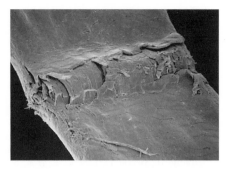

Figures 2 and 3. Scanning electron microscopy: very flattened hairs with severe damage of the cuticle or absence of it, longitudinal grooves and irregular crests with images of trichoschisis

Discussion

The most important finding of TTD is low sulfur content of the hair determined by X-ray microanalysis, amino acid analysis or electron dispersive analysis [1]. This abnormality must be associated with at least one of the following findings: trichoschisis, alternating light and dark bands by polarizing microscopy, or absent or severely damaged hair cuticle by scanning electron microscopy [2]. The finding of a single, isolated hair is not sufficient to establish the diagnosis of TTD.

TTD is associated with an heterogeneous spectrum of neuroectodermal disorders with an autosomic recessive pattern of heritance. The range of clinical phenotypes associated with TTD is not well known, and the plethora of eponyms and acronyms (Pollit syndrome, Tay syndrome, Sabinas syndrome, Amish Brittle Hair, BIDS, IBIDS, PIBIDS, SIBIDS, ONMRS) in published reports causes confusion rather than enlightenment [3]. A pragmatic method for categorizing the patients in subgroups by severity was proposed by Van Neste *et al.* [4].

To our knowledge there are no previously reported cases of TTD associated with urinary malformation. Our patient presented a rare complex urologic malformation consisting of a right hydronephrosis with an ureteral duplicity and a left pyelocalicial ectasia. Ectodermal disorders are congenital diseases with the main manifestations expressed in tissues of ectodermal origin. However, ectodermal dysplasias usually accompagnied mesodermal and rarely endodermal dysplasias. During embryogenesis, tissue organization involves all germ layers [2].

The presence of hypercalciuria and elevated IgE level in urine have not been previously described with correlation to ectodermal abnormality.

It will be important to analyze other tissues of TTD patients besides the hair and skin for amino acid composition and DNA excision repair since the basis of the sulfur matrix protein defect, and the role of DNA repair proteins remain the most fascinating questions of this heterogeneous disorder.

References

1   Price VH, Richard BO, Ward WH, Jones FH. Trichothiodystrophy. Arch Dermatol. 1980; 116: 1378-1384
2   Itin PH, Pittelkow MR. Trichothiodystrophy: review of sulfur-deficient brittle hair syndromes and association with the ectodermal dysplasias. J Am Acad Dermatol. 1990; 22: 705-717
3   Tolmie JL, Berker D, Dawber R, *et al.* Syndromes associated with trichothiodystrophy. Clin Dysmorphol. 1994; 3: 1-14
4   Van Neste D. Trichothiodystrophy: Recent advances. Eur J Pediatr Dermatol. 1991; 1: 45-50

A structural defect in the fibre cuticle of hair resulting from a deficiency in the enzyme branched chain 2-oxo acid dehydrogenase

L.N. Jones[1] and D.E. Rivett[2]

[1]CSIRO Division of Wool Technology, Belmont, Victoria 3216, Australia
[2]CSIRO Division of Biomolecular Engineering, Parkville, Victoria 3052, Australia

Introduction

Mammalian hairs consist of spindle-shaped cortical cells surrounded by multiple layers of flattened rectangular cuticle cells. The hydrophobic nature of mammalian hair can be explained if the cuticle surface is coated with long chain fatty acids. Recent research has shown that not only does the cuticle surface of mammalian hair consist of a heavily acylated protein but that the surface lipid component is dominated by the unusual anteiso fatty acid, 18-methyleicosanoic acid (C_{21a}) [1-4].

A deficiency in the enzyme, branched 2-oxo acid dehydrogenase leads to the accumulation of valine, leucine and isoleucine and the derived α-ketoacids (Maple Syrup Urine Disease, MSUD) which would lead to defects in the synthesis of branched-chain fatty acids derived from the branched-chain amino acids [5]. In hair from MSUD patients the C_{21a} should be absent, with a potential malformation in the fibre cuticle (FCU). We have presently characterized the chemical and structural effects on hair shafts in MSUD. The location and function of C_{21a} in human hair fibres is discussed.

Materials and methods

Hair samples
Two samples of human scalp hair, approximately 100 mg each, were obtained from patients diagnosed with Maple Syrup Urine Disease.

Lipid analysis
After removal of solvent (chloroform/methanol) extractable lipids, the covalently bound fatty acids were removed and alkylated according to Negri et al. 1991 [4].

Transmission electron microscopy

Hair samples (control and MSUD) were reduced in 0.5 M thioglycollic acid (pH 5.6) for 3h, washed and immersed in 2% w/v osmium tetroxide for 72 hours. After dehydration they were embedded in Spurr's medium. Sections were post stained with 0.5% w/v uranyl acetate and Reynolds' lead citrate.

Results and discussion

Studies using transmission electron microscopy have shown that the structural defect in MSUD hair appears to be confined to the β-layers of FCU cells (Fig. 1). These β-layers comprise the so-called fibre cuticle surface membrane (FCUSM) [7].

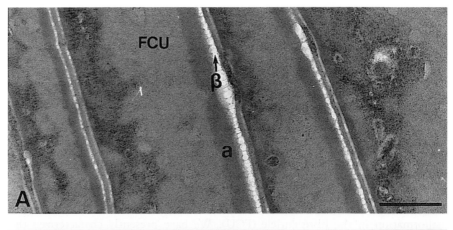

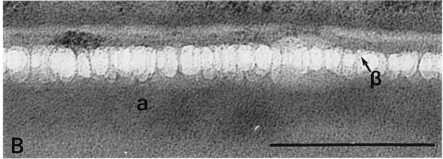

Figure 1. Micrographs showing defect in FCU of hairs from MSUD patients. The defect is confined to the surface β-layers (β) shown in A. In B the surface defect is shown in greater detail. The a-layer is denoted (a). Bars equal 100nm.

Other observations have indicated that the structural fault was located in the β-layers in the upper surface of FCU cells while the β-layers on the underside of FCU cells were not affected. This observation argues for a difference in the composition of FCU surface membranes with respect to the upper and lower surfaces.

In recent studies the formation of the FCUSM in mammalian hair follicles was monitored using energy-filtered transmission electron microscopy [7]. The findings demonstrated that the original presumptive FCU plasma-membrane on the upper surface was disrupted during cuticle cell development while the plasma membrane on the underside was essentially maintained intact throughout the differentiation process. The emerging FCUSM (outer surface) was derived from newly synthesized intercellular laminae. The currently observed defect in MSUD is in agreement with these conclusions.

The most obvious difference in the ratio of covalently bound fatty acids between MSUD hair and normal hair is the 90% or more reduction in C_{21a} and the 3-fold increase in C20: 0 in the MSUD hair (Table 1). Eicosanoic acid (C20: 0) is usually a relatively minor constituent of the bound fatty acids in hair fibres (comprising approximately 5%) but in MSUD hair it is one of the major fatty acids, 15-19% of the total, and appears to some extent to replace C_{21a}. In MSUD hair there appears to be a general increase in all of the linear saturated fatty acids, particularly 16: 0, 18: 0 and 20: 0 with the increase in the latter being the most pronounced.

One of the major physical differences between eicosanoic acid (C20: 0) and 18-methyleicosanoic acid (C_{21a}) is in the melting points. The introduction of a methyl group lowers the melting point from 77°C for the former to 56°C for the latter. The loss of C_{21a} in the cuticle membrane and its replacement with C20: 0 would possibly affect the fluidity of the membrane, leading to greater stiffness or rigidity and possibly loss of adhesion between the cells. We suggest that C_{21a} has a specific structural role in the fibre, a concept which is reinforced by the finding of significant amounts of this uncommon fatty acid covalently linked to the cuticle of the hair fibres from most mammals [8].

Hence, in this context the observed structural defect associated with the β-layers of FCU cells in hair from MSUD patients correlates with disruption in the synthesis of C_{21a}. We can consequently conclude that in normal hair the C_{21a} is present in the outer β-layers of FCU cells.

Table 1

Percentage (mol) of major covalently bound fatty acids in MSUD and normal hair

Fatty acid	MSUD Hair (Patient 1)	MSUD Hair (Patient 2)	Normal Hair	
C14: 0	3.6	5.7	7.6	3.2
C15: 0	1.5	2.3	4.6	2.4
C16: 1	1.6	2.4	3.3	1.3
C16: 0	38.0	38.5	33.5	27.8
C17: 0br	0.6	0.6	3.2	4.5
C17: 0	3.0	3.0	4.1	3.6
C18: 1	2.7	7.0	3.1	2.6
C18: 0	20.8	17.3	12.0	10.4
C19: 0br	0.1	0.0	1.4	2.0
C20: 0br	0.0	0.0	1.3	1.8
C20: 0	18.8	15.6	5.6	5.2
C21: 0a	1.8	1.6	17.8	31.7
C21: 0	1.1	1.3	0.8	1.3
C22: 0	3.3	2.6	0.9	1.1
C24: 0	3.2	1.9	0.8	1.0
Total (µg/mg)	201	178	147	139

A potential benefit derived from this work could be the use of hair ultrastructural studies in conjunction with analysis for C_{21a}, or a ratio of C_{21a} to C20: 0, in the hair of patients as an extra diagnostic tool for MSUD.

References

1   Kopke V and Nilssen BJ. Text. Inst. 1960; 51: T1398-T1413
2   Evans DJ, Leeder JD, Rippon JA and Rivett DE. Proc. 7th Int. Wool Text. Res. Conf. Tokyo. 1985; 1: 135-142
3   Wertz PW and Downing DT. Lipids. 1988; 23: 878-881
4   Negri AP, Cornell HJ and Rivett DE. Aust. J. Agric. Res. 1991; 42: 1285-1292
5   Zhang B, Healy PJ, Zhao Y, Crabb DW and Harris RA. J. Biol. Chem. 1990; 265: 2425-2427
6   Negri AP. PhD Dissertation. Royal Melbourne Inst. of Technology. 1993
7   Jones LN, Horr T and Kaplin IJ. Micron. 1994; 25: 589-595
8   Peet DJ, Wettenhall REH and Rivett DE. Comp. Biochem. Physiol. 1992; 102B: 363-366

Generalized congenital hypotrichosis and male pseudohermaphroditism

J.-J. Stene[1], J.-P. Chanoine[2], G.E. Piérard[3], D. Van Neste[4] and M. Song[1]

[1]Department of Dermatology, Hôpital Universitaire St-Pierre, U.L.B., Brussels, Belgium
[2]Department of Pediatrics, HUDERF, U.L.B., Brussels, Belgium
[3]CHU Liège, Belgium
[4]Skin Study Center, Skinterface, Tournai, Belgium

Case report

O.H. was born in 1979 from Aramean parents originating from the same village though unrelated. Around the sixth week of pregnancy, the mother took without success abortive drugs of unknown composition. Neither parents nor the seven other children showed any abnormality.

In 1984, sexual ambiguity was diagnosed for the first time (Fig. 1). There were high testicles located in the labia majora, a 30 x 13 mm penis and perineoscrotal hypospadias with a rudimentary vagina. Uterus and ovaries were absent. We found a normal male 46 XY karyotype. Gonadotrophin secretion and

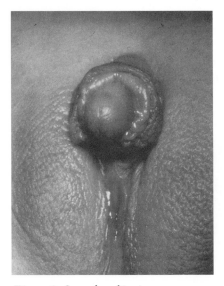

Figure 1. Sexual ambiguity

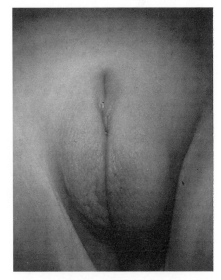

Figure 2. After surgical correction

levels of testosterone and dihydrotestosterone were within normal limits. Since the child has always been regarded as a girl, a surgical procedure was considered. This included castration, clitoridoplasty and vaginoplasty (Fig. 2).

Later on associated abnormalities were diagnosed: in 1993, we noted generalized congenital hypotrichosis (Fig. 3). There were thin and sparse vellus hairs on the scalp, no eyebrows, rare and short eyelashes, and absence of hair on the rest of the body except for thin vellus hairs on the wrist's back and on the proximal part of the forearms. A few apparent comedos were found on the nose.

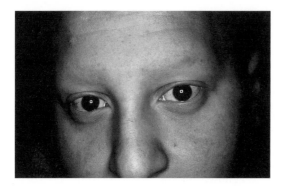

Figure 3. Hypotrichosis

Additional investigations

Histology of the scalp showed rare hair follicles (Fig. 4) with trichomalacia and increased apoptosis (Figs. 5 and 6).

A biopsy was taken from genital skin and fibroblasts were cultured. The latter showed normal 5α-reductase activity and a normal hormone-receptor affinity.

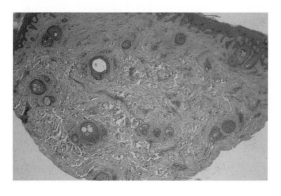

Figure 4. Rare hair follicles

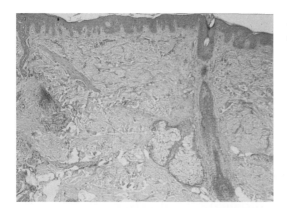

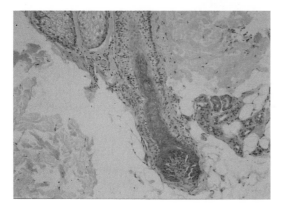

Figures 5 and 6. Trichomalacia and apoptosis

Discussion

Some cases associated hypogonadism and alopecia had been reported in the literature [1-3]. However, up to our knowledge, the association of pseudohermaphroditism and congenital hypotrichosis affecting all hair areas including the scalp is as yet unreported. Should these two observed abnormalities be regarded as two separate genetic mutations occurring simultaneously or is there a common physiopathological pathway leading to this complex phenotype, is an unresolved question.

Given the normal 5α-reductase activity and the normal hormone-receptor affinity, pseudo-hermaphroditism could be explained by a more peripheral androgen resistance i.e. distal to the receptor. The ingestion by the mother of an abortive preparation (combination of estrogens-progestogens?) around the 6th week of pregnancy could be at the origin of the abnormality in the sexual differentiation of the internal and external genitalia. This is indeed a key period for the embryogenesis of the genitalia. Whether it is also the case for hair follicles

42

is unknown. Indeed at the 6th week of estimated gestational age (EGA) the embryonic skin is a simple epithelium consisting of periderm and basal cells resting on a «generic» basement membrane i.e. one that lacks skin-specific antigens [4]. However, one must be close to the period of intense gene-regulation and many other changes (stratification of the epidermis, maturation of basement membrane, nerve and blood vessel migration,...) that are intimately associated with hair follicle induction resulting in hair germs around the 80th day of EGA [4]. Therefore a sudden change in hormonal levels during this critical period might result in an irreversible defect in the morphogenesis of the hair follicles. Vice-versa this raises the question of the possible role played by estrogens and/or androgens or androgen-like compounds, at a precise moment, during the induction of certain key-characteristics that can be retained by the mature hair follicle enabling it to initiate and maintain the growth of hair.

Acknowledgements

We would like to thank Dr Vamos (Hôp. univ. Brugmann, Brussels, Belgium) for the cultures of fibroblasts and Drs Ch. Sultan (CHU Montpellier, France) and I. Mowszowicz (Hôp. Necker, Paris, France) for performing the assay for 5α-reductase activity and hormone-receptor affinity. We are grateful to Dr Fr. Collier (Dpt of Surgery, HUDERF, Brussels, Belgium) for the pictures of the external genitalia.

References

1   Crandall BF, Samec L, Sparkes RS. J Pediatr. 1973; 82: 461-465
2   Al-Awadi SA, Farag TI, Teebi AS. Am J Med Genet. 1985; 22: 619-622
3   Johnston K, Golabi M, Hall M. Am J Med Genet. 1987; 26: 925-927
4   Holbrook KA, Minami SI. N Y Acad Sci. 1991; 842: 167-196,

Colour plate I

Hair research for the next millenium
D.J.J. Van Neste and V.A. Randall (Eds)

Spiny hyperkeratoses in a renal transplant recipient. A novel side effect of cyclosporin A

J. Izakovic, S.A. Büchner and P.H. Itin

Department of Dermatology, University Hospital, Basel, Switzerland
(Chairman: Prof. Dr. Theo Rufli)

Introduction

Cyclosporin A today is one of the most frequently used immunosuppressive drugs worldwide for preventing the rejection of transplanted organs. The hitherto reported side effects are mainly focused on the appendices of the skin, especially hair follicles and sebaceous glands [2, 5, 8, 10, 19, 22, 26, 34, 36, 40]. Best established are hypertrichosis, gingival hyperplasia, acne, keratosis pilaris, hyperplasia of sebaceous glands, epidermal cysts and folliculitis.

In our case we report an unusual generalized hyperplasia of hair follicles and sebaceous glands, which, to our knowledge has never been observed before with such a marked expression. In our opinion, this side effect can be attributed to cyclosporin A with a high degree of probability, since our patient did not receive neither prednisolone nor azathioprine at the time of appearance of his cutaneous symptoms.

The spontaneous regression of the skin alterations after stepwise reduction of cyclosporin A leads us to the assumption of a dose-dependency.

Materials and methods

Case report

In 1980, the now 31-year-old patient was treated for a membranoproliferative glomerulonephritis with terminal renal insufficiency, which was presumably due to a streptococcal infection earlier in his lifetime. The treatment at that time consisted of prednisolone and cyclophosphamide. In 1992, the patient underwent a peritoneal dialysis and received a renal transplant 4 months later. The initial immunosuppression consisted of methylprednisolone 1000 mg on the first day followed by a daily reduction of the dosage by 50 percent. After the third postoperative day he was switched to an oral treatment of prednisolone 30 mg daily with a subsequent stepwise reduction to zero over several weeks. In parallel, an immunosuppressive therapy with cyclosporin A, with an initial dosage of 260 mg intravenously on the first day rising to 400 mg orally on a twice daily basis later on, was initiated. Under this dosage the patient remained in a stable state with regard to the transplant function.

The first skin alterations showing some papules and cysts appeared 7 months after initiation of the immunosuppressive therapy.

Skin status

Initially, skin-coloured to whitish peri-follicular papules of a few millimeters diameter could be found on the central parts of the patient's face. Those papules, to a lesser extent, were also located on all other regions of the body except for the scalp, palm of hands and plant of feet. About two months later, the patient presented a different skin alteration with hair-like, hyperkeratotic spines, which originated from hair follicles. These alterations were mainly distributed on the patient's trunk, the extensor surfaces of his limbs and on his face. Very noticeable and unique was the involvement of the eyelids and the nostrils. All of these 2 to 4 mm long brush-like hyperkeratoses could be extracted or pressed out easily and some of them broke readily at their base. There was no hypertrichosis in this patient.

Histopathologic and scanning electron microscopic findings

The epidermis was hyperkeratotic with some acanthosis. The lumina of the hyperplastic sebaceous gland follicles were markedly widened and showed a substantial keratinization disorder with embedded eosinophilic clots of keratin. Along with their migration to the surface, these keratin clots formed a digitate, hair-like spine. The scanning electron microscopy photographs revealed that these «spines» appear to have a hair-like lamellar keratinous organization (Fig. 1). In the dermis there was a fairly visible perivascular lympho-histiocytic infiltrate.

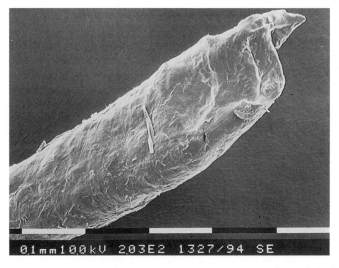

Figure 1. Scanning electron microscopy examination of one of the hair-like "spines"

Therapy and follow-up

Therapeutic attempts with topical ointments of metronidazole or tretinoin failed and were, therefore, discontinued after rather a short period of time. A planned systemic therapy with isotretinoin has been refused by the patient, because of reduction of the dosage of cyclosporin A by the nephrologists and some concomitant tendency to involution of the skin disorder. With the continuous reduction of the cyclosporin A - intake from 400 mg to 175 mg twice a day - always under a good renal function - the patient showed a nearly complete regression of the hyperkeratotic «spines» as well as of the sebaceous gland hyperplasia in a time span of three months. A relapse or an additional cutaneous manifestation could not be observed hitherto.

Discussion

Our patient shows a new cutaneous side effect of cyclosporin A. Clinically similar disorders have already been reported in different settings and with different concomitant diseases without being classified as drug induced side effects [9, 13, 16-18, 28, 32, 35, 41]. Reports concerning the cutaneous side effects of cyclosporin A already in the past had been targeted at the follicular bound keratinization disorders, mainly the hypertrichosis, since these are the most frequent side effects, appearing at a rate of up to 95 % [2, 10, 21-23, 26, 34, 36]. Other frequent side effects include follicular hyperkeratoses, keratosis pilaris and porokeratosis [2, 5, 10, 22, 34, 40].

In addition, there are a number of reports on porokeratoses associated with digitate hyperkeratoses, but none of them had any relation either to the follicle nor were they induced by cyclosporin A - treatment [18, 24, 30, 32, 45]. The multiple spiny brush-like hyperkeratoses described by Feldmann and Harms [16] belong to that group, although it seems that this disorder possibly represents an entity with an autosomal dominant mode of inheritance of it's own. If the macroscopic morphologic findings are compared, the alterations seen in our patient are closely related to the last mentioned case, although similar clinical descriptions, not always associated with the hair follicle, have already been published in the past under different names [1, 4, 11, 18, 39, 41, 43, 44]. Such digitate keratoses had been reported in a 15 months old child [15].

Follicular spiny hyperkeratoses appear less frequently in the literature. Some great similarities (documented in Table 1) do exist with our case as well from the clinical [9, 17, 28, 31, 35] as from the histopathologic point of view [3, 9, 14, 17, 28, 38].

Acne vulgaris, as an example of the possible affection on sebaceous glands, may also represent a remarkable side effect of cyclosporin A [10, 34, 40]. More seldom are descriptions of epidermal cysts [2, 8, 36]. Viral warts, herpes simplex and herpes zoster are examples of the frequent viral infections associated with immunosuppression by cyclosporin A [2, 5, 8, 10, 22, 34, 40]. Furthermore,

Table 1. Digitate hyperkeratoses associated with hair follicles

Clinical description	Localization/distribution	Associated disease
Spiny hyperkeratosis	Upper parts of back and chest, arms, neck	None reported
Lichen spinulosus-like eruptions	Ventral aspects of upper trunk, face, arms	HIV-positive
Generalized lichen spinulosus	Extensor surfaces of fingers, toes, knees	HIV-positive
«Paraneoplastic follicular spicules»	Face, nose, scalp	Multiple myeloma
Pityriasis rubra pilaris	Face, neck, upper trunk	Pityriasis rubra pilaris
«Spines» in connection with «disseminated superficial actinic porokeratosis»	Back	«Disseminated superficial actinic porokeratosis»
«Kératose pilaire spinulosique diffuse»	Cheeks, chin, upper lip, eyelids, scalp, to a lesser extent on trunk and limbs	Reticulosarcoma
«Hyperkératose piliforme disséminée familiale»	Trunk, limbs, chest, flanks, shoulders	None reported
«Transient post-inflammatory digitate keratoses»	Trunk, shoulders, buttocks, thighs	Not specified inflammatory skin diseases
Hairlike hyperkeratoses	Face, trunk, limbs	Immunosuppression with cyclosporin A after renal transplantation

Pathohistological characteristics	Particularities	Authors
Compact, concentric, orthohyperkeratotic horny spicules, discrete acanthosis of the epidermis, no dermal infiltrate	Horny spicules very well attached and difficult to extract	[17]
Parakeratotic horny spicules chronic perifolliculitis eosinophils dermal fibrosis	Horny spicules easy to extract	[35]
Parakeratotic horny spicules perifollicular and perivascular lymphocytic infiltrate		[13]
Orthoparakeratotic horny spicules intercellular eosinophilic material in epidermis and eosinophilic masses in hair follicles no dermal infiltrate	Horny spicules easy to scratch off cryoglobulinemia IgG-deposits in intercellular spaces between keratinocytes	[9]
Follicular hyperkeratosis follicular and perifollicular parakeratosis dermal perivascular lymphocytic infiltrate	Responded to 3-months systemic therapy with Isotretinoin	[28]
Follicular horny spicules in central areas of the superficial actinic porokeratoses	Cornoid lamellae in the hair follicles	[38]
Hyperkeratotic horny spicules dermal lymphohistiocytic infiltrate with few eosinophils		[31]
Hyperparakeratotic horny spicules papillary edema with mucinosis hypotrophic hair follicles perivascular lymphocytic infiltrate	Familial occurrence	[3]
Follicular and non-follicular spiny keratoses acanthosis, hypergranulosis single cell cornifications discrete perifollicular lymphocytic infiltrate	Follicular and non-follicular keratoses side by side in the same patient spontaneous healing within one month	[14]
Hairlike hyperkeratoses hyperplasia of sebaceous glands hairfollicles filled with eosinophilic material discrete perivascular lymphohistiocytic infiltrate	Dose-dependency	Izakovic et al.

several malignant skin diseases such as spindle cell or basal cell carcinomas and malignant melanoma have to be mentioned as possibly associated with cyclosporin A treatment [2, 5, 34]. Other dermatoses, like striae rubrae, are rather infrequent [8].

Gingival hyperplasia seems to be the most frequent mucosal side effect of cyclosporin A [2, 5, 8, 21-23, 36, 40].

Our reported case of a hyperkeratotic skin disorder under the influence of a cyclosporin A treatment can also fit into a series of etiologically significant observations where endogenous or exogenous dysregulations of the immune response may lead to different clinical and histopathological types of hyperkeratoses. The reason may be in an underlying general disease that affects the immune system, for example an infectious disease like lung tuberculosis [20] or AIDS [13, 27, 35] or a malignant neoplasia [25, 29]. Yet more frequently a hyperkeratotic skin disorder represents a side effect of a therapeutic intervention, where different immunosuppressants such as prednisolone, azathioprine or cyclosporin A have been used [6, 33, 37]. Immunosuppression induced by radiotherapy or UV-irradiation represent other, potentially synergistic, trigger mechanism for the breakout of a keratosis [7, 11, 42]. In 1990, Carmichael and Tan [12] reported spiny hyperkeratosis surprisingly induced by etretinate.

In our case there is a clear-cut pathogenetic correlation between the development of hairy hyperkeratoses with the intake of cyclosporin A. Our patient developed his skin alterations after a high dose standard therapy was initiated and the symptoms were regressive after the dosage was reduced. In our opinion, hairy hyperkeratoses should be included in the spectrum of possible side effects of cyclosporin A.

References

1   Aloi FG, Pippione M, Molinero A. Porokeratotic minute digitate hyperkeratoses. In: Wilkinson DS, Mascaro JM, Orfanos CE (eds) Clinical dermatology: The World Congress of Dermatology. Case collection. Schattauer, Stuttgart. 1987; pp 184-185

2   Assalve D, Simonetti S, Fiorella S, Calandra P. Alterazioni cutanee osservate in 64 trapiantati renali. Ann It Derm Clin Sper. 1988; 42: 255-262

3   Aufgang A Hyperkératose piliforme disséminée familiale. Ann Dermatol Syphil. 1972; 99: 381-390

4   Balus L, Donati P, Amantea A, Breathnach AS. Multiple minute digitate hyperkeratosis. J Am Acad Dermatol. 1988; 18: 431-436

5   Barr BBB, McLaren K, Smith IW, Benton EC, Bunney MH, Blessing K, Hunter JAA. Human papilloma virus infection and skin cancer in renal allograft recipients. Lancet. 1989; I: 124-129

6   Bencini PL, Bianchini E, Crosti C. Porocheratosi e terapia immunosoppressiva. Presentazione di un ulteriore caso e revisione della letteratura. Giorn It Derm Vener. 1988; 123: 39-40

7   Bencini PL, Crosti C, Sala F. Porokeratosis: immunosuppression and exposure to sunlight. Br J Dermatol. 1987; 116: 113-116

8   Bencini PL, Montagnino G, Sala F, De Vecchi A, Crosti C, Tarantino A. Cutaneous lesions in 67 cyclosporin-treated renal transplant recipients. Dermatologica. 1986; 172: 24-30

9   Bork K, Böckers M, Pfeifle J. Pathogenesis of paraneoplastic follicular hyperkeratotic spicules

in multiple myeloma. Follicular and epidermal accumulation of IgG dysprotein and cryoglobulin. Arch Dermatol. 1990; 126: 509-513

10 Bunney MH, Benton EC, Barr BB, Smith IW, Anderton JL, Hunter JAA. The prevalence of skin disorders in renal allograft recipients receiving cyclosporin A compared with those receiving azathioprine. Nephrol Dial Transplant. 1990; 5: 379-382

11 Burns DA. Post-irradiation digitate keratoses. Clin Exp Dermatol. 1986; 11: 646-649

12 Carmichael AJ, Tan CY. Digitate keratoses - a complication of etretinate used in the treatment of disseminated superficial actinic porokeratosis. Clin Exp Dermatol. 1990; 15: 370-371

13 Cohen SJ, Dicken CH. Generalized lichen spinulosus in an HIV-positive man. J Am Acad Dermatol. 1991; 25: 116-118

14 Cox NH, Ince P. Transient post-inflammatory digitate keratoses. Clin Exp Dermatol. 1989; 14: 170-172

15 Daudén E, Vanaclocha F, Gil R, Iglesias L. Generalized spiny hyperkeratosis with neurosensory deafness. In: Panconesi E (ed) Dermatology in Europe. Proceedings of the 1st Congress of the European Academy of Dermatology and Venereology. Blackwell Scientific Publications, Oxford. 1991; pp 607-608

16 Feldmann R, Harms M. Multiple filiforme Hyperkeratosen. Hautarzt. 1993; 44: 658-661

17 Fölster-Holst R, Christophers E. Filiforme Keratose. Hautarzt. 1994; 45: 484-488

18 Frenk E, Mevorah B, Leu F. Disseminated spiked hyperkeratosis. An unusual discrete nonfollicular keratinization disorder. Arch Dermatol. 1981; 117: 412-414

19 Gebhart W, Schmidt JB, Schemper M, Spona J, Kopsa H, Zazgornik J. Cyclosporin-A-induced hair growth in human renal allograft recipients and alopecia areata. Arch Dermatol Res. 1986; 278: 238-240

20 Gimenez-Arnau A, Camarasa JG. Palmar filiform or spiny hyperkeratosis associated with pulmonary tuberculosis. J Europ Acad Dermatol Venereol. 1994; 3: 400-406

21 Gupta AK, Brown MD, Ellis CN, Rocher LL, Fisher GJ, Baadsgaard O, Cooper KD, Voorhees JJ. Cyclosporine in dermatology. J Am Acad Dermatol. 1989; 21: 1245-1256

22 Halpert E, Tunnessen WW, Fivush B, Case B. Cutaneous lesions associated with cyclosporine therapy in pediatric renal transplant recipients. J Pediatr. 1991; 119: 489-491

23 Harper JI, Kendra JR, Desai S, Staughton RCD, Barrett AJ, Hobbs JR. Dermatological aspects of the use of cyclosporin A for prophylaxis of graft-versus-host disease. Br J Dermatol. 1984; 110: 469-474

24 Itin PH. Porokeratosis plantaris, palmaris et disseminata mit multiplen filiformen Hyperkeratosen und Nageldystrophie. Hautarz. 1995; 46: 869-872

25 Kaddu S, Soyer HP, Kerl H. Palmar filiform hyperkeratosis: a new paraneoplastic syndrome? Br J Dermatol. 1994; 131: 74 (Suppl.)

26 Kahan BD, Flechner SM, Lorber MI, Golden D, Conley S, Van Buren CT. Complications of cyclosporine-prednisone immunosuppression in 402 renal allograft recipients exclusively followed at a single center for from one to five years. Transplantation. 1987; 43: 197-204

27 Kanitakis J, Misery L, Nicolas JF, Lyonnet S, Chouvet B, Haftek M, Faure M, Claudy A, Thivolet J. Disseminated superficial porokeratosis in a patient with AIDS. Br J Dermatol. 1994; 131: 284-289

28 Koehn GG. Dramatic follicular plugging in pityriasis rubra pilaris. J Am Acad Dermatol. 1990; 23: 526-527

29 Luelmo-Aguilar J, Gonzalez-Castro U, Mieras-Barcelo C, Castells-Rodellas A. Disseminated porokeratosis and myelodysplastic syndrome. Dermatology. 1992; 184: 289

30 Moulonguet-Michau I, Bazex J, Franck N, Alibert M, Blanchet-Bardon C, Civatte J, Dubertret L. Hyperkératoses multiples minuscules. A propos de 2 observations. Ann Dermatol Venereol. 1991; 118: 615-618

31 Nazzaro P, Argentieri R, Balus L, Bassetti F, Fazio M, Giacalone B, Ponno R. Syndrome paranéoplasique avec lésions papulo-kératosiques des extrémités et kératose pilaire spinulosique diffuse. Ann Dermatol Syphil. 1974; 101: 411-413

32 Nedwich JA, Sullivan JJ. Disseminated spiked hyperkeratosis. Int J Dermatol. 1987; 26: 358-361

33 Neumann RA, Knobler RM, Metze D, Jurecka W. Disseminated superficial porokeratosis and immunosuppression. Br J Dermatol. 1988; 119: 375-380

34 O'Connell BM, Abel EA, Nickoloff BJ, Bell BJ, Hunt SA, Theodore J, Shumway NE, Jacobs PH. Dermatologic complications following heart transplantation. J Heart Transplant. 1986; 5: 430-436

35 Resnick SD, Murrell DF, Woosley J. Acne conglobata and a generalized lichen spinulosus-like eruption in a man seropositive for human immunodeficiency virus. J Am Acad Dermatol. 1992; 26: 1013-1014

36 Richter A, Beideck S, Bender W, Frosch PJ. Epidermalzysten und Follikuliditen durch Cyclosporin A. Hautarzt. 1993; 44: 521-523

37 Ross M, Goodman MM, Barr RJ, Liao SY. Multiple eruptive benign keratoses associated with cyclosporine therapy for psoriasis. J Am Acad Dermatol. 1992; 26: 128-129

38 Shumack SP, Commens CA. Disseminated superficial actinic porokeratosis: A clinical study. J Am Acad Dermatol. 1989; 20: 1015-1022

39 Shuttleworth D, Graham-Brown RAC, Hutchinson PE. Minute aggregate keratoses - a report of three cases. Clin Exp Dermatol. 1985; 10: 566-571

40 Sobh MA, Abdel Hamid IA, Saad HM, Eid MM, Abdel Razic MM, Elshamy S, Ghoniem MA. Dermatologic complications in renal transplant recipients versus uraemic patients under maintenance hemodialysis treatment. J Europ Acad Dermatol Venereol. 1992; 1: 217-223

41 Vaillant L, De Muret A, Arbeille B, Morere JP, Muller C, Lorette G. Hyperkératose filiforme diffuse. Ann Dermatol Venereol. 1991; 118: 891-894

42 Vestey JP, Hunter JAA, Mallet RB, Rodger A. Post irradiation conical keratosis. J Royal Soc Med. 1989; 82: 166-167

43 Wilkinson SM, Wilkinson N, Chalmers RJG. Multiple minute digitate keratoses: a transient, sporadic variant. J Am Acad Dermatol. 1994; 31: 802-803

44 Yoon SW, Gibbs RB. Multiple minute digitate hyperkeratoses. Arch Dermatol. 1975; 111: 1176-1177

45 Zarour H, Grob JJ, Andrac L, Bonerandi JJ. Palmoplantar orthokeratotic filiform hyperkeratosis in a patient with associated Darier's disease. Classification of filiform hyperkeratosis. Dermatology. 1992; 185: 205-209

The multiple faces of trichonodosis

F.M. Camacho and M.A. Muñoz

Department of Medical-Surgical Dermatology, Facultad de Medicina, Hospital Virgen Macarena, Avda. Dr. Fedriani s/n, 41071 Sevilla, Spain

Introduction

Trichonodosis is characterized by the presence of real «knots» or «half knots» on the hair shaft [1]. Even though these trichological findings are frequent, few reports have been published since it was first described by Galewsky and McLeod [2-6].

Trichonodosis is classified into two types: the first one shows isolated knots with abnormal hair growth and diffuse alopecia on the frontal region and vertex. It mainly affects girls from early infancy and is characterized by scalp hyperhydrosis and diffuse alopecia on the frontal region and vertex. Hair growth is usually abnormal with short and twisted hairs with longitudinal fissures and fractures of cortex and cuticular cells [7]. Only one knot is seen near the free end of the hair. In these cases no similar condition was reported in their families [8]. The second type includes acquired knots induced by mechanical or physical forces [1]. It is very common and is defined by the presence of one or several knots along the scalp hairs, pubic vellum and others hairs of the body.

There are different patterns of presentation:
1. One or several knots along the hairs.
2. Pseudoknots or half knots.
3. Tangles of hair.

Materials and methods

Case reports

We illustrate 4 types of trichonodosis observed in our dermatology practice in several patients. It is not the objective of this paper to comment on the diseases where these kinds of hair dysplasias appear.

Illustrations

Figure 1 shows a typical simple knot. It should be distinguished from the «pseudo- knots» (Fig. 2) where you cannot find a real knot. The knot-like images seen in the microscopy are due to the superposition of the twisted hair and are not a real knot. Figure 3 illustrates a double knot. Figure 4 shows a tangle of hair.

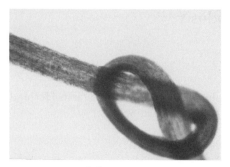

Figure 1. Simple knot

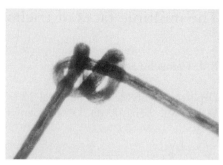

Figure 2. Simple knot (right) with pseudo-knot (left)

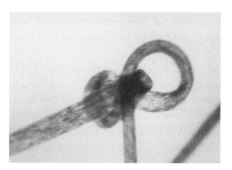

Figure 3. Double knot

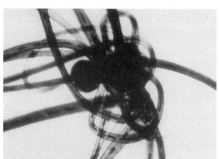

Figure 4. Tangle of hair

Discussion

Recently, there were three cases of patients presenting twisted and coiled hairs that tended to form real tangles of hair [9] rather than knots.

Some authors think that this is a new syndrome being acquired or hereditary, apparently via autosomic dominance, or that this would just be the result of repeated massages on the area, as occurs in the «induced trichonodosis» [10]. Other authors think that this condition is similar to «neuropathic plica» [11]. The familial condition described by Itin et al. could simply be a familial predisposition to develop knots and twisted hairs. It remains unclear why the five cases described by Itin developed this special type of tangle trichonodosis only on the right side of the back [12].

References

1   Dawber RPR. Knotting of Scalp Hair. Br J Dermatol. 1974; 91: 169-173
2   Whiting DA. Hair shaft defects. In: Olsen EA (ed), Disorders of hair growth. Diagnosis and treatment. New York, McGraw-Hill Inc. 1994; 91-137

3   Camacho F, Ferrando J. Hair shaft dysplasias. Int J Dermatol. 1988; 27: 71-80

4   Whiting DA. Structural abnormalities of the hair shaft. J Am Acad Dermatol. 1987; 16: 1-2

5   Pfister R, Driban N. Estudios de anomalias del tallo piloso con el microscopio electrònico Scanning. 2 Parte. Trichorrhexis nodosa, Trichoclasia, Trichoptilosis. Pelo en bayoneta. Med Cut. 1973; 7: 27-34

6   Jarret A, Johnson E, Spearman RJC. Abnormal hair growth in man. In: Jarret A (ed), The Physiology and Pathophysiology of the Skin. Londres, Academic. Press Inc. 1977; 1516

7   Forslind B. Queratina y queratinizacion del pelo. Aspectos bioquimicos y biologicos. In: Camacho F and Montagna W (Eds). Tricologia. Madrid. Biblioteca Aula Médica Ed. 1996; 51-68

8   Zhu W-Y, Xia M-Y. Trichonodosis. Pediatr Dermatol. 1993; 10: 392-393

9   Itin PH, Bircher AJ, Lautenschlager S, Zuberbühler E, Guggenheim R: A new clinical disorder of twisted and rolled body hairs with multiple, large knots. J Am Acad Dermatol. 1994; 30: 31-35

10 Resnik KS. Twisted and rolled body hairs. J Am Acad Dermatol. 1994; 31: 1076

11 Trüeb RM. Trichonodosis neurotica and familial trichonodosis. J Am Acad Dermatol. 1994; 31: 1077

12 Itin PH, Bircher AJ, Lautenschlager S. Reply. A new clinical disorder of twisted and rolled body hairs with multiple, large knots. J Am Acad Dermatol. 1994; 31: 1077-1078

Mycobacterium Fortuitum masquerading as dissecting cellulitis of the scalp

V.C. Fiedler[1], S. Alaiti[1] and S.G. Ronan[1, 2]

[1]Department of Dermatology, University of Illinois at Chicago, USA
[2]Department of Pathology, University of Illinois at Chicago, USA

Introduction

Mycobacterium Fortuitum is a facultative rapid-growing mycobacterium (group IV Runyon classification). This organism is ubiquitous and can commonly be found in soil and in water supplies. There have been several reports of *Mycobacterium Fortuitum* infection following trauma, surgery or injections. Here we describe a case of cutaneous *Mycobacterium Fortuitum* infection mimicking dissecting cellulitis of the scalp.

Case presentation

A 29 year old black man presented in October 1994 complaining of treatment resistant painful scalp nodules and cysts, and hairloss for eighteen months. Past treatments included prolonged courses of oral antibiotics and topical and intralesional steroids all without improvement. Past medical history is significant for alopecia areata of the beard area. He was on no medications.

Examination of the scalp revealed alopecia and multiple tender nodules and cysts as well as a few pustules and many firm papules over the occipital scalp (Fig. 1).

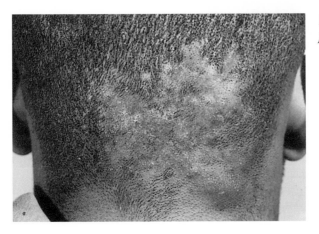

Figure 1. Patient at presentation

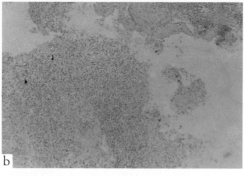

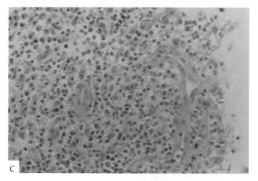

Figure 2 (a, b, c). Abscess in the deep reticular dermis surrounded by histiocytes, lymphocytes and granulation tissue

Laboratory studies including CBC, electrolytes, kidney and liver function tests, and urinalysis were normal. Bacterial culture grew few coagulase negative staphylococcus aureus. Fungal and mycobacterial cultures were negative. Chest X-ray was normal. PPD was negative, anergy battery was positive. Scalp biopsy showed an abscess in the deep reticular dermis surrounded by histiocytes, lymphocytes and granulation tissue (Figs. 2 a, b and c). Ziehl-Neelsen stain was negative for acid-fast organisms.

A diagnosis of dissecting cellulitis of the scalp was made and the patient was started on a trial of high dose isotretinoin (80 mg/day), low dose prednisone

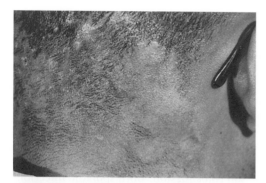

Figure 3. After 2 months of therapy with isotretinoin, oral and intralesional steroids

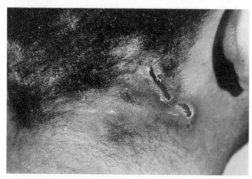

Figure 4. After one month of therapy with amikacin and ciprofloxacin

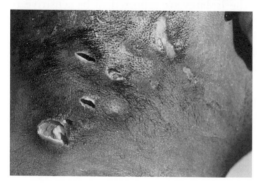

Figure 5. After four months of therapy with clofazimine and ciprofloxacin

(20 mg/day), as well as occasional intralesional steroids for two months with no improvement (Fig. 3).

Two additional cultures eventually grew *Mycobacterium Fortuitum* which was sensitive to amikacin, ciprofloxacin and clofazimine. The cysts were incised and drained and he received a 30 day course of intravenous amikacin along with oral ciprofloxacin (Fig. 4). The initial lesions and the alopecia continue to improve with an ongoing course of clofazimine and ciprofloxacin; however he continues to develop new abscesses in the neck requiring incision and drainage (Fig. 5). The purulent material obtained from these abscesses has grown *Mycobacterium Fortuitum*.

Discussion

Mycobacterium Fortuitum and *Mycobacterium Chelonae* are the major pathogens in Runyon group IV (rapidly growing mycobacteria) [1]. They are acid-fast rods that resemble diphteroids on gram stain. On primary isolation they require 2 to 30 days for growth. These ubiquitous organisms survive nutritional deprivation and extremes of temperature.

Most human infections with *Mycobacterium Fortuitum* are acquired by inoculation during accidental trauma, surgery or injections. Incubation periods vary from 1 week to 2 years, but most infections occur within one month. There is no evidence for person to person transmission. Both sporadic infections and outbreaks have been described in healthy individuals as well as in immunocompromised patients.

Cutaneous infection with *Mycobacterium Fortuitum* may resemble pyogenic abscesses with an acute inflammatory reaction and suppuration [2], or may progress slowly with chronic inflammation, ulceration, sinus tract formation and exudates that resemble sporotrichosis. The course of the disease is highly variable. In most cases the disease is relentlessly progressive, however spontaneous resolution has been reported. The infection may heal leaving significant scarring.

Mycobacterium Fortuitum is usually resistant to classical antituberculous therapy; however, it may be sensitive to amikacin [3], ciprofloxacin [4] and sulfonamides [5]. Less than half of the isolates are reported to be sensitive to doxycycline [3]. As yet, there have been no reported controlled trials defining optimal treatments for *Mycobacterium Fortuitum*. Single drug therapy should be avoided to reduce the emergence of drug resistance. Selection of chemotherapeutic agents should be guided by drug sensitivity testing. Some authorities recommend surgical removal of all tissues involved, as much as feasible and debridement [6]. Because of continued development of new lesions despite long term antibiotic therapy, our patient required surgical intervention as well.

Conclusions

Atypical mycobacterial infection may mimic dissecting cellulitis of the scalp. It is important to consider atypical mycobacterial infection in the pathogenesis of chronic recalcitrant cutaneous disease. The mode of inoculation is not known in this case. Treatment of cutaneous mycobacterial infection may require medical and surgical treatments as in our patient.

References

1 Sanders Jr WE, Horowitz EA. Other mycobacterium species. In: Mandell GL, Douglas RG, Bennett JE, eds. Principles and practice of infectious diseases. New York: Churchill Livingstone Inc. 1990

2 Carey MJ, Maclaren HM, Miller MV: A cutaneous infection with *Mycobacterium Fortuitum*. Ann-Emerg-Med. 1994; 23(2): 347-349

3 Dalovisio JR, Pankey GA, Wallace RJ, *et al.* Clinical usefulness of amikacin and doxycycline in the treatment of infection due to *Mycobacterium Fortuitum* and *Mycobacterium Chelonae*. Rev Infect Dis. 1981; 3: 1068-1074

4 Garcia-Rodriguez JA, Gomez Garcia AC: *In-Vitro* Activities of Quinilone against Mycobacteria. J Antimicrob Chemother. 1993; 32 (6): 797-808

5 Tice AD, Solomon RJ. Disseminated *Mycobacterium Chelonae* infection: response to sulfonamides. Am Rev Rerfir. 1979; 120: 197-201

6 Rappaport W, Dunington G, Norton L, *et al.*: The surgical management of atypical mycobacterial soft-tissue infections. Surgery. 1990; 108: 36-39

©1996 Elsevier Science B.V. All rights reserved.
Hair research for the next millenium
D.J.J. Van Neste and V.A. Randall (Eds)

Safety of long term therapy with 3% and 5% topical minoxidil in female androgenetic alopecia

C. Boeck[1], J. Parker[1], J. Shank[2] and M. Hordinsky[1]

[1]Clinical Research Division, Department of Dermatology, University of Minnesota, 420 Delaware Street SE, Minneapolis, Minnesota 55455-0392, USA
[2]Metropolitan Dermatology and Cutaneous Surgery, P.A., 2050 Merrimac Lane, Plymouth, MN 55447, USA

Introduction

Little is known about the long term safety of topical minoxidil in the management of female androgenetic alopecia. In this study, we investigated the safety of long-term therapy with topical 3% minoxidil (up to 156 weeks) 1 cc b.i.d. in 34 patients followed by topical 5% minoxidil (up to 300 weeks); 1cc b.i.d. in 23 patients with female androgenetic alopecia (14 to 63 years of age). In addition, we examined at baseline whether or not systemic endocrine dysfunction was present in a subset of women (20 pre-menopausal; 2 post-menopausal) along with age-and sex-matched controls.

Materials and methods

Patient population

This study was approved by the University of Minnesota Committee for Use of Humans in Research. Thirty-three caucasian women and one black woman between the ages of 14 and 63 with Grade I, II, or III androgenetic alopecia (Ludwig classification) participated in this study [1]. All but two of the patients were pre-menopausal. Patients enrolled were those with an ideal weight and height.

To exclude patients with ovarian or adrenal gland disease, a subset of 22 women, 20 pre-menopausal and 2 post-menopausal, also participated in a baseline evaluation of their endocrine status. Two months prior to entry, the pre-menopausal patients and age-and sex-matched controls were asked to record their daily basal body temperature in order to determine time of ovulation. The following endocrine parameters were then assessed pre and post ovulation: DHEA-S, prolactin, progesterone, follicle stimulating hormone, luteinizing hormone, free and total testosterone.

Protocol M/7410/0044 was a long-term, open-label 48-week study in which thirty-four patients with female androgenetic alopecia received 3% topical minoxidil solution, 1 cc applied twice daily. Patients were evaluated monthly the first six months, and then every two months. This period was followed by an Addendum tò Protocol M/7410/0044 which was a long-term, open-label, 96 week extension (108 week extension for 3 patients) of the above protocol. Patients were evaluated monthly the first three months and then every three months. This addendum was followed by Protocol M/7410/0153 a long-term, open-ended, open-label, continuation study of protocol M/7410/0044. Patients received an increase in dose of topical minoxidil solution from 3% to 5%, 1 cc applied twice daily and were evaluated monthly the first three months and then every three months.

The following safety parameters were assessed at each visit: blood pressure, pulse, weight and local tolerance. Erythema, stinging/burning, itching, dryness/scale, folliculitis were assessed utilizing a 4-level scale (none, mild, moderate and severe). The following parameters were initially measured every six months, then every twelve months: electrocardiograms, serum minoxidil levels, urine analysis, complete blood counts, clinical chemistries including alkaline phosphatase, total bilirubin, calcium, chloride, cholesterol, creatinine, glucose, phosphorus, potassium, total protein, BUN, SGOT, sodium, thyroxine, TSH, uric acid (CPK and LDH if SGOT was increased). Safety was also evaluated by noting any emergent medical condition(s) during study participation and comparing any changes in conditions from baseline.

Results

Patient population
Twenty-four patients completed Protocol M/7410/0044 (up to 156 weeks of topical therapy with 3% minoxidil) and were enrolled in Protocol M/7410/0153. Of the ten patients who did not proceed to Protocol M/7410/0153, five patients were lost to follow-up, two discontinued their participation because of lack of efficacy, two requested to discontinue their participation, and one patient discontinued her participation because of a non-serious medical event. All but one patient completed Protocol M/7410/0153. This patient developed mild mitral regurgitation unrelated to the use of topical minoxidil and was asked to discontinue her participation in this study.

Endocrine Studies
All 20 pre-menopausal patients and matched controls documented normal basal body temperature charts and demonstrated the ability to ovulate. Except for one pre-menopausal patient who had an elevated DHEA-S level of 474 m/dL (20-430), no significant endocrine laboratory abnormalities were found in either the patients or controls.

Safety Parameters

Blood pressure, pulse, weight, electrocardiograms, clinical chemistries, urine analysis and complete blood counts: no significant adverse experiences related to the use of topical minoxidil were documented during the duration of this study. The mean range of the serum minoxidil levels was less than 10 ng/ml throughout the study. In Protocol M/7410/0044, the minoxidil level ranged from 0.9 ± 0.9 to 1.2 ± 1.6 ng/ml and in Protocol M/7410/0153 from 1.5 ± 2.4 to 2.4 ± 2.6 ng/ml. Erythema, stinging, burning, dryness, scaling and itching were experienced by some participants in both studies (Tables 1 and 2). Although two patients, a 63-year-old white female and her 31-year-old daughter, complained of severe itching in protocol M/710/0044 and one, the 63-year-old female also had severe dryness/scale, no study participant was terminated because of drug intolerance.

Table 1

Greatest severity of symptom scores reported by patients (absolute numbers (#) and relative percentage (%) of patients) in 3% topical minoxidil treatment period: protocol M/7410/0044 and addendum

Symptom	None #	None %	Mild #	Mild %	Moderate #	Moderate %	Severe #	Severe %	Total #	Total %
Erythema	20	58.8	11	32.4	3	8.8			34	100
Stinging/burning	29	85.3	3	8.8	2	5.9			34	100
Itching	16	47.1	13	38.2	3	8.8	2	5.9	34	100
Dryness/scaling	7	20.6	20	58.8	6	17.6	1	2.9	34	100
Folliculitis	26	76.5	5	14.7	3	8.8			34	100

Table 2

Greatest severity of symptom scores reported by patients (absolute numbers (#) and relative percentage (%) of patients) in 5% topical minoxidil treatment period: protocol M/7410/0153

Symptom	None #	None %	Mild #	Mild %	Moderate #	Moderate %	Severe #	Severe %	Total #	Total %
Erythema	11	47.8	10	43.5	2	8.7			23	100
Stinging/burning	21	91.3	2	8.7					23	100
Itching	9	39.1	11	47.8	2	8.7	1	4.3	23	100
Dryness/scaling	1	4.3	16	69.6	6	26.1			23	100
Folliculitis	17	73.9	6	26.1					23	100

64

The development of transient hypertrichosis was the major medical condition which occurred during the study. This hypertrichosis was considered to be most likely related to the use of topical minoxidil. Prominent hair growth occurred primarily in the preauricular areas or on the arms of 12 (11 pre-menopausal/1 post-menopausal) women during Protocol M/7410/0044 and in 10 of 24 women in Protocol M/7410/0153 (Fig. 1). In this and other cases, the hypertrichosis was decreased by altering the drug application schedule from 1 cc b.i.d. to 1 cc q.d. When the facial hypertrichosis persisted and dark terminal hairs began to develop above the upper lip and on the forearms of the post-menopausal patient, her endocrinologic status was reevaluated, detecting a rising serum testosterone level (Fig. 2). The patient was referred for further evaluation. Bilateral ovarian hilar cell hyperplasia was identified following a total abdominal hysterectomy and oophorectomy [2].

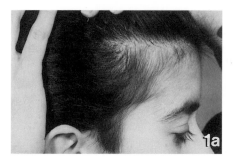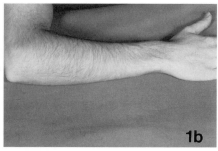

Figure 1. (a) Facial hypertrichosis and (b) elongation of hairs on the right arm and hand of a 26-year-old white female who participated in this study.

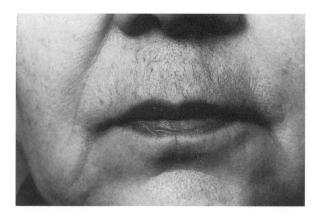

Figure 2. Dark, terminal hairs above the upper lip of a 63-year-old white female developed during the first year of this study. This patient was subsequently diagnosed with bilateral ovarian hilar cell hyperplasia.

Conclusions

No major or serious complications related to the long-term use of either 3% or 5% topical minoxidil were seen in this study. The most common complications included transient hypertrichosis and mild to moderate scalp erythema, itching, dryness or scaling. There is no known potential for minoxidil to pharmacologically induce ovarian or adrenal tumors but the potential for developing ovarian or adrenal gland disorders does exist in women [3, 4]. Clinically, affected patients may present with hirsutism or hair loss. Therefore, it is appropriate to obtain baseline endocrine studies prior to initiating long term therapy with topical minoxidil for female androgenetic alopecia. Having these results will establish a baseline as well as exclude women with androgenetic alopecia who have ovarian or adrenal gland disease.

Acknowledgements

This work was supported by a grant from the Upjohn Company. We would also like to acknowledge a close colleague, Richard (Dick) Key, from the Upjohn Company who passed away this year, 1995. Dick introduced us to the enjoyment of clinical research and supported our efforts for many years.

References

1   Ludwig E. Classification of the types of androgenetic alopecia (common baldness) occurring in the female sex. Br J Dermatol. 1977; 97:247-254
2   Hordinsky MK, Shank J. Three percent topical minoxidil therapy for female androgenetic alopecia. Clin Dermatol. 1988; 6:213- 217
3   Jacobs JP, et al. Use of topical minoxidil therapy for androgenetic alopecia in women. Int J Dermatol. 1993; 32: 758-762
4   DeVillez R, et al. Androgenetic alopecia in the female. Arch Dermatol. 1994; 130: 303-307

Quantitative estimation of hair growth: comparative changes in weight and hair count with 5% and 2% minoxidil, placebo and no treatment

V.H. Price[1] and E. Menefee[2]

[1]Department of Dermatology, University of California, San Francisco, 350 Parnassus Avenue, Suite 404, San Francisco, California 94117, U.S.A.
[2]Trichos Research, 5313 Rosalind Avenue, Richmond, California 94805, U.S.A.

Introduction

We previously recommended total hair mass (weight) from a defined scalp area as the primary estimator for hair growth [1]. The efficacy of a hair growth promoting agent can be established in 24 weeks by comparing the total hair mass (weight) of hair grown in a small, carefully maintained area on the scalp in subjects given either a hair growth promoter or a placebo. However, assessing the effect of a treatment on retarding the hair loss process requires a much longer time (at least two years), with the hair mass measurements also being made on a similar group of subjects receiving no treatment.

In this study, quantitative estimation of hair growth was recorded for 120 weeks for a group of men with androgenetic alopecia. Our purpose was to compare the effect of 5% and 2% topical minoxidil solution and placebo, in a random, double-blind protocol, on both hair growth promotion and on retardation of the hair loss process, using total hair weights and counts. After 96 weeks, treatment was stopped, although the hair growth measurements were continued for 24 additional weeks. Concurrently, a group of men with androgenetic alopecia received no treatment and their hair growth was compared with the treated groups over the same 120 week period. This group was perforce not part of the blind study.

Materials and methods

Subject selection

Eligible subjects for this study were men of ages 18 to 40 with androgenetic alopecia as evidenced by frontal/parietal thinning defined by the Hamilton scale as Type III or IV. They had to be in good health, and have dark, undyed hair, with no grey or white hair. Exclusion criteria included use of topical minoxidil within the previous six months, use of any investigational drug within the previous six months, concomitant use of steroids, vasodilators, antihypertensives, calcium channel blockers, antiepileptic drugs, cytotoxic agents, «hair restorers», other medications that could influence hair growth, or prior participation in a topical minoxidil study. Pre-enrollment laboratory studies included a complete blood count with differential, urinalysis with microscopic examination, liver function tests, lactic dehydrogenase, calcium, phosphorus, creatinine, uric acid, blood urea nitrogen, serum electrolytes, thyroxine and thyroid-stimulating hormone. These studies, as well as an electrocardiogram, and chest X-ray if not taken in the prior six months, all had to be normal to qualify for eligibility in the study. Thirty six men aged 24 to 40 qualified for the study and signed an informed consent.

Scalp site selection and sampling frequency

A representative site was selected on the thinning frontal/parietal scalp. Hair in the designated area was carefully hand clipped under magnification on the screening visit (designated as week -6) and at six week intervals thereafter, for a total of 120 weeks. No treatment was given during the first six weeks, so that the sample collected at the end of this interval represented baseline growth (week 0). For the men assigned to one of the treated groups, treatment was started on the second visit (week 0) and continued for 96 weeks. After 96 weeks, treatment was stopped and hair clippings were continued at six week intervals for 24 additional weeks. Concurrently, the group of untreated men had their hair clipped with the same method every six weeks for 120 weeks.

Marking and clipping procedure

During the screening (week -6) clipping, a template consisting of a plastic sheet with a 1.2 cm^2 hole was placed over the selected site. All hairs within the template square were pulled through it, with the help of a magnifying lamp to ensure that only hair originating within the square was included. The hairs were grasped and hand clipped to ca. 1 mm length with small straight surgical scissors. Four small dots were then placed in the corners of the square with a fine ball point pen. After removing the template, the four corners were permanently marked using ink and the Spalding and Rodgers marking apparatus.

On subsequent visits at six week intervals, the plastic template was laid in exact correspondence with the permanent markings, and the hair in the marked square carefully hand clipped and collected under magnification in the manner previously described [1].

Measurement method

Hair samples were degreased in Freon TF and dried. The total hair sample was spread out on a grid and counted. Hairs with pointed tips were separated from those with blunt or cut tips for the counting procedure. The hair sample was then placed in the chamber of an analytical balance having 0.01 mg readability. After conditioning for at least 1 hour in the balance chamber, the ambient relative humidity was recorded, and the samples weighed. Sample weights were corrected to a standard humidity of 65% [1].

Protocol

Following their hair clipping on the second visit, 27 subjects were assigned test solutions which were either a solution of 2% minoxidil (in a vehicle of 20% v/v propylene glycol, 60% ethanol, and water) or 5% minoxidil (in a vehicle of 50% v/v propylene glycol, 30% ethanol, and water), or the vehicle solution referred to as placebo. The subjects were assigned the test solutions in a randomized, double-blind manner as follows: 9 men received 5% topical minoxidil solution, 8 men received 2% topical minoxidil solution, and 10 men received placebo. They were instructed to apply 1 ml of the assigned solutions with a metered dropper twice daily to the frontal/parietal scalp, beginning at the clipped site. Applications were made with the scalp dry, spread with one finger tip, and then allowed to dry without a hair dryer. After 96 weeks, treatment was stopped and the hair growth measurements were continued for 24 additional weeks. Nine additional men with similar hair thinning were followed concurrently without treatment for 120 weeks.

All 36 subjects were well matched in age, duration and extent of alopecia, and original target area hair density. To avoid accidental hair cutting in the test site, hair cuts for the purpose of hair styling were permissible only during the 7 days following a clipping procedure.

During the study, vital signs, medical events, and skin tolerance were monitored, and serum minoxidil levels, hematology and blood chemistries were measured.

Results

Thirty two subjects completed the entire 120 week study. One untreated subject withdrew at week 6, two treated subjects (assigned to 2% minoxidil solution and placebo) withdrew at week 48 because of scheduling problems, and one treated subject (assigned to 2% minoxidil solution) dropped out at week 96 because he did not wish to stop treatment.

Figures 1 and 2 show the percent change in mean weight and the percent change in mean number of hairs in the 4 groups over the 120 weeks.

Discussion

During the 96 weeks of treatment, the 5% and 2% minoxidil groups showed a substantially greater hair mass from baseline compared to the placebo and untreated groups. The 5% minoxidil group showed the greatest increase in percent change in mean weight, the 2% minoxidil group also showed an increase, but it was smaller than the 5% minoxidil group. On the other hand, the placebo and untreated groups seemed much alike in their response, showing a steady decrease in hair mass from baseline over the 120 weeks. After treatment was stopped at week 96, the 5% and 2% minoxidil groups showed a rapid loss of hair mass. By 24 weeks after stopping treatment the hair mass was similar among the minoxidil-treated groups and the placebo and untreated groups. The percent change in mean number generally paralleled the percent change in weights. The weights tend to greater accuracy since the somewhat uncertain number of very small hairs affect the number count, but has little effect on the weight.

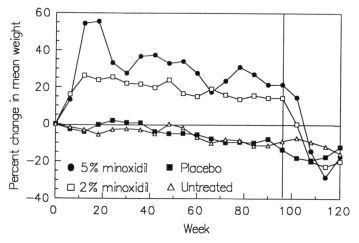

Figure 1. Percent change in mean weight per cm²

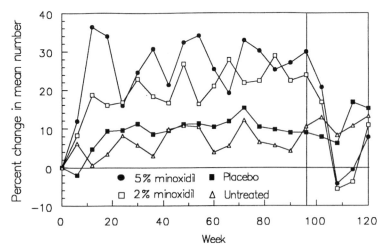

Figure 2. Percent change in mean number per cm²

In addition to the total hair count, hairs with pointed tips were separately counted from those with blunt or cut ends. A large increase in the number of pointed hairs in the treated samples was noted, especially during the early treatment intervals. A surge in hair weight was similarly observed in the first 20 weeks after initiating treatment. These increases were most prominent in the 5% group (Figs. 1 and 2), and are due to the known effect of minoxidil initiating anagen growth. The initial surge was followed by a period of shedding, by a smaller surge, and so on, with eventual diminishing of these periodic responses. The large variations shown represent true temporal changes and not experimental error.

These observations demonstrate that 5% and 2% topical minoxidil solutions promote hair growth and retard the hair loss process over 96 weeks, with the 5% topical minoxidil solution having the greater efficacy. Although a slight decrease in hair mass was seen over a long period, minoxidil maintained weight production at a high level compared to the placebo and untreated groups, which had about a 7% to 8% per year decrease in hair mass.

Acknowledgements

We thank The Upjohn Company for continued support and encouragement. We are grateful to Cathy Cortez, Andrea Menefee, and Lita Regezi for technical assistance.

Reference

1   Price VH, Menefee E. Quantitative estimation of hair growth. I. Androgenetic alopecia in women: effect of minoxidil. J Invest Dermatol. 1990; 95: 683-687

Effect of an antimicrobial lotion on androgenetic alopecia-related inflammation

G.E. Piérard[1], C. Piérard-Franchimont[1], N. Nikkels-Tassoudji[1], A.F. Nikkels[1] and D. Saint-Léger[2]

[1]Department of Dermatopathology, CHU Sart Tilman, B-4000 Liège, Belgium
[2]L'Oréal Research Laboratories, F 92117 Clichy, France

Introduction

Few histological observations deal with the aetiopathogeny of androgenetic alopecia (AGA). Only rare publications clearly report inflammatory infiltrates in AGA [1-4]. What role such inflammatory reaction may play in the AGA scene is still obscure (Fig. 1).

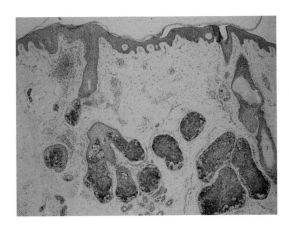

Figure 1. Typical histologic al view of AGA with miniaturized hairs, large sebaceous glands and dense periadnexal infiltrate

One of the possible causative factors of such an inflammatory reaction, the resident flora of the scalp skin has been poorly documented. This skin site is permanently colonized by a rather stable microflora: Propionibacterium spp, Staphylococcus spp, Malassezia spp [5, 6]. Among these, the latter makes the scalp one of its privileged ecological niche.

The aim of this work was two-fold:

1) To quantify through immunohistological observations the presence and localization of inflammatory reactions in AGA, as compared to non-involved sites.

2) To ascertain the participation of the resident flora of the scalp in the inflammatory scenario.

Materials and methods

Patients

Twenty men (age range 26-48) showing AGA patterns III (n = 12) to IV (n = 8), according to Hamilton's classification, were enrolled in the study. They gave their informed consent about the nature and protocol of the assay.

Treatment

The subjects were instructed to apply a lotion containing 0.25 % piroctone olamine (Octopirox®, Hoechst) and 0.3 % trichlosan (Irgasan®, Ciba-Geigy) in ethanol: water (40:60 V/V). daily These compounds exert potent antifungal (piroctone olamine) and antibacterial (trichlosan) activities. Volunteers received a non-medicated mild shampoo (shampooing doux Galenco) to be used during the whole study and excluded any other scalp care product. The treatment period lasted 18 months, the subjects being enrolled between August 1992 and April 1993.

Monthly subjective evaluations

- Self assessment questionnaires (severity of seborrhea, pruritus, dandruff, hair loss, ...)
- Self assessment of daily hair loss through visual examination of transparent envelopes containing known amounts of hairs (10 to 120).

Quantitative objective evaluations

Hair (quarterly evaluations):
- Trichograms (> 80 hairs) were carried out. The index of Hair Cycle Disturbance (HCD) was calculated in % following $(C + T/A) \times 100$, where C, T and A represent the number of hair in catagen, telogen and anagen phases, respectively.
- Hair density was evaluated through standardized photographs (Dermaphot®, Heine).

Histology (at 6-month intervals):
- Punch biopsies were performed and processed under classical procedures for immunochemistry and morphometric purposes, using antibodies to CD45, CD45R, CD45RO, L1 antigen (Mac 387), EMA and IgG. Isotype-matched controls were carried out to exclude non-specific binding of primary antibodies.

Statistics

Paired Student t-test and analysis of variance (ANOVA) for changes in time were used to detect significant effects of treatment.

Results

Self-evaluations of the hair-loss by the subjects followed a logarithmic ($r = -0.56$, $p < 0.01$) trend in improvement during the long term applications of the lotion (average 5.5 ml/day/subject). Self-assessment questionnaires indicated that scalp pruritus resolved as quickly as the first month of treatment and was barely noticeable for the rest of the study. The tolerance of the lotion was excellent for all subjects. No side effect was recorded.

A progressive decrease of the AGA severity was also evidenced by the clinical photographs and the HCD index. A negative logarithmic correlation ($r = -0.64$, $p < 0.01$) was found between HCD index and duration of treatment. Compared to the baseline HCD index (48.6 ± 15.6), a significant ($p < 0.05$) improvement was reached at month 6 (37.8 ± 13.3) and maintained afterwards.

At entry to the study, CD45-positive lymphocytes and CD45RO-positive T cells (about 90 %) admixed with rare Mac 387-positive monocytes were abutted to each infrainfundibulum of transitional hairs. They were almost absent in the non-alopecic area of the same subjects. The density of these cells significantly decreased with time in the transitional area (Fig. 2). CD45R-positive cells were not found in the infiltrates. Though difficult to quantify, the presence of IgG deposits, which were detected close to clumps of M. ovalis in 9 of the 20 subjects at the beginning of the study, were no longer present after 6 and 12 months of treatment.

At entry and throughout the study, image analysis of serial sections of the sebaceous glands, well contrasted by EMA staining, indicated a significant ($p < 0.001$) inverse correlation between their area and the diameter of their associated hair shafts. The average size of sebaceous glands and the mean hair shaft diameter remained unchanged during the study.

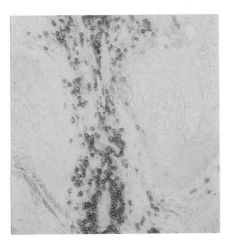 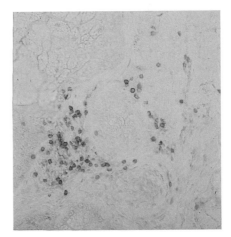

Figure 2. CD45RO-positive T lymphocytes before (A) and after (B) a 18-month treatment with the lotion.

Discussion

The present study confirms the presence of an inflammatory infiltrate in AGA-transitional scalp regions, as compared to non-involved sites. A vast majority of these cells belong to memory CD45RO-positive T cells. They are specifically found in the transitional area, infiltrating the upper isthmal portion of the hair follicle close to the secretory duct opening of the sebaceous gland. In the same anatomical region, IgG were observed in some subjects, indicating that these antibodies may be turned against well localized antigens which might be related to M. ovalis.

The influence of inflammatory reactions on the AGA hair cycle status was studied through a long time application of a cosmetically acceptable lotion with antifungal and antibacterial properties. Basically, a significant decrease in some immuno-inflammatory aspects and consequent changes in the hair cycle were suggested by clinical photographs and trichograms. These positive findings were in apparent contradiction with the absence of improvement in the morphometric measurements of hair shaft diameter on transverse histological sections. In fact, morphometric analysis was performed on all hairs without distinction between terminal, transitional and vellus types. The range of diameter of these hairs was so broad that no difference was seen in time. On the other hand, the calculation of the HCD index on transitional hairs proved to be more informative.

With regard to the sebaceous glands, we confirm some previous observations by which they were found enlarged in AGA. In our study, we found that the larger the glands, the thinner their associated hair shafts are. The size of the sebaceous glands, however, remained unchanged with treatment, implying that the decrease in the inflammatory infiltrate had little influence if any compared to their androgenic stimulation.

Though non-controlled, the present work gives support for a close connection between the follicular alterations in AGA and immuno-inflammatory aspects which seem, for a part, initiated by the scalp microflora. The latter, though non pathogenic, has been clearly shown to be potent elicitors of the immune response in other skin diseases [6]. In such scenario, immunological status might well represent an important factor in modulating the hair cycle and the various expressions of AGA.

References

1   Lattanand A, Johnson WC. J Cutan Pathol. 1975; 2: 58-70
2   Kligman AM. Clin Dermatol. 1988; 6: 108-118
3   Young JW, Conte ET, Leavitt ML, Nafz MA, et al. J Am Osteopath Ass. 1991; 91: 765-771
4   Jaworsky C, Kligman AM, Murphy GF. Br J Dermatol. 1992; 127: 239-246
5   Saint-Léger D, Kligman AM, Stoudemayer TJ. J Soc Cosmet Chem. 1989; 40: 109-117
6   Piérard-Franchimont C, Arrese JE, Piérard GE. Eur Acad Dermatol Venereol. 1995; 4: 14-19

©1996 Elsevier Science B.V. All rights reserved.
Hair research for the next millenium
D.J.J. Van Neste and V.A. Randall (Eds)

Topical application of retinoic acid (RA) induces hair casts (HCs) formation

M. Barbareschi, A. Angius and F. Greppi

Institute of Dermatological Sciences IRCCS, University of Milan, Via Pace, 9, 20122 Milano, Italy

Introduction

Hair casts (HCs) were probably first described in 1897 by Grindon [1] with the term of «Ecbolic Folliculitis». In 1957 Kligman [2] renamed them «Hair Casts». In 1983, Scott and Roenigk [3] suggested classification of HCs according to keratin or non-keratin material ensheathing the hair shaft. Today many authors [4-7] distinguish two types of HCs: the first one, previously considered to be rare, is reported in young girls without primary abnormality of the scalp; the second is quite frequent and is secondary to scalp diseases such as psoriasis, Darier's disease or lichen plano-pilaris. In order to avoid confusion, Keipert [5] proposed to call «peripilar keratin casts» the idiopathic form of HCs while «parakeratotic hair casts» are those HCs associated with parakeratotic scalp diseases. The pathogenesis of HCs is not clearly understood. The observation of HCs formation in patients treated topically with RA is an interesting finding that might provide some insight into HCs' pathogenesis.

Materials and methods

Case reports

Two patients (males aged 27 and 30 years) who suffered from androgenetic alopecia were treated with a solution containing 1% minoxidil associated with 0.025% RA, after a period of treatment with topical minoxidil alone. The solutions were applied twice daily. During application of minoxidil HCs were not observed. However, after a few months of treatment by minoxidil associated with RA both patients developed HCs in the treated zone. HCs appeared as small gray-white elements, measuring few millimeters in length. A few hairs were collected and examinated with a scanning electron microscope (SEM 505 Philips).

Ultrastructural examination

At ultrastructural level HCs appeared to have an irregular shape. Some ones had a regular diameter, extending into a few millimeters long cylinders (Fig. 1), while others were much shorter and had a polyhedric shape (Fig. 2). Some ensheathed more than one hair shaft (Fig. 3). The ensheathed shafts showed a regular cuticular pattern. At higher magnification, HCs appeared to be constituted by flattened horny cells. The constitutive elements had polyhedric shape and a pronounced surface roughness (Fig. 4). The free edges of those cells had a tendency to protrude outwards. Neither bacteria nor fungi were detected.

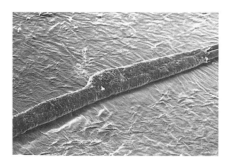

Figure 1. Long and cylindrical hair cast (x32)

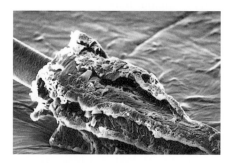

Figure 2. Short polyhedric cast ensheathing a single hair shaft (x110)

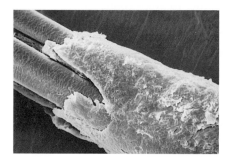

Figure 3. Multiple hair shafts ensheathed by a single cast (x110)

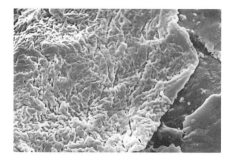

Figure 4. High power view of horny cells forming the cast (x237)

Discussion

Hair casts (HCs) are usually localized at some centimeters from the scalp where they move freely along the hair shaft. Up to now many reports in the literature focused on the classification of hair casts and speculated about their pathogenesis. Hence, Kligman [2] suggested that undissolved keratinized internal root sheath and parakeratosis of the infundibulum were predisposing factors. Taieb [4] did not find infundibular parakeratosis but showed presence of keratinized inner root sheath in the casts. Zhang [8] explained this phenomenon as a consequence of frequent tractions on hair shafts leading to parakeratosis of the inner and outer root sheath cells over the infundibulum. Other authors suggested that an individual predisposition was necessary to develop HCs.

Our observations refer to patients who developed HCs after topical application of all-trans retinoic acid solution. There is evidence in the literature that systemic administration of etretinate may cause alopecia characterized by reduction of the duration of the anagen phase and increased telogen shedding. The latter would be secondary to reduction of adhesiveness between the hair shaft and the immediately adjacent hair follicle structures [9]. On the contrary, experimental models and clinical studies demonstrated that a local stimulus mediated by retinoic acid had a positive effect on follicular cell proliferation [10, 11]. The action of retinoids at nuclear level results in mRNA- and protein synthesis. This hypothesis seems to suggest that retinoids first stimulate proliferative processes resulting in some cell accumulation. The 'excess' would be subsequently eliminated via HCs formation. If this hypothesis proves correct topically applied retinoids would represent a useful tool to experimentally induce HCs. Moreover some supposed pathogenetic mechanisms such as «hair traction» may at least lead to hyperproliferative stimulus and HCs formation confirming the former hypothesis.

This view would be in contrast with Taieb's proposal to treat HCs with topically applied retinoids [4].

References

1   Grindon J. J Cutan Genitourin Dis. 1897; 15: 256-259
2   Kligman AM. Arch Dermatol. 1957; 75: 509-511
3   Scott JS, Roenigk HH. J Am Acad Dermatol. 1983; 8: 27-32
4   Taieb A, Surlève-Bazeille JE, Maleville J. Arch Dermatol. 1985; 121: 1009-1013
5   Keipert JA. Arch Dermatol. 1986; 122: 927-930
6   Mainardi L, Carminati G, Menni S, Croci S, Caputo R. G Ital Dermatol Venereol. 1988; 123: 565-566
7   Bayerl C, Moll I. Hautarzt. 1993; 44: 37-39
8   Zhang W. Clin Exper Dermatol. 1995; 20: 202-207
9   Berth-Jones J, Hutkinson PE. Br J Dermatol. 1995; 132: 367-375
10 Bazzano G, Terezakis N, Attia H, Bazzano A, et al. J Invest Dermatol. 1993; 101: 138S-142S
11 Bazzano GS, Terezakis N, Galen W. J Am Acad Dermatol. 1986; 15: 880-883; 890-893

Physical aspects
and hair transplantation techniques

©1996 Elsevier Science B.V. All rights reserved.
Hair research for the next millenium
D.J.J. Van Neste and V.A. Randall (Eds)

Workshop report on:

Physical methods for human hair evaluation

B. Forslind, H. Baden and H. Ogawa

B. Forslind

Physical methods for evaluation of hair disease and disorders are generally restricted to transmission electron microscopy (TEM) and scanning microscopy (SEM) for imageing subcellular abnormalities and topographic changes respectively. For elemental analysis on bulk samples of hair spectrographic techniques have been utilized frequently. In the past a great number of works dealing with hair elemental analysis has been performed to test the feasibility of different techniques to biological material. In spite of the fact that a great number of investigations are done each year, little concern has unfortunately been taken to ensure that the biological material has been collected under optimal conditions. It has been shown that contamination constitutes a serious problem in elemental hair analysis and that the virgin, uncontaminated part of the hair fibre is the intrafollicular part plus one or two millimeters protruding over the scalp surface. Single hair fibre analysis is therefore a recommended approach when elemental analysis is desired, but enough material should be investigated to account for variations in elemental content of fibres from the same location and individual. Particle probe techniques are especially advantageous since they give simultaneous recordings of all physiologically interesting and contaminating elements. This allows evaluation of hair growth physiology and monitoring of elemental extrusion of elements, e.g., toxic metals.

H. Baden

Major strides have been made in the understanding genetic diseases through techniques of molecular biology. Physical methods, however, may provide clues or clarify diagnostic problems. Trichothiodystrophy is a rare disease of hair showing alternating light and dark bands by polarizing microscopy (PM). This results from lack of matrix protein and misalignment of keratin filaments. A patient with arginosuccinic aciduria had fragile hair and banding by PM. Scanning electron microscopy (SEM) revealed periodic longitudinal grooves of the surface. With proper diet, the hair became normal. The uncombable hair syndrome presents a hair unable to lie flat and results from the shaft having a triangular shape. A child presented unruly sparse hair, not triangular in shape.

SEM showed hairs with an abnormal cuticle that kept the shafts apart. These are examples demonstrating the value of physical methods (e. g., SEM) in understanding shaft abnormalities.

R. Tsuboi, R. Ueki and H. Ogawa

Several methods have been reported for the quantitative analysis of human scalp hair loss including photography, counting of fallen hairs, counting newly grown hairs, trichogram and phototrichogram. The phototrichogram uses a photographic technique to measure hair elongation by recording two photographs of a specified area within a specified period. The method has an advantage in being non-invasive and allowing quantitative analysis during long observation periods. Our phototrichogram method has been used to the study female diffuse alopecia of unknown origin. Hairs in an area of 1 cm^2 were clipped with scissors and a photograph was recorded at a fixed distance using an optical microscope and a video recorder. This first photographic recording was designated as hairs at time 0 hours. Another photograph of exactly the same area was recorded 48 hours later at the same fixed distance. Computer based image analysis was performed using NIH image software. The rate of hair growth was given in mm/day, while anagen hair ratio was calculated as the percentage of hairs having growth rates greater than 0.2 mm/day. Hairs clipped for the phototrichogram were collected and the diameter of the hairs, expressed in mm, was measured at three different points using a micrometer. Patients with the diagnosis of diffuse alopecia of unknown origin had reduced hair density and/or hair growth rate when compared to the normal individuals suggesting the heterogeneity of the disorder.

RJ. Trancik

The process of evaluating hair growth has evolved rapidly in recent years primarily because of the development of agents which affect hair regrowth. Methods are needed that are accurate, reproducible, non-invasive, and could be used in large scale clinical trials. Various methods that have been used to evaluate hair regrowth, a technology still considered in its infancy, were reviewed and discussed. The feasibility of their applications in clinical research was also presented. Through continued modification and refinement, improved methods are certain to be developed.

Clinical methods for determining the efficacy of hair growth products

Method	Invasive	Accurate	Reproducible	Easy to perform	Permanent record
Biopsy	yes	+++	yes	yes, but	yes
Hair pull	yes	±	no	yes	yes
Trichogram	yes	+	yes	yes	yes
Hair count	no	+	yes, but	no	yes
Phototrichogram	no	++	yes	yes, but	yes
Hair weight	no	+++	yes	no	yes
Global	no	±	?	yes	yes
Questionnaire	no	?	?	yes, but	yes

B. Forslind

The problems of hair diameter measurements were discussed. Several options were suggested: measurements in the SEM, optical diffraction techniques using HeNe-laser light which provides a very high accuracy (better than 0.05 µm), or image analysis on optical microscope images of cross sections of fibres in bundles compacted by thermosensitive crimp-plastic tubes. Caucasian fibres as a rule have an eliptic cross section and tend to show the widest diameter when the fiber is lying flat on the support. Making a hair-pin loop will show the smallest diameter at the bend.

Microanalysis: application in hair study

A. Rossi, L. Daniele, P. Bonaccorsi, S. Giustini and S. Calvieri

Department of Dermatology, University of Rome «La Sapienza», Italy

Introduction

During our years of study on hair pathology we concluded that a better knowledge of hair chemical composition could help us in understanding of hair pathology. To this end, we tried to elaborate an easy and reliable method for detecting the presence of chemical elements on the hair shaft. Microanalysis is not a new technique because it was already well known in the field of mineral engineering when we hypothesized its application in the study of hair shaft. Microanalysis allows researchers to demonstrate the presence of chemical elements (oligoelements) along the hair shaft surface and to contemporaneously observe the sample under scanning electron microscopy, immediately correlating the morphological data with the biochemical findings. Moreover, the only processing procedures required are those necessary for scanning electron microscopy. Microanalysis is an analytical investigation which allows for a quali-quantitative analysis of sample surface. The sample, excited by an electron beam, releases different types of radiation itself: type II and back scattered electrons used for vision, and X-rays used for microanalysis. X-rays are used to determine and to localize the presence of the different oligoelements on hair shaft surface. They are captured by a probe and transferred into a computer which processes these data and plots the presence of the different oligoelements. Samples of hair shaft from 20 healthy subjects were studied. The aim of our study was to establish the pattern of oligoelement in normal hair surface, in order to give a basis for the research on hair pathologies. Moreover X-ray maps give us the topographic distribution of the different oligoelements on hair shaft surface. All this information can help us to interpret some morphological alterations often found in microscopical studies (eg trichothiodystrophy). In normal hair, keratins have a regular and periodic distribution. X-ray map support can be of great value in determining the presence of oligoelements on normal hair surface.

Materials and methods

Samples of hair shaft from 20 healthy and black haired subjects, ranging from 6 to 70 years of age, were examined. Samples were taken from various scalp zones with titanium scissors. Samples were always taken and preserved in the same conditions of heat and humidity. Each sample was examined for 1cm of length. Samples were fixed, dehydrated and then carbonized with an Evaporizator Balzers SCD 040, observed under a scanning electron microscope Philips 515S and analysed by means of a microanalysis system Edax 9800. Slides obtained from light and polarized microscopy and from scanning electron microscopy were then reversed on a Photo-CD. The digital image elaboration has been made with the support of a personal computer 486 DX2 66Mhz, 8M Ram, 420M HD, video board 24-bit (true color), digitalizer board Matrox IP-8, Photo-CD unit reader, software for image analysis and processing AnalySIS 2.0, iPhoto Plus 1.0.

Results

All samples examined under scanning electron microscopy showed a normal morphology, i.e. the cuticle was normally inbricated. The spectrum of the qualitative examination showed peaks of Na, Mg, Si, P, S, Cl, K, Ca, Fe. On the basis of this spectrometric qualitative analysis, we performed a quantitative analysis which showed the presence of high S, Ca and Cl contents, with mean percentage values of 91.95%, 1.97% and 1.17% respectively. The other oligoelements were present in traces with mean percentage values ranging from 0.14% to 0.97%. Because of the significative presence of S, Cl and Ca, we decided to make X-rays maps of those oligoelements. These maps have been overlapped over the SEM hair image to visualize the oligoelements distribution along the hair shaft. Sulphur X-ray map showed an homogenous periodic distribution of this oligoelement along the examined hair shaft surface. Cl and Ca were less significantly represented but equally homogeneously distributed.

Conclusions

Our results supply us with the oligoelements composition of the surface of the cuticle of normal hair shaft, whereas X-rays maps documented their statistical distribution along hair shaft surface. The presence of oligoelements is easily explained in some cases (S, Na, K, Fe, P), more difficult to interpret in other cases. Although further studies and wider statistics are probably necessary, we are confident of our data reliability because they were confirmed in all patients. On the other hand an influence of environmental, dietary and lavorative factors between different populations and also within the same geographic areas, must be taken into account. To this end, it is in our programs to study samples coming from other countries and from different work categories. It would also be interesting to find out which chemical differences do exist between dark and blond hair because of the different melanin they contain. Moreover, the reproducibility of our study is confirmed by the results we obtained in another study conducted on hair affected by trichothiodystrophy. In fact, in this case, results obtained by microanalysis significantly differed from those obtained from healthy subjects. The present study represents the starting point for the study of different hair pathologies. In our opinion, the possibility to correlate morphological and chemical information could give interesting information for understanding of the pathogenesis of several hair defects.

References

1   Calvieri S. Trichothiodystrophy. G Ital Dermatol Venereol. 1993; 128: 17-26
2   Itin PH, Pittlelkow MR. Trichothiodystrophy: review of sulphur/deficient brittle hair syndromes and association with ectodermal dysplasias. J Am Acad Dermatol. 1990; 22(5): 705-717
3   Curstedt T, Johansson J, Barros-Soderling J, et al. Low molecular-mass surfactant protein type I. The primary structure of a hydrophobic 8-kDa polypeptide with eight half-cystine residues. Eur J Biochem. 1988; 172: 521-525
4   Gillespie JM. The structural proteins of hair: isolation, characterization and regulation of biosynthesis. In: Goldsmith LA. Ed. Biochemistry and physiology of the skin. Oxford University Press, Oxford, 1983; pp 475-510
5   Shrestha KP, Schrauzer GN. Trace elements in hair: a study of residents in Darjeeling (India) and San Diego, California. Science Total Env. 1989; 79: 171-177
6   Wilhelm M. Ohnesorge FH, Lombeck I, Hafner D. Uptake of aluminium, cadmium, copper, lead and zinc by human scalp hair and elution of the absorbed metals. J Analytic Toxical. 1989; 13: 17-21
7   Fenton DA, Morris IW, Kendal MD. Energy-dispersive X-ray microanalysis (EDAX): a method to access the elemental composition of hair. Clin Exp.Dermatol. 1988; 2: 46-47
8   Samani SB, Kiprawi AZ, Ismail RB. Mercury determination in hair of malaysian fisherman by neutron activation analysis. Biol Trace Elem Res. 1994 fall; 43-45: 435-441
9   Contiero E, Folin M. Trace elements nutritional status. Use of hair as a diagnostic tool. Biol Trace Elem Res. 1994 Feb; 40(2): 151-160
10 Lamand M, Favier A, Ineau A. Determination of trace elements in the hair: significance and limitations. Ann Biol Clin. Paris. 1990; 48(7): 433-442
11 Calvieri S, Zampetti M, Corbo A, et al. Risultati preliminari dell'impiego in un sistema di microanalisi del capello in pazienti affetti da Tricotiodistrofia. G Ital Dermatol Venereol. 1988; 123: 583-585
12 Rossi A. La microanalisi degli oligoelementi: un sistema di indagine nella patologia degli annessi. Suppl Dermotime. 4/1995; VI-XI

©1996 Elsevier Science B.V. All rights reserved.
Hair research for the next millenium
D.J.J. Van Neste and V.A. Randall (Eds)

Elemental analysis of hair: what techniques can be used and what information can be obtained ?

B. Forslind

EDRG Medical Biophysics, MBB Karolinska Institute 171 77 Stockholm, Sweden

Introduction

Bulk or single fibre analysis - the sampling problem

The human scalp hair fibre is fully consolidated one millimeter above the midbulb level [1]. It is conceivable that physiologically important elements are more or less effectively trapped by binding to proteins in the consolidated fibre. In consequence, the overall elemental composition will reflect the status of the particular hair follicle at growth. Longitudinal studies of the elemental distributions in hair follicles support this tentative argument [2]. Analysis of a virgin part of the hair fibre, i.e within the 2-3 mm from the root of plucked hair fibres, provide the information sought for with minimal interference due to contamination and extraction imposed on the fibre by the environment (including any cosmetic activity).

The sampling area is important as individuals with a heredity for androgenetic alopecia (AnA) may have a conspicuously increased number of telogen follicles in coronal and frontal areas long before the typical pattern of hair loss becomes obvious. The temporal region chosen in our studies represents an area with normal anagen/telogen ratio. Also, it was shown [2] that different areas of the scalp may indeed reveal different elemental contents.

Bulk analyses and single hair fibre analysis

Spectrographic methods either utilize «bulk» specimens or single fibres. In the first case, e.g. AAS, NAA, 50-200 mg of material is needed for the analysis [3], in the second method, e.g., particle probes, a few millimeters of a single fibre provide a satisfactory volume for analysis.

Spectrographic methods generally require standards for absolute quantitation [2], therefore no quantitation will be better than that allowed by the standard, i.e. the stoichiometric composition of the chosen standard. In addition, it should be emphasized that most bulk methods are completely destructive in contrast to single strand analyses.

Particle probe analyses of single hair fibres

Particle probe techniques involve excitation of the elements contained in the irradiated cross section volume by impinging on elementary particles. In wave length dispersive X-ray (WLDX) analysis and energy dispersive X-ray analysis (EDX) the sample is irradiated with a beam of electrons [2]. As a secondary effect the excited elements will emit characteristic X-ray quanta. WLDX analysis only allows single energy (quantum) analysis whereas EDX provides an energy spectrum recording several elements simultaneously. The sensitivity of the EDX is high, i.e levels down to 200 ppm (parts per million, e.g. $\mu g/g$) can be detected and only a very small area of the specimen is irradiated. The methods can be thought of as essentially non-destructive. The X-ray microanalysis performed in the STEM (scanning transmission electron microscope) requires that the specimen is a thin section, usually <6 μm and it is possible to discern details of the morphology to allow a precise localization of the probe within a cellular or even a subcellular compartment. Bulk specimens are analyzed and viewed in SEM (scanning electron microscope) mode, and effectively the spatial resolution is less than in the STEM mode.

Since protons are approximately 2000 times heavier than electrons the stopping power of the material under analysis is much less than for electrons. Therefore protons will produce virtually no background radiation directly and PIXE-(particle induced X-ray emission) analysis has a sensitivity that can be brought down to at least 1 ppm for elements of $Z>12$ [2]. For light elements PIXE essentially gives information from the surface of the object and therefore the form of the hair fibre under analysis may influence the results [4].

The great advantage of the EDX and PIXE techniques is the simultaneous recording of all elements (of interest). Quotients (or ratios) of specific elements have proven to be of value for assessment of biological activity and function [5].

X-ray fluorescence analysis (XRF) of single hair fibres

A new X-ray fluorescent technique for trace element analysis of small sample volumes (<1-2 mm^3) was recently introduced [6]. It achieves a high radiation flux on the specimen by focusing X-rays from a conventional industrial X-ray tube using a conical capillary which concentrates the beam onto the object specimen. The secondary fluorescent X-rays are collected by an energy dispersive system which has a sensitivity range from $Z>11$, i.e. elements heavier than Na and the technique gives high sensitivity, down to 1 ppm for certain elements, e.g. Mn, Fe, Ni, Cu, and Zn [6]. Little, if any, specimen preparation is needed except for removal of obvious surface contamination by rinsing or other means. Being a non-vacuum, «open system» method, it allows control of humidity and temperature when desired. With respect to sensitivity the XRF technique compares well to the PIXE analysis technique [4, 6] and can be optimized for a number of specific analysis tasks by selective choice of the excitation wavelength (X-ray tube), i.e. anode material, e.g. Mo, Cr *etc.* The effectiveness per dose unit in producing secondary X-ray quanta appears higher for primary excitatory X-rays than for the same dose of particles with EDX and PIXE. A notable advantage of this technique is that it is truly non-destructive when normal exposure times are used and the reproducibility is high, which has been shown by repeated analyses of hairs.

Results

A compilation of our single fibre data is presented in Tables 1 and 2. All analyses were done in triplets [4,6]. The PIXE analysis was done 5 mm from the root end and already here effects of contamination through cosmetic and other sources are noted, e.g. in conspicuous variation in the Ca and Cl values. The XRF values are given as median values because there are skew distributions of the primary data which is deemed to be related mainly to varying cross sections of the fibres under analysis. Especially the characteristic fluorescent X-rays originating from elements with low atomic number, e.g., $Z < 17$, will suffer some «self-absorption» in the specimen material and this results in recording of too low elemental content data.

Table 1.
Elemental content (dry weight) of human hair fibres (x 3) obtained from the temporal region of 103 healthy caucasian probands [4].

Table 2.
Median values of elemental content ($\mu g/g$ dw) of root and consolidated hair fibre (x 3) from 10 healthy probands [6]

PIXE analysis		XRF analysis		
Element	Content (dry weight)	Element	Root	Fibre
^{15}P	n.d.	^{15}P	4861	9
^{16}S	0.049 ± 0.008 g/g	^{16}S	6689	22.2272*
^{17}Cl	3.3 ± 2.2 mg/g	^{17}Cl	1958	534
^{19}K	n.d.	^{19}K	11.938	0.4
^{20}Ca	330 ± 240 $\mu g/g$	^{20}Ca	274	217
^{30}Zn	170 ± 50 $\mu g/g$	^{30}Zn	114	101

*The low ^{16}S value (0,022 µg/g dry weight) is due to self absorption of the low energy $S_{K\alpha}$ characteristic X-ray-radiation as discussed elsewhere {6}.

Conclusions

EDX, PIXE and XRF analysis of sulfur and trace elements in hair fibres for pathological diagnosis is still in its cradle. In order to be able to take full advantage of these techniques we are in great need of data from large populations, more precise than those given by previous work [3]. Such data should be obtained in conjunction with blood analyses whenever possible for assessment of body status in relation to the hair analysis. No doubt, elemental analysis represents a promising approach to understand the physiology of keratin formation both in the normal and pathological case. In conjunction with biochemical techniques, e.g., electrophoresis and immunological methods it furthermore represents an additional way to understand the phenomena of hair growth and the disturbances involved in the process of cell differentiation and hair formation in the hair follicle.

References

1   Forslind B, Lindström B, Swanbeck G. Microradiographic and autoradiographic studies of keratin formation in the human hair. Acta Dermatovener (Stockholm). 1970; 51: 81-89
2   Forslind B. X-ray microanalysis of the integument. In P Ingram, JD Shelburne, VL Roggli (eds). Microprobe analysis in medicine, Hemisphere Publ. Corp, New York. 1989; Ch 11: pp 207-218
3   Iyengar GV, Kollmer WE, Bowen HJM. The elemental composition of human tissues and body fluids. A compilation of values for adults. Verlag Chemie, Weinheim, New York. 1978; pp 51-54
4   Forslind B, Li HK, Malmqvist KG, Wiegleb D. Elemental content of anagen hairs in a normal caucasian population. S tudies with PIXE. Scanning Electron Microscopy. 1986; I: 237-241
5   Forslind B, Malmqvist KG, Wiren K. Genetic diseases, hair structure and elemental content. In GE Rogers et al.: The Biology of Wool and Hair, Chapman & Hall, London & New York. 1988; pp 275-285
6   Stocklassa B, Aransay-Vitores M, Nilsson G, Wiegleb D, Forslind B. The elemental content of human hair fibres. Accepted for publication in Scanning Microscopy. 1994

Microanalysis: study of hair affected by trichothiodystrophy

A. Rossi, L. Daniele, P. Bonaccorsi, M. Carlesimo and S. Calvieri

Department of Dermatology, University of Rome "La Sapienza", Italy

Introduction

Trichothiodystrophy (TTD), or sulphur deficient brittle hair, is a clinical marker for a neuroectodermal symptom complex that usually features mental and physical retardation and may also include nail dystrophy, ichthyosis, ocular and dental anomalies and decreased fertility. The hallmark of this entity is the tiger tail appearance of affected hair under polarized microscopy, consisting of bright and dark alternating bands along the hair shaft. Because of reduced sulphur containing aminoacids, TTD represents a good experimental model for evaluation of the reliability of this relatively new and poorly known technique. Microanalysis allows researchers to demonstrate the presence of chemical elements (oligoelements) along the hair shaft surface and to contemporaneously observe the sample under scanning electron microscopy (SEM). An electron beam released by the scanning electron microscope, excites the surface under examination which releases many electrons itself. While some of these electrons are used for vision on SEM, the others are captured by a probe and transferred into a computer. The computer processes these data and plots the presence of the different oligoelements. It is also possible to create X-ray maps which demonstrate the presence of oligoelements molecules on the sample surface. We tried therefore to interpret the morphological data connected with the tiger tail appearance from a chemical point of view. The oligoelements most abundant in normal hair are calcium and sulphur. Hair affected by TTD was therefore tested for these two oligoelements.

Materials and methods

Samples from 7 children affected by various varieties of TTD, ranging from 3 to 11 years of age were examined. Samples were taken from various scalp zones with titanium scissors. Each sample was examined for 1cm of lenght, in light microscopy, polarized microscopy by means of a Leitz Laborlux 12. Samples were then fixed, dehydrated and then carbonized with a Evaporizator Balzers SCD 040, observed under a scanning electron microscope Philips 515S and analyzed by means of a microanalysis system Edax 9800. Slides obtained from light and polarized microscopy and from scanning electron microscopy, were then reversed on a Photo-CD. The digital image elaboration has been made with the support of a personal computer 486 DX2 66Mhz, 8M Ram, 420M HD, video board 24-bit (true color), digitalizer board Matrox IP-8, Photo-CD unit reader, software for image analysis and processing AnalySIS 2.0, iPhoto Plus 1.0.

Results

The qualitative examination that we performed by means of microanalysis on normal hair, showed the presence of Na, Mg, Si, P, S, Cl, K, Ca and Fe. On the basis of this spectrometric qualitative analysis, we performed a quantitative study which showed the presence of an high percentage of S, ranging between 89% and 98% ; Cl and Ca were present in percentages ranging between 1% and 3% ; the other oligoelements were present in traces. Because S and Ca were the most abundant oligoelements in normal hair, we decided to study their distribution in both normal and pathological samples by means of X-Ray map. Thank to a computerized system of digital image elaboration we could correlate information coming from scanning electron microscopy, light and polarized microscopy and microanalysis. Our results showed that whereas Ca and S were homogeneously represented along normal hair shaft, in pathological samples S concentration resulted reduced and Ca was absent in some of the examined tracts. Data coming from our system of image overlapping showed that calcium was absent in tracts corresponding to dark bands while it was normally present in light bands.

Conclusions

By means of X-rays maps we were able to evaluate the distribution of oligoelements under consideration (S, Ca). Moreover, thank to our image analysis system, which allows to overlap image of the same sample obtained in light and polarized microscopy, in scanning electron microscopy and X-ray maps we were able to correlate morphological and chemical informations. From these data we found that whereas in normal hair sulphur was highly and homogeneously distributed along hair shaft surface, in hair affected by TTD sulphur representation is, as expected, reduced. Moreover it is interesting to observe calcium behaviour. In normal sample it was present in percentages ranging from 1% to 3% and was homogeneously distributed, whereas in pathological samples it was present only in some of the examined tracts. More precisely, the data coming from image analysis showed that calcium was absent in dark bands, but was normally present in bright bands. Although it is difficult to find a pathogenetic explanation of these results, at least where calcium is concerned, we can hypothesize that this distribution of calcium and sulphur, different from that found in normal hair, could be responsible for the morphological alteration found in hair affected by TTD. It is in our programm to conduct studies on a wider statistics and to study the distribution of other oligoelements.

References

1   Calvieri S. Trichothiodystrophy. G Ital Dermatol Venereol. 1993; 128: 17-26
2   Itin PH, Pittlelkow MR. Trichothiodystrophy: Review of sulphur/deficient brittle hair syndromes and association with ectodermal dysplasias. J Am Acad Dermatol. 1990; 22(5): 705-717
3   Curstedt T, Johansson J, Barros-Soderling J, *et al.* Low molecular-mass surfactant protein type I. The primary structure of a hydrophobic 8-kDa polypeptide with eight half-cystine residues. Eur J Biochem. 1988; 172: 521-525
4   Gillespie JM. The structural proteins of hair: Isolation, characterization and regulation of biosynthesis. In: Goldsmith LA (Ed). Biochemistry and physiology of the skin. Oxford University Press, Oxford. 1983; pp 475-510
5   Shrestha KP, Schrauzer GN. Trace elements in hair: A study of residents in Darjeeling (India) and San Diego, California. Science Total Env. 1989; 79: 171-177
6   Wilhelm M, Ohnesorge FH, Lombeck I, Hafner D. Uptake of aluminium, cadmium, copper, lead and zinc by human scalp hair and elution of the absorbed metals. J Analytic Toxicol. 1989; 13: 17-21
7   Fenton DA, Morris IW, Kendal MD. Energy-dispersive X-ray microanalysis (EDAX): A method to access the elemental composition of hair. Clin Exp Dermatol. 1988; 2: 46-47
8   Samani SB, Kiprawi AZ, Ismail RB. Mercury determination in hair of malaysian fisherman by neutron activation analysis. Biol Trace Elem Res. 1994; 43-45: 435-441
9   Contiero E, Folin M. Trace elements nutritional status. Use of hair as a diagnostic tool. Biol Trace Elem Res. 1994 Feb; 40(2): 151-160
10 Lamand M, Favier A, Ineau A. Determination of trace elements in the hair: significance and limitations. Ann Biol Clin Paris. 1990; 48(7): 433-442

A simple apparatus to obtain the stress-strain curve of the hair shaft

A. Tosti[1], B.M. Piraccini[1], C. Misciali[1], R. Zannoli[2], G. Testoni[2], B. Berardi[2] and M. Baccolini[2]

[1]Department of Dermatology, University of Bologna, Via Massarenti, 1 40138 Bologna, Italy
[2]Department of Medical Physics, University of Bologna, Italy

Introduction

The study of biomechanics of the hair shaft is useful in studying several hair diseases [1-6].

The evaluation of the mechanical characteristics of hair shaft requires sophisticated and complex instruments, which are not always accessible for the majority of the researchers working in the hair field [6]. In many cases the specimens are sent to central laboratories specialized in the study of wool hair, which is very complex and wastes much time.

At the Department of Dermatology of the University of Bologna, a very simple and inexpensive apparatus (Fig. 1) was developed in order to overcome the described difficulties.

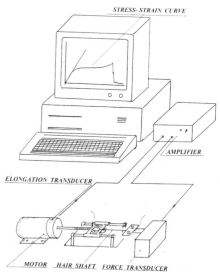

STRESS-STRAIN CURVE

AMPLIFIER

ELONGATION TRANSDUCER

MOTOR   HAIR SHAFT FORCE TRANSDUCER

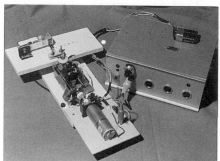

Figure 1. General view of the apparatus. The available apparatus comprises three parts:
- Load cell with amplifier;
- Mechanical stretching apparatus;
- Computer interface and dedicated software.

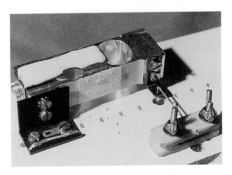

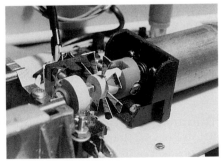

Figure 2. Load cell with amplifier   *Figure 3. Mechanical stretching apparatus*

Materials and methods

Hair specimens are obtained from the scalp of volunteers using forceps placed close to the scalp in order to avoid a permanent deformation of the hair shaft.

Load cell with amplifier (max load 600 grams, sensitivity 0.1 grams) (Fig. 2)

The load cell is a strength transducer, which converts strength in electrical signals directly proportional to the applied load. Tensile stress is applied by an electrical engine, which drives, through a precision worm-screw, a slide connected to the first clamp which fixes the specimen. The second clamp is directly linked to the load cell for the real time evaluation of the applied strength.

Mechanical stretching apparatus (Fig. 3)

The stretch is evaluated by the rotation of a paddle wheel that is found in front of a photoelectric cell. This then counts the number of the lapses, which is proportional to the shift of the slide. The maximum slide shift is 40 mm and the resolution in the evaluation of the stretch is 0.06 mm.

Computer interface and dedicated program

Used for execution, storage and analysis of procedures. Electric signals proportional to applied force and stretch are sent to a personal computer through a 12 bits A/D converter and hardware interface. Dedicated software was developed to control the acquisition, the calculation, the elaboration and the storage of the data.

A strength-stretch curve is displayed in real time on the PC monitor and can be analyzed to obtain the stress-strain curve and to calculate elastical parameters like the Young modulus and the break-point stress.

Stress is calculated measuring the cross-section of the hair. We performed this measurement in two ways: by an electron microscope (0.1 micron resolution) or by light microscope photographs with a definite magnification measuring hair shaft diameter with a simple ruler.

Results

We performed preliminary experiments to test the linearity of the measuring system using a small spring with a constant elasticity of 25 gr/cm. The stress-strain curve was in this case a perfect straight line.

Young modulus is evaluated by a linear fitting of the values in the elastic region of the stress-strain curve and is represented by the angular coefficient of the interpolation straight line.

Normal hair shaft stress-strain curve (Fig. 4): in the elastic region (20-25% strain) the linear fitting and the evaluation of the Young modulus are shown. Break-point stress and maximum strain are displayed.

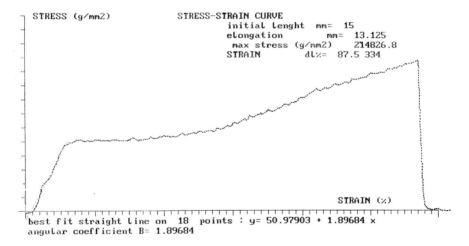

Figure 4. Normal hair shaft stress-strain curve

Discussion

The purpose of this paper is to provide a simple and inexpensive system for the analysis of the hair shaft mechano-elastic properties, which can be used by the dermatologist himself in both scientific research and clinical routine. Obtained values are perfectly comparable when we use an electron microscope and/or a light microscope to evaluate the cross-section of the hair shaft. The whole measuring procedure is very simple: tools and devices used are easily found and not expensive. Data elaboration, evaluation of the stress, calculation of the Young modulus with a minimum squared linear fitting method and data storage are all simple to perform. Nevertheless the system is characterized by precise results. The complete construction of a stress strain curve requires no more than five minutes and our system can analyze a large number of specimens and can be used not only in scientific research, but also in clinical routine.

References

1   Korostoff E, Rawnsley HM, Shelley WB. Normalized stress-strain relationship in human hair perturbation by hypothyroidism. Br J Dermatol. 1970; 83 Jubilee Issue: 27-36
2   Goldsmith LA, Baden HP. The mechanical properties of hair. Chemical modifications and pathological hairs. J Invest Dermatol. 1971; 56: 200
3   Swanbeck G, Nyren J, Juhlin L. Mechanical properties of hairs from patients with different types of hair disease. J Invest Dermatol. 1970; 54: 248
4   Nikiforidis G, Balas C, Tsambaos D. Mechanical parameters of human hair: possible application in the diagnosis and follow-up of hair disorders. Clin Phys Physiol Meas. 1992; 13: 281-290
5   Nikiforidis G, Balas C, Tsambaos D. A method for the determination of viscoelastic parameters of human hair in relation to its structure. Skin Pharmacol. 1993; 6: 32-37
6   Nikiforidis G, Balas C, Tsambaos D. Viscoelastic response of human hair cortex. Med Biol Eng Comput. 1992; 301: 83-88

Scanning electron microscopy details in bubble hair

J. Ferrando[1], T. Solé[1], R. Grimalt[1] and A. Dominguez[2]

[1]Department of Dermatology, Faculty of Medicine, Hospital Clinic. Villarroel 170, 08036 Barcelona, Spain
[2]Unit of Electron Microscopy, University of Barcelona, Spain

Introduction

Bubble hair (BH) is a recently identified acquired hair shaft abnormality characterized by patches of coarse hair in the occipital and/or parietal areas with broken hair, a few centimeters from the scalp. Microscopic examination reveals the presence of multiple bubble-like areas in the hair. All four published cases are women [1-3].

A BH-like defect has been reproduced experimentally by overheating hair with a hair-drier. Bubbles contain air but no liquid [2].

Materials and methods

We studied under the scanning electron microscope (SEM) the first case of BH localized in the frontal area of a male.

Results

The SEM study shows:
- Alternating dilatations of the hair shaft corresponding to the bubble-like areas and cavities (Fig. 1).
- Longitudinally disposed fissures of the hair shaft near orifices at the hair surface (Figs. 2 and 3).
- Irregular distal fractures exposing the hair cortex with multiple inner cavities i.e. «Swiss cheese-like» appearance of the broken hair edge (Fig. 4).
- Minor cavities with dilatations of the hair cuticule (Fig. 4).

Discussion

BH is an acquired hair defect caused by dry heating. This results in wide and multiple dilatations within all constitutive layers of the hair shaft including the

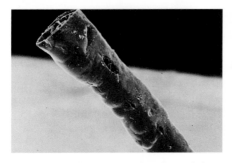

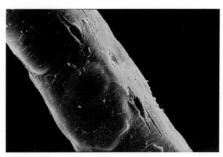

Figure 1. Dilatations and orifices of the hair shaft.

Figure 2. Longitudinally disposed fissures nearby the orifices.

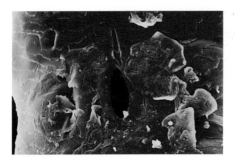

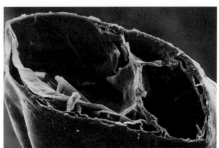

Figure 3. Close-up of figure 2

Figure 4. «Swiss cheese-like» appearance of the cortex and minor cavities inside the cuticular layer.

hair cuticule. Ambiant air enters the bubbles through the damaged cuticle. The weakened shaft breaks prematurely in the absence of any underlying structural hair defects.

Our case report is the first study of BH affecting the frontal area in a male. We also report for the first time the presence of fissures, orifices and dilatations of the cuticule.

References

1   Brown VM, Crounse RG, Abele DC. An unusual new hair shaft abnormality: «bubble hair». J Am Acad Dermatol. 1986; 15: 1113-1117

2   Detwiler SP, Carson JL, Woosley JT, Gambling TM, Briggaman RA. Bubble Hair. Case caused by an overheating hair dryer and reproducibility in normal hair with heat. J Am Acad Dermatol. 1994; 30: 54-60

3   Elston DM, Bergfeld WF, Whiting DA, McMahon JT, Dawson DM, Quint KL, Muhlbauer JE. Bubble hair. J Cutan Pathol. 1992; 19: 439-444

©1996 Elsevier Science B.V. All rights reserved.
Hair research for the next millenium
D.J.J. Van Neste and V.A. Randall (Eds)

Phototrichogram: an entirely automated method of quantification by image analysis

F. Chatenay, M. Courtois, G. Loussouarn and C. Hourseau

Laboratoires de Recherche Appliquée et Développement L'Oréal, 92117 Clichy Cedex, France

Introduction

The phototrichogram (PTG) was developed to monitor the principal parameters of hair growth. After shaving a small scalp area, it is possible to observe the growth of hair after 2 or 3 days and evaluate the number in telogen, the number in anagen, their growth rate and diameter [1-3]. If the same scalp area is observed at regular intervals, the evolution of these parameters as well as the succession of hair cycles can be monitored. PTG's computerized approaches have already been attempted [4, 5], allowing semi-automated analysis but still a number of technical difficulties remain unsolved [6]. The use of the PTG technique in clinical studies of hair care products needs a huge number of photos for analysis, for this reason we sought to develop a completely automated program for PTG analysis.

Materials and methods

130 volunteers, 18 to 55 years old, with androgenetic alopecia (Hamilton grade II to V) were treated under double-blind conditions daily for 3 months. Half the group received the active product (hair treatment lotion), the other half receiving the placebo.

On each subject a PTG was performed on the same scalp area (1 cm²) at time 0, 6 and 14 weeks.

The photographs were taken under standard conditions with a reflex camera (Olympus + macro lens + ring flash). The analysis of a PTG is accomplished on the basis of 3 slides (Fig. 1):

- the 1st after shaving, at a length of 0.7 mm.
- the 2nd after a 2nd shave, which cuts the hair down to scalp level
- the 3rd, 2 days after hair growth.

The slides are digitalized, stored on optical disk and submitted to morphometric analysis using the image analyzer Quantimet 570 Leica. On each slide, analysis is made on an area of 0.4 cm².

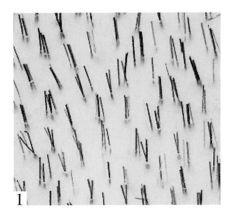
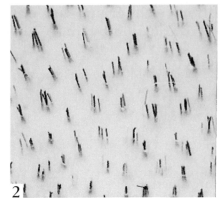
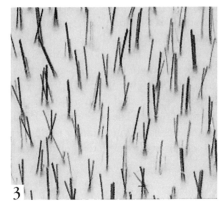

Figure 1. Photos 1 and 2: day 0 (light shave followed by close shave); Photo 3: after 2 days

The analysis consists of the following steps

Image matching

The automatic comparison of images requires that the 2 images correspond very precisely. Despite every effort on positioning when the shot is taken, no two slides of the same area can ever be perfectly superimposed. An automated correction, carried out according to an algorithm developed by M. Herbin and A. Venot A [unpublished data], ensures hair by hair matching of the PTGs of the same scalp area.

The correction consists of a two-dimensional translation, a rotation and a homothetic transformation. The photo at day 0 is the reference used for correction of all the PTGs of the same area carried out subsequently.

Identification of the hairs

A set of binary and grey level morphological transformations of the images is performed. These transformations consist on the one hand of differentiating between hairs and scalp, eliminating scalp imperfections and, on the other hand, of carrying out binary detection whose threshold and specificity are progressively refined to detect all the hairs and only the hairs. The comparison between the three photos allows the hair count (photos 1 and 2), the identification (x, y position) and the characterization (anagen or telogen phase) of each hair, the measurement of the rate of growth and, if necessary, of the diameter (photos 2 and 3).

Validation of automatic counts

The validation of automatic counts of hairs in anagen and telogen was carried out by assessing the equivalence of the results of the automated method to those obtained by visual observation by a group of experts. In all, 336 phototrichograms were analyzed visually and by computer. The criteria laid down were densities of anagen and telogen hairs and % of hairs in telogen.

The correlation between the visual and computerized counts for each of the parameters is very good (r = 0.99). The differences between the visual and computerized results were calculated (Table 1). These differences, compared with the degree of variability arising from visual hair counts shows the equivalence of the 2 visual and computerized systems of counting (p < 0.0001).

A second way of assessing the method was to examine product efficacy results from the clinical study depending on which data were used: computerized measurements or visual readings.

The reduction in % telogen in the active group by comparison with the placebo group after 6 weeks' treatment demonstrated the positive effect of treatment, and demonstrated it in an equivalent fashion with the 2 methods of counting (Table 2). The overall density did not vary in a significant manner in the course of treatment, whichever counts were chosen.

The repeated measures analysis of variance shows that the response to treatment measured by the two counting techniques was identical, with a p value of less than 5 %.

Table 1.

Comparison of visual and computerized counting

	Anagen	Telogen	Telogen %
δ*	1.33	-0.99	0.02
$\pm 2\sigma$**	± 3.44	± 3.10	± 2.79

* δ = *difference (computerized - visual)*
** *the 95% confidence intervals can be calculated as* $\delta \pm 2\sigma$ *according to the variability from visual counts*

Table 2.
Comparison of the 2 methods: changes in telogen % in the course of treatment

	Visual counting		Computerized counting	
	6 weeks	14 weeks	6 weeks	14 weeks
Active group	-0.5	4.6	-0.7	5.0
Placebo group	2.9	4.1	2.8	4.1
Significance	S	NS	S	NS

Discussion

In the light of these results, the automated method of quantification of phototrichograms by image analysis is as effective as the eye of a trained observer.

It provides the main parameters of hair growth (density, telogen-anagen ratio, growth rate and cycle monitoring). This method offers the advantage over visual detection of being more reliable (no visual fatigue), and extremely time-saving (all the operations after photography are performed without human intervention) when wide-ranging analysis of phototrichograms have to be performed.

As with all techniques based on photography, the quality of the photos is of paramount importance. In particular the contrast between hair and scalp is an important factor. The use of video images might overcome some of the drawbacks of still photography: real time visualization and digitalisation of the images. This seems to us the next step worth investigating in this field.

If computerized measurement of hair diameter, currently being assessed, is added to the technique described, this automated analysis will cover, in a reliable and accurate manner, all the significant parameters of hair growth.

References

1   Saitoh M, Uzuka M, Sakamoto M. J Invest Dermatol. 1970; 54: 65-81
2   Fiquet C, Courtois M. Cutis. 1979; 3: 975-984
3   Courtois M, Loussouarn G, Hourseau C, Grollier J.F. Br J Dermatol. 1995; 132: 86-93
4   Pelfini L, Fideli D, Speziali A, Vignini M. Int J Cosmetic Sciences. 1987; 9: 1-11
5   Hayashi S, Miyamoto I, Takeda K. Br J Dermatol. 1991; 125: 123-129
6   Van Neste D. Dermatology. 1993; 187: 233-234

Hair research for the next millenium
D.J.J. Van Neste and V.A. Randall (Eds)

The detection of pores and holes in hair by electron microscopy

J.A. Swift

Department of Textiles & Fashion, De Montfort University, The Gateway, Leicester, LE1 9BH, U.K.

Introduction

The routes for diffusion and the sites occupied by dyestuffs and other water-soluble materials in keratin fibres such as human hair and sheep's wool, are of commercial interest. Current wisdom is that the so-called non-keratins of the cortex (i.e. the inter-macrofibrillar matrix and nuclear remnants) and cuticle (endocuticle) are key structures through which primary diffusion occurs. Further it has been suggested that initial access for aqueous-borne materials into the fibres takes place within the plane of the cell membrane complex (CMC) which separates the cells of the hair from each other [1]. More specifically it has been suggested that the intercellular cement or delta-layer, which is the centrally-located lamina of the CMC, swells in water and that this provides the primary route for transport [1]. Large holes and fissures in damaged hair have been revealed with phosphotungstic acid (PTA) [2] but, since this heteropolyacid is approximately 2.0 nm in diameter [3] it was inappropriate for «probing» fine diffusion pathways. In this paper a much smaller precipitated silver sulphide (Ag_2S) probe has been used to investigate aqueous diffusion processes in human hair with the aid of the electron microscope and, amongst other things, this has revealed that the delta-layer is not a major diffusion pathway.

Materials and methods

Long hair of approximately 400 mm length from a 30-year old woman was chosen for this study. The best description of the subject's hair was that it was «normal average» and in a style which was straight and freely hanging to the waist. No harsh treatments such as permanent waving, bleaching, or dyeing had been used nor did the subject use any styling aids. There was an abundance of «split ends» indicating that a modicum of natural weathering had taken place. It had been subjected to a routine of shampooing three times per week (which included the use of a hair dryer) and brief combing 4 or 5 times per day.

The hair was treated according to the method of Sotton [4]. In this it was subjected to 100 atmospheres pressure of hydrogen sulphide for 24 hours, then vented to atmospheric pressure, immediately immersed in 0.1N silver nitrate solution for 1 hour and finally rinsed in fresh changes of distilled water over a period of 24 hours. Each hair sample was blotted dry on tissue, then allowed to dry in air and embedded in Spurr's resin. Thin transverse and longitudinal sections were cut and mounted on grids for direct examination in the transmission electron microscope (TEM) at 80 keV. In addition the blocks from which the sections had been cut were glued with their smoothed surface uppermost to a mounting stub, coated with a thin layer of carbon and then examined in a scanning electron microscope (SEM) by secondary electron emission using a primary electron beam of 10 keV energy.

Results and discussion

The deposition of Ag_2S in hair by the present methods provided for dramatic results from the electron microscope. The Ag_2S probe was capable of occupying very much smaller holes in the hair's structure than does PTA. Whilst it is not possible to be specific about the minimum size of these holes, one imagines them to be the order of 0.5 nm. The presence of Ag_2S in a given structure implies that the silver ion has gained access from the outside of the hair. More importantly one should consider that if a given internal component of the hair swells significantly in water, then it will have a greater capacity for Ag_2S being deposited in it than will structures which swell to a lesser degree. In other words the density of the precipitate could be indicative of local capacity for aqueous swelling.

SEM observations

This approach was a convenient way for assessing the pattern of silver diffusion into the hair. In Figure 1 one notes the fractal-like nature of the diffusion channels extending from the hair's surface, the lack of Ag_2S at the center of the hair and a region of lower Ag_2S content at the periphery of the cortex. We have no immediate explanation for this latter effect.

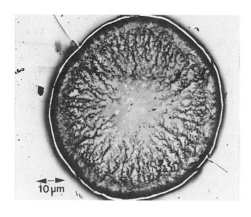

Figure 1. Transversely-cut face through an Ag_2S-treated hair approx. 200 mm from its root-end and examined in the SEM. The contrast in the photograph has been inverted; now consistent with regions containing silver being black.

TEM observations

Dense deposits of Ag_2S were clearly visible under the TEM and silver was also present at a much lower level which enabled most of the principal structures of the hairs to be discerned (Fig. 2). This latter staining seems likely to be attributable more to the binding of silver to such groups as cystine, than it is to the presence of Ag_2S.

Ag_2S is deposited in significantly-large amounts in the endocuticle and in the non-keratin components of the cortex (inter-macrofibrillar matrix, nuclear remnants and intracellular envelope) indicating that these are the structures which swell most in water and that they are the major routes for the aqueous diffusion of the silver ions into the hair. Ag_2S was not found in the keratin composite of the macrofibrils except in severely weathered parts of the hair, where some peripheral penetration was observed.

Very little Ag_2S was found within the bounds of the cell membrane complex (CMC) of either the cuticle or the cortex (Fig. 2). That this structure was not continuously occupied by a dense deposit of Ag_2S provided key evidence that the main route for aqueous diffusion had <u>not</u> occurred within the plane of the intercellular cement of the CMC as was commonly supposed [1]. Diffusion rather seemed to have taken place perpendicularly through adventitious holes in the CMC, though what characterizes these specific regions remains to be seen.

In relatively undamaged hair, the principal route to diffusion through the hair's surface was *via* the exposed edges of the cuticle cells and then further mainly within the plane of the endocuticle to the junction of each cuticle cell

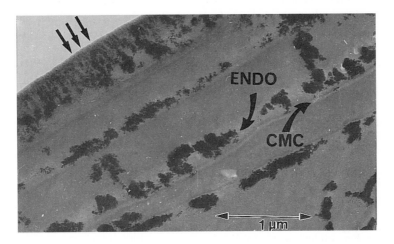

Figure 2. Transmission electron micrograph of a transverse section through a moderately weathered part of a hair. Note the presence of silver in the endocuticle (ENDO) but general lack of it in the cell membrane complex (CMC) of the cuticle and the fine pattern of diffusion which has occurred through the cuticle's outer damaged surface (arrowed).

with the cortex. Such a process, where the CMC at this boundary will be a major barrier to diffusion, provides an explanation for the phenomenon of «ring dyeing» encountered with many types of dyestuff and notably with those of large molecular size.

In weathered hair, diffusion also took place *via* a network of fine channels extending from the outer exposed surface of the scales, through the A-layer and exocuticle and into the endocuticle (Fig. 2). Further perpendicular penetration through the next underlying cell membrane complex seemed to be hindered. Direct penetration through the surface of the first cuticle cell could indicate that the hair's outer barrier of lipid, covalently-bound to the underlying A-layer, has been either removed or has undergone chemical degradation.

Conclusions

The precipitation of silver sulphide into hair and the subsequent examination of sections of the fibres in the transmission electron microscope has enabled us to identify the principal routes for aqueous diffusion and to identify the swelling potential of the hair's different internal components. We demonstrate that it is the non-keratin components of the hair shaft which provide the major routes for aqueous diffusion and it appears these structures swell to the greatest extent. More specifically diffusion does not occur within the plane of the cell membrane complex but rather traverses this structure perpendicularly through occasional adventitious holes. Whereas in undamaged hair initial access to the hair's inner structure seems to be gained through the edges of the cuticle cells and into the endocuticle, in the case of weathered hair the A-layer and exocuticle of the outermost cuticle cells now appear to be pervious.

Acknowledgements

Grateful thanks are due to Dr Michel Sotton of Institut Textile de France for impregnating various samples of hair by the silver sulphide technique.

References

1   Leeder JD, Rippon JA, Rothery FE, Stapleton IW. Proc 7th Internat Textile Res Conf Tokyo. 1985; 5: 99-108
2   Swift JA. Proc 3rd Internat Wool Textile Res Conf Paris. 1965; 1: 265-272
3   Keggin JF. Proc Roy Soc A. 1934; 144: 75-100
4   Sotton M. C R Acad Sci Ser B. 1970; 270: 1261-1265

Scanning electron microscopy changes induced by hair cosmetic procedures

R. Grimalt[1], J. Ferrando[1], R. Fontarnau[2], J.M. Capdevila[1] and J.M. Mascaro[1]

[1]Department of Dermatology, Faculty of Medicine, Hospital Clinic. Villaroel 170, 08036 Barcelona, Spain
[2]Unit of Electron Microscopy, University of Barcelona, Spain

Introduction

Cosmetic products are used by the consumer for the primary purpose of cleansing and beautification of the skin, hair and nails. Because these keratinizing structures continue to grow and are influenced by endogenous and exogenous environmental changes, the cosmetic products employed for beautification are used repetitively and frequently to maintain the desired appearance.

Hair cosmetics represent one of the most important classes of cosmetics that are used by the consumer. They can be divided into categories according to their chemical formulations and action properties including cleansers, manageability, increasers softeners, thickeners, curlers, straighteners and color additives or color removers. Since these cosmetic products employ both chemical formulations and physical modalities, there is a risk at anytime of temporary adverse effects on hair fibers and scalp skin. These adverse effects appear primarily as a result of misuse of hair cosmetics on damaged hair and of the poor compliance to instructions of application.

Particularly worrisome to the consumer as well as the dermatologist is the appearance of alopecia after a cosmetic procedure applied on the scalp.

The «straighteners» usually based on thioglycollic acid rearrange sulphide-bonds and produce a permanent straightness of the hair. When these products are used incorrectly or over-used, they may produce different degrees of morphological changes on the hair surface, leading, in intensive cases, to partial alopecia.

Materials and methods

The affected hair of three females with clinical changes due to hair cosmetic procedures were studied by scanning electron microscopy.

Results

The alterations were predominantly found in the cuticula and varied from minimal changes to a severe damage, including the total loss of the cuticula.

The alterations found were the following:
- Saw-margins of the cuticular cells
- Fissuring of the cuticular cells
- Cuticular detachment
- Orifices of different sizes in the cuticular cell body
- Presence of amorphous material adhering to the surface
- Total loss of the cuticular layer

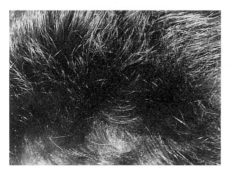

Figure 1. Macroscopic hair alterations after a chemical cosmetic procedure

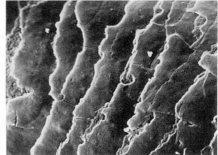

Figure 2. Saw-margins and fissuring of the cuticular cells

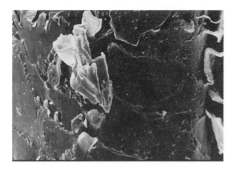

Figure 3. Cuticular detachments

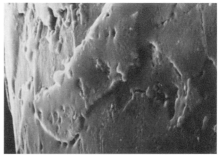

Figure 4. Orifices in the cuticular cell body

Discussion

Relaxers and straighteners are caustic substances, with their pH strictly regulated, and all commercial products carry specific instruction regarding application. This states that the procedure should be performed no more than once in 8 weeks, to a maximum duration of 20 minutes, and only on new growing hair.

The reasons for such strict regulations are that the ultrastructural rearrangement increases the fragility of the hair shaft, and that the caustic nature of the agents will cause damage to the scalp.

The time of onset of the alopecia after the cosmetic procedure varies depending on the severity of the insult, the application of additional cosmetic procedures and even other weathering factors.

Despite the precise instructions included in all these products, they are frequently ignored by the users. Therefore, as long as individuals desire to conform with the dictates of fashion, the misuse of these chemical agents will continue. Recognition of chemically induced alopecia is important, in order that clinicians may provide appropriate advice on the avoidance of such irritants.

The abuse and malpractice of physico-chemical hair treatments with cosmetic purposes induce mostly cuticular changes which leave the cortex unprotected and exposed.

These changes are similar to those seen in states of malnutrition, hypotrichosis congenita, dysplasic syndromes and those provoked by weathering factors.

References

1   Nicholson AG, Harland CC, Bull RH, Mortimer PS, Cook MG. Chemically induced cosmetic alopecia. Br J Dermatol. 1993; 128: 537-541
2   Bergfeld WF. The side effects of products on the scalp and hair. In: Hair Research, ed. Orfanos, Montagna, Stüttgen. Berlin: Springer-Verlag. 1981; 507-511

©1996 Elsevier Science B.V. All rights reserved.
Hair research for the next millenium
D.J.J. Van Neste and V.A. Randall (Eds)

Ceramides in hair: practical approach using sphingoid long-chain bases as determined by GC/MS

G. Kaba, G. Hussler, M.A. Lefebvre and N. Goetz

L'Oréal Research Laboratories Department of Analytical Chemistry
1 avenue E. Schueller 93600 Aulnay-sous-Bois France

Introduction

Ceramides are a class of polar lipids that are essential to the protection of the cuticle. They may represent one of the constituents of the extracellular matrix which is located between the cuticle and the cortex cells. The abundant production of neutral lipids (free-fatty acids, squalene, cholesterol, waxes, triglycerides, etc.) by the sebaceous glands attached to the hair follicles and their transfer to the skin and hair has an effect of diluting these ceramides and making their detection and identification more difficult. Despite several previous descriptions [1-3], the precise composition of the ceramides and especially the identification of the parent bases within human and mammalian hair lipids are still unknown. In a previous study [5] we analyzed the free ceramides; i.e., non-covalently bound to the protein matrix, that were isolated by the liquid extraction of 1.3 kg of hair followed by silica-gel column liquid chromatography. They were identified by GC/MS and are principally related to ceramide classes II and V according to the classification by Wertz and Downing [4] in which the long-chain base was predominantly sphinganine [5]. Their weak concentrations in the hair extracts (0.01% of the total amount of hair) increase the difficulty of their detection and identification. In order to ascertain their possible use as a marker in relation to gender and hair types, it was necessary to develop another approach suitable for the analysis of only a few grams of hair. This approach was based upon the distribution of the long-chain bases.

Materials and methods

All solvents used were of analytical grade. Methanol, hexane and diethyl oxide were purchased from S.D.S. (Peypin, France). Hydrochloric acid, 37%, was obtained from MERCK (Darmstad, Germany), sodium hydroxide from PROLABO (Manchester, England) and anhydrous sodium sulfate from CARLO ERBA (Milan, Italy). Deionized water was obtained by an in-house deionizing system. Trimethylsilylimidazole (TMSI) and N-methyl-N-bis-trifluoroacetamide (MBTFA) were supplied by PIERCE (Rockford, IL, USA). Sphinganine

(D,L-*erythro*) and sphingenine (D-*erythro*) were from SIGMA (Saint Louis, MO, USA).

Hair collection

Samples of human hair were collected from five Caucasian men, one Caucasian woman, five Japanese men and two African men. The hair samples from each subject had received no cosmetic treatments such as permanent waving or hair dyeing prior to sampling. The hair samples were washed with a commercial shampoo preparation and rinsed with tap water.

Hydrolysis of the hair

A lock of hair from each subject weighing about two grams was submitted to an acidic methanolysis in 35 ml of a mixture of methanol/hydrochloric acid in a ratio of 86/14 v/v at 80°C for seven hours. After cooling, 20 ml of deionized water was added and the neutral lipids were removed with a hexane extraction (3×40 ml). The aqueous phase was adjusted to pH 12 with 5N sodium hydroxide. The free sphingoid bases were recovered with diethyl oxide (2×40 ml) and filtered through sodium sulfate. An aliquot (20 ml) of this fraction was subsequently dried under a nitrogen stream.

Derivatization of the long-chain bases

Two derivatization reagents were used simultaneously: MBTFA to convert the amino functions to N-trifluoroacetyl derivatives and TMSI to convert the hydroxy functions to trimethylsilyl derivatives. The solution resulting from the addition of 500 μl each of MBTFA and TMSI to the dried fraction above was heated at 105°C for 45 min.

Capillary gas chromatography-mass spectrometry

The analyses were performed on a Hewlett Packard 5890 Series II gas chromatograph (Hewlett Packard Instruments, Palo Alto, CA, USA) equipped with a Finnigan Ion Trap Detector (Finnigan MAT, San Jose, CA, USA). A 30m×0.32mm×0.25 μm PTE™ 5 fused silica capillary column (Supelco Inc., Bellefonte, PA, USA) was used for the chromatographic separation. Injections were performed *via* split mode at a ratio of 1:20 at 300 °C. Helium was used as the carrier gas at a flow rate of 0.8 ml min^{-1}. The column temperature was programed from 150 °C to 270 °C at 4 °C min^{-1} and held at the final temperature for 10 min. The Ion Trap Detector was scanned from 40 to 650 amu in 1 sec. The source and transfer line were set to 220 °C and 260 °C, respectively. The emission current for EI ionization was 50 μA and the electron multiplier was set to 1500 V.

Mass spectra of the derivatized long-chain bases

The EI mass spectra of the four major derivatized long-chain bases (peaks 1-4) showed the following characteristic fragment ions:

$[M-CH_3]^+$ (1 to 4%, peaks 1 to 4), $[M-CH_3-Me_3SiOH]^+$ (1 to 14%, peaks 1 to 4), $[C_{15}H_{29}-CH-OSiMe_3]^+$ (m/z 311, 100%, peaks 1 and 2), $[C_{15}H_{31}-CHO-SiMe_3]^+$ (m/z 313, 63%, peak 3), $[C_{17}H_{35}-CHO-SiMe_3]^+$ (m/z 341, 52%, peak 4), $[CH_2-OSiMe_3]^+$ (m/z 103, 6 to 14%, peaks 1 to 4), $[SiMe_3]^+$ (m/z 73, 60 to 100%, peaks 1 to 4).

Results

The methodology used for obtaining and analyzing the long-chain bases of ceramides was the same as that used in our laboratory for the analysis of the sphingoid bases from the glucoceramides of natural plant extracts. As described in the experimental part, it consisted of an acidic hydrolysis of two grams of natural hair. This method does not affect the covalently bound ceramides which can be obtained by performing a basic hydrolysis [3, 6]. This acidic hydrolysis does not change the distribution of the long-chain bases in comparison to the distribution of the original ceramides. This very important criterion has been verified by analyzing the long-chain bases obtained from an acidic hydrolysis of the isolated free ceramides from 1.3 kg of hair and a two gram lock of the same hair: the quantities and distributions of the long-chain bases were identical in the two cases. The two main advantages of this method are listed below:

- the formation of hydrochlorated bases that are easily separated from the bulk mixture of compounds present on the hair fiber,

- a one-step derivatization of these long-chain bases and their identification by GC/MS.

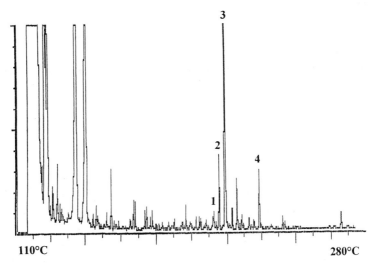

Figure 1. Total ion current trace of the derivatized long-chain bases from a sample of European hair.

Figuge 1 shows the long-chain base distribution of a fraction obtained by an acidic hydrolysis of two grams of European hair and derivatized with a mixture of MBTFA and TMSI. The mass spectra of the major components eluted in the 200 °C to 240 °C temperature range (peaks n° 1 to 4) revealed a fragmentation pattern characteristic of sphinganine and sphingenine derivatives. The identification of these long-chain bases was achieved *via* a coelution with sphingenine and sphinganine reference compounds and a comparison of their mass spectra.

This methodology was then applied to a number of various hair types in order to evaluate the distribution of the four major long-chain bases characteristic of the hair as described above. The relative amounts of each type of long-chain base in the hair of different genders and hair-types were determined by GC/MS using the surface of the chromatographic peaks (TIC trace). These relative amounts are presented in Table 1 (sphingenine is the sum of the *cis* and *trans* isomers, peaks 1 and 2, respectively).

Table 1.

% Relative amounts of the main long-chain bases of free ceramides in different hair-types

| | European hair | | African hair | Japanese hair |
	M	F	M	M
Sphingenine (Peaks 1+2)	10	20	15	12
Sphinganine (Peak 3)	80	70	80	82
Eicosasphinganine (Peak 4)	10	10	5	6

It is clear from the above results that a uniform pattern of these bases exists in all of the hair samples studied with a prevalence of saturated over unsaturated long-chain bases. This is different from that found in the bases of the ceramides of *Stratum Corneum* [4].

Conclusion

A new methodology giving a direct analysis of the long-chain bases of free ceramides was developed and is well adapted to very small sample sizes of hair. Moreover, it correlates very well to the free ceramides naturally found in the hair. The application of this method enabled us to describe the distribution of these bases in different types of hair. A more precise determination of the composition of human-hair free ceramides will lead to a better understanding of the behavior of the hair fiber under various hair-care and conditioning situations.

Acknowledgements

The authors thank C. Comparon for the gas chromatographic analyses, M. Kaba and E. Monteil for providing the hair samples and D. Good for reviewing the manuscript.

References

1   Mix MA, Wertz PW, Downing DT. Comp Biochem Physiol. 1987; 86B: 671-673
2   Wertz PW, Downing DT. Lipids. 1988; 23: 878-881
3   Wertz PW, Downing DT. Comp Biochem Physiol. 1989; 92B: 759-761
4   Wertz PW, Downing DT. J Lipid Res. 1983; 24: 759-765
5   Hussler G, Kaba G, Franois AM, Saint-Léger D. I.J.C.S. 1995; 17: 197-206
6   Robson KJ, Stewart ME, Michelsen S, Lazo ND, Downing DT. J Lipid Res. 1994; 35: 2060-2068

Small lipid nanoparticles: a new delivery system of lipophilic agents to hair and scalp

F. Zülli and F. Suter

Mibelle AG, Biochemistry, Bolimattstrasse 1, CH 5033 Buchs, Switzerland

Introduction

The formulation of lipophilic agents in hair care products is unsatisfactory. Conventional oil-in-water emulsions or alcoholic hair tonics which are usually used to deliver lipophilic agents to hair and scalp perform poorly. They leave hair feeling sticky and greasy. In addition, only a low affinity of the substances to hair is observed.

In our laboratory, we have employed a new system to deliver hydrophobic agents to hair and scalp. The system consists of small water dispersible lipid nanoparticles. The vesicles are formed by a monolayer of phospholipids encapsulating a tiny oil core carrying lipophilic agents.

Compared to liposomes (Fig. 1) (optimal carrier for water-soluble drugs), the pay-load of lipophilic substances by nanoparticles is much higher. Nanoparticle preparations are quickly gaining wide recognition in the cosmetic field [1]. They are also used as parenteral emulsions [2] and in a few other pharmaceutical products.

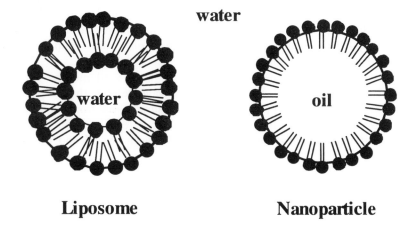

Figure 1. Structural comparison of liposomes and lipid nanoparticles

Materials and methods

Preparation of Nanoparticles

Nanoparticles are prepared by high pressure homogenization using a Microfluidizer® [3]. Phospholipids from soy oil containing the substance of interest and water are mixed to form a predispersion. Multiple cycles through the homogenizer at 1200 bar are performed to obtain a homogeneous preparation of small vesicles.

The composition of nanoparticle preparations can vary: lecithin (1-15%), triglycerides (1-60%), active ingredients (0-40%), water (25-95%) and alcohol (0-20%).

The size of the vesicles can be influenced by the concentration of ethanol or glycerol during the preparation and has a great impact on the properties of the dispersion [4]. Nanoparticles composed of natural phospholipids have a negative surface charge (zetapotential-30 mV). By the addition of the cationic lipid stearylamine, the zetapotential of the vesicles are reversed to +50 mV, resulting in an enhanced affinity of the particles to hair and scalp.

Characterization

The parameters used to characterize lipid nanoparticles are optical appearance, particle size and size distribution, lamellarity, trapped volume and stability (leakage). The optical appearance of nanoparticle preparations is influenced by the size of the vesicles. Preparations of particles with diameters above 150 nm are white, even in diluted dispersions. Preparations containing particles of 100 nm become opaque. A further reduction of the particle size to below 60 nm results in clear transparent dispersions of oil-in-water. The particle size, as well as the particle size distribution can be determined by photon correlation spectroscopy. However, freeze fracture electron microscopy (EM) has been used to characterize the size and shape of the lipid particles exactly. Our calculations regarding the trapped volume of nanoparticle preparations in relation to the lecithin concentration confirmed the assumption that only one monolayer of phospholipids surrounds the oil cores.

Nanoparticles are stable at room temperature for several months without changes in the mean size of the particles. Leakage tests with encapsulated Safranin T (a lipophilic cation [5]) showed a very slow release from the vesicles. Yet the barrier function of the phospholipid shell is less important than the partition coefficient of the encapsulated agent between the oil and the water phase.

Results

Small nanoparticles carrying different active agents of cosmetic or pharmaceutical interest can be prepared using the sophisticated technology of microfluidization. Lipophilic ingredients become water-dispersible by their complete encapsulation in the oil core of small vesicles. Preparations of the particles can easily be sterilized by heat treatment or filtration. Active ingredients like vitamins, sunscreens, fragrances and essential oils have been incorporated in consumer products without additional surfactants or solubilizers. Phospholipids from soy are well tolerated emulsifiers which have a high affinity to the skin [6]. To target these particles to hair, the phospholipid shell can be dotted with cationic molecules resulting in nanoparticles with a positive zetapotential (Table 1). In our *in vitro* experiments (Fig. 2), using UV filters as active agents, we showed that these positively charged particles have a one hundred fold higher affinity to hair compared to untreated negatively charged nanoparticles.

Table 1.
Preparation of anionic and cationic nanoparticles containing a sunscreen.
Uvinul T 150® is a totally water insoluble UV-B filter with an extremely high extinction coefficient. The preparation of positively and negatively charged nanoparticles containing this sunscreen results in convenient formulations for hair and skin care products.

Product	Zetapotential	Particle size
Nano-Lipobelle® UV-F4 2% Lecithin, 6% Uvinul T 150®	-32.5 mV	148.3 nm
Nano-Lipobelle® UV-F9 ditto +0.5% Stearylamine	+49.9 mV	117.5 nm

Conclusions

Lipid nanoparticles are an ideal carrier system for the transport and the protection of lipophilic substances for topical applications in cosmetics and dermatology. The preparations have a low viscosity and are not greasy. In addition, nanoparticles have a high affinity to the skin and enhance the bioavailability of the encapsulated agents. Thus the topical treatment of the scalp is of special interest due to an already high percutaneous absorption rate [7]. With the preparation of positively charged nanoparticles, a highly improved targeting to hair can be obtained.

To summarize, nanoparticles offer new promising possibilities for the utilization of lipophilic agents in advanced hair care preparations.

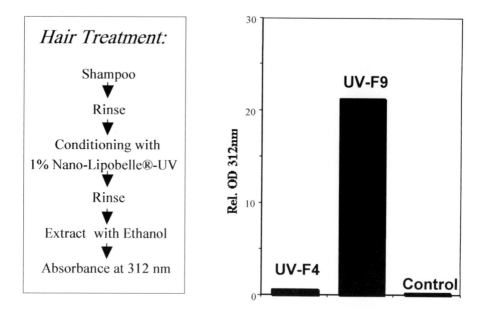

Figure 2. Hair treatment with UV-filters encapsulated in positively and negatively charged nanoparticles

References

1   Brunke RA, Charlet E. Seifen, Oele, Fette, Wachse. 1991; 14: 514-517
2   Washington C, Davis SS. International Journal of Pharmaceutics. 1988; 44: 169-176
3   Mayhew E, Lazo R, Vail WJ, King JAM, Green AM. Biochimica et Biophysica Acta. 1984; 775: 169-174
4   Zülli F, Suter F. Proceed Intern Symp Control Rel Bioact Mater. 1994; 21: 459-460
5   Bally MB, Hope MJ, Echteld CJA, Cullis PR. Biochimica et Biophysica Acta. 1985; 812: 66-76
6   Artmann C, Röding J, Ghyczy M, Pratzel HG. Parfümerie und Kosmetik. 1990; 5: 326-327
7   Wester, Maibach. In: Percutaneous Absorption. Bronaugh & Maibach, eds. New York: Marcel Dekker. 1989; 111-118

©1996 Elsevier Science B.V. All rights reserved.
Hair research for the next millenium
D.J.J. Van Neste and V.A. Randall (Eds)

Histological changes in rat vibrissal follicles after electrolysis and the optimum length of time to apply the current

K. Tezuka[1], M. Nakamura[2] and K. Katsuoka[1]

[1]Department of Dermatology, Kitasato University School of Medicine, Sagamihara, Japan
[2]Chigasaki Tokushukai Medical Center, Chigasaki, Japan

Introduction

The aim of electrolysis is the permanent hair removal of unwanted hair by an electric current. However, regrowth occurs if the current is too weak to cause sufficient destruction of the hair follicle. On the other hand, if the current is too excessive, the hair follicle will be destroyed but scarring may occur. Therefore, what is required to achieve permanent hair removal is that the current should be applied for an appropriate length of time.

In this study, we have attempted to determine the optimum length of time for application of the electric current to achieve the permanent hair removal of rat vibrissae. Further, we also have examined the histological changes that occur in vibrissal follicles due to electrolysis.

Materials and methods

The vibrissae of anesthetized Sprague-Dawley rats were removed by electrolysis. The modalities we used were thermolysis (HR-5000, IME Co., Ltd., Japan) and the blend (Ultrablend, Clareblend Inc., U.S.A.).

The following 4 graded times were studied: 2, 4, 6 and 8 sec in thermolysis and 10, 20, 30 and 40 sec in the blend. Vibrissal regrowth was then counted at 2, 4, and 10 weeks after electrolysis and the vibrissal follicles were biopsied 10 weeks after electrolysis. For controls, vibrissal regrowth was followed in other rats who had undergone vibrissal plucking by tweezers. The regrowth rate was calculated from the following formula: (number of regrown vibrissae/number of vibrissae given electrolysis)×100.

Results

Length of time for electrolysis

It was found that 2 sec of thermolysis and 10 sec in the blend was too short, since almost all of the vibrissae regrew in the same manner as in the controls. However, 8 sec of thermolysis and 40 sec in the blend was decidedly too long, for at 2 weeks after electrolysis excessive redness was still present, and at 10 weeks, there was no regrowth at all in the treated area, even of short hairs that had not been subjected to electrolysis.

As shown in Table 1, on comparing regrowth of vibrissae subjected to 4 and 6 sec of thermolysis and 20 and 30 sec in the blend, it was found that the regrowth rate of vibrissae given 6 sec of thermolysis was lower than that of vibrissae given 4 sec of thermolysis. Even so, 4 sec of thermolysis was decided to be more appropriate, since there was also a slight loss of short hairs around the treated vibrissae in the 6 sec rat. As for the blend, it was found that 30 sec was more appropriate, as the rate of regrowth was lower than in rats given the 20 sec blend.

Table 1.
Regrowth rate of vibrissae after electrolysis (%)

	2 weeks	4 weeks	10 weeks
Control (plucking)	62.5	100.0	100.0
T 4 sec	8.3	16.6	20.8
T 6 sec	8.3	8.3	12.5
B 20 sec	20.8	33.3	45.6
B 30 sec	12.0	21.0	36.0

T: thermolysis, B: the blend

Histology

Successful electrolysis

At 10 weeks after 4 sec of thermolysis, dermal papilla and hair matrix were still present in the lower vibrissal follicles. Also, epithelial cysts that showed no hair-growth capability were formed (Fig. 1). This also was seen in the blend.

Over treatment

At 10 weeks after 40 sec in the blend, the same characteristics were seen as described above, except for excessive capsular damage and damage to the surrounding dermis and epidermis (Fig. 2). This clearly indicated that the 40 sec blend was far too strong.

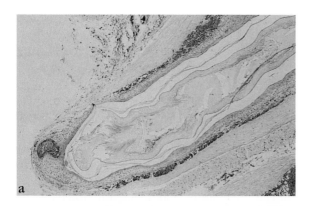

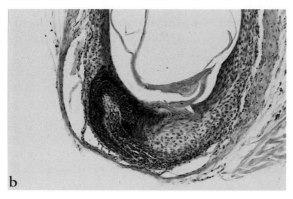

Figure 1 (a-b). Vibrissal follicles at 10 weeks after the 4-sec thermolysis which shows successful electrolysis

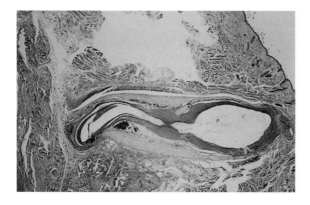

Figure 2. Vibrissal follicles at 10 weeks after the 40 sec blend which shows over treatment

130

Discussion and conclusions

When using electrolysis for hair removal, it is important that no prolonged inflammation or scarring occur; these requirements are not simple to achieve.

In this rat vibrissal study, in attempting to determine the appropriate duration of the electrical flow, we found that 4 sec of thermolysis and 30 sec in the blend were the most appropriate values, both of which are from two to three times longer than for the electrolysis of human hair.

With regard to human hair, the regrowth rate after electrolysis is estimated to range from 15% to 20% [1-4]. Thus, the vibrissal regrowth rate after electrolysis at the above time lengths was found to fall within this range.

In a future project, we intend to examine morphological differences in electrolysis-treated vibrissal follicles which should achieve permanent hair removal and which should cause hair regrowth, and also intend to determine the potential for hair regrowth by the depth of follicular damage using the appropriate time lengths confirmed by this study.

References

1   Behrman HT. JAMA. 1960; 172: 1924-1931
2   Chernosky ME. Tex Med. 1971; 67: 72-78
3   Spoor HJ. Cutis. 1978; 21: 283, 286-287
4   Wagner RF Jr, Tomich JM, Grande DJ, Boston MA. J Am Acad Dermatol. 1985; 12: 441-449

Colour plate III

©1996 Elsevier Science B.V. All rights reserved.
Hair research for the next millenium
D.J.J. Van Neste and V.A. Randall (Eds)

Workshop report on:

What is new in scalp cosmetic surgery?

P. Pouteaux[1] and D. Van Neste[2]

[1]Rue Cler 15, F- 75007 Paris, France
[2]H.A.I.R. Technology®, Avenue du Prince Héritier 31, B-1200 Bruxelles, Belgium

The technique of mini- and micro-grafts has been considered as one of the best improvements in hair-transplantation surgery (Fig. 1). Two or 3 sessions of about 500 grafts provide a sufficient volume of hair in the bald area and can result in a natural and undetectable hair-line [1]. The technique has been made easier and safer by the use of new and disposable instruments [2-4].

Extensive sessions, transplanting up to 3000 grafts in a single session employing a large medical team, working 8 to 10 hours under local anaesthesia, could be highly dangerous and the stress involved would seem to outweigh the therapeutic benefits.

Laser surgery, used to make slits to insert grafts into the recipient area, must be reserved for those experienced to this technique. As yet there is no conclusive

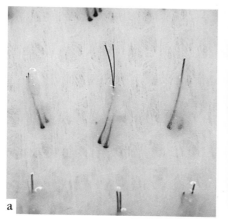 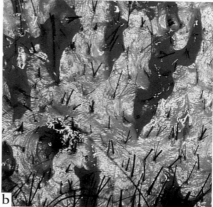

Figure 1: Micrograft preparation for cosmetic scalp surgery
Preparation of micrografts for a session of hair transplantation in a human subject with male pattern baldness (a). The micrografts are inserted in slits made amidst existing scalp hair follicles (b). (From 7 with permission)

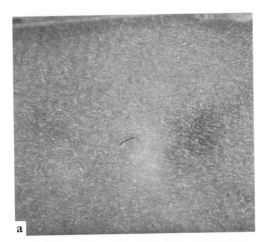

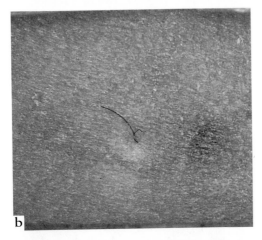

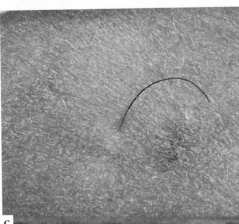

Figure 2: Cosmetic surgery techniques applied in the research laboratory (modified after [6])

Specimen preparation, skin incision and micrograft implantation has been performed onto nude mice in a similar way as shown in figure. 1. This results in «hairy islands» producing 1 up to 3 human hairs in the nude mouse skin (tattoos serve as site markers). This serial photography, performed 3 months after grafting onto nude mice, illustrates a single hair growing from a micrograft placed just between the two tattoos: (a) immediately after clipping, (b) 4 days later and (c) 15 days later. When hair follicles were horizontally sectionned, there was always less hair growth (lower two thirds of the follicle) or no growth at all when the lower third of the follicle was engrafted (Caroline Tételin personal communication).

evidence of substantial advantages of this method compared with the classical steel punch or other mechanical techniques.

The other possibilities for the treatment of baldness, intending to reduce the area of baldness, cannot create a natural and soft hair-line on the forehead. Hence, they should be limited to the vertex. Scalp reductions, with or without extenders or scalp-liftings, reducing the density of the occipito-temporal site, impair the results of eventual grafting into the forehead, which is cosmetically the most aesthetically important part of the scalp.

From basic research data, cosmetic surgeons hypothesized that, by cutting the follicles at different levels close to the bulge, it should be possible to obtain 2 hairs from a single one [5], thereby doubling the amount of donor follicles.

D. Van Neste and co-workers (Fig. 2) have tested this interesting hypothesis [6, 7], but agree with Limmer *et al.* [5] that such microscopic work is unrealistic for a surgical application [5].

References

1   Pouteaux P. Le traitement de la calvitie par minis et microgreffes. La revue de chirurgie esthétique de langue Française. 1994; 76: 39-41
2   Pouteaux P. De nouveaux instruments pour la transplantation de cheveux. Journal de médecine esthétique et de chirurgie dermatologique. 1994; 83: 149-153
3   Pouteaux P. Les auto-greffes du cuir chevelu, utilisation du bistouri à 3 lames. Bulletin de la Société Française de chirurgie dermatologique. 1993; 2: 6-11
4   Pouteaux P. The use of the three-bladed scalpel in hair-transplant surgery. The American Journal of Cosmetic Surgery. 1995; 2: 103-106
5   Limmer BL, Razmi R, Davis T, Stevens C. Relating hair growth theory and experimental evidence to practical hair transplantation. The American Journal of Cosmetic Surgery. 1994; 11: 305-310
6   Van Neste D. The growth of human hair in nude mice. Clinics in North America. D. Whiting (Ed), in press
7   Van Neste D. Production de cheveux humains au laboratoire: où en sommes-nous en 1995? Journal d'Actualités Dermatologiques Belges. 1995; 23: 22-30

Colour plate V

Regeneration of the human scalp hair follicle after horizontal sectioning: implications for pluripotent stem cells and melanocyte reservoir

J.C. Kim, M.K. Kim and Y.C. Choi

Department of Immunology, School of Medicine, Kyungpook National University, Dongin Dong 101, Taegu 700-422, Korea

Introduction

The growth of hair follicle, sebaceous gland, and epidermis is known to be intimately related. Chase [1] postulated in 1954 that upper outer root sheath of the follicle contains a population of pluripotent stem cells capable of not only forming the follicle, but also the epidermis and sebaceous gland. Some earlier observations support this hypothesis [2, 3].

Particularly insightful work on this problem by Cotsarelis et al. [4] led to the discovery that follicular cells retaining ^{3}H-thymidine were located in the bulge region close to the insertion of the arrector pili muscle. These data along with previous histological findings [5], make the bulge a tempting candidate as the site of the follicular stem cells. Kobayashi et al. [6] also reported that in the rat vibrissa, keratinocyte colony-forming cells are highly clustered in the bulge. Upon the examination of the human scalp hair follicle, Yang et al. [7] reported that keratinocytes from the bulge area indeed have a longer in vitro life span than cells of the lower follicle, sebaceous gland, and even the epidermis, supporting the hypothesis that, as in rodents, the stem cells reside in the bulge. However, Rochat et al. [8] have demonstrated that a large number of keratinocyte colony-forming cells is clustered at a region below the midpoint of the human scalp hair follicle. This region lies deeper than the site of insertion of the arrector pili muscle. The exact distribution of the stem cells within the human scalp hair follicle is not known with certainty.

Therefore, we have performed transplantation experiments of human scalp hair follicle after horizontal sectioning to locate the follicular stem cells.

Materials and methods

We removed human hair follicles from the occipital scalp by microdissection. Implants were prepared from follicles as follows:
- the upper one-third and lower two-thirds of the follicle were obtained by horizontal section just below the pilosebaceous junction,

- the upper and lower halves of the follicle were obtained from a transverse cut at the middle portion of the follicle,

- the upper two-thirds and lower one-third of the follicle were obtained from the transection of the follicle at the lower one-third of the follicle.

Both upper and lower follicle grafts were transplanted onto the forehead or leg using Choi hair transplanter [9]. Histologic examinations were performed for each successive biopsy after grafting. Biopsy samples were fixed in buffered formalin, paraffin-embedded, and sections were stained with hematoxylin-eosin.

Results

Eight months after grafting, 13 of the 20 grafted upper two-thirds, 25 of the 30 grafted lower two-thirds, 10 of the 25 grafted upper half, 4 of the 15 lower half follicles have regenerated complete hair follicles. However no hair follicle was regenerated from the grafted lower one-third and upper one-third follicle. The regenerated hairs from upper follicle implants were thinner than those from lower follicle implants (Fig. 1a).

A histological examination, 8 months after grafting, showed that the regenerated hair follicle from the upper half follicle implant revealed the presence of a reformed dermal papilla, a matrix, and active melanocytes. The reformed

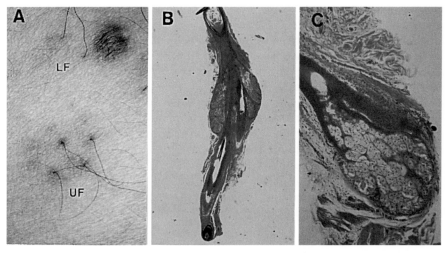

Figure 1. A: Surface view of the leg, 8 months after grafting upper and lower 1/2 grafts. UF: regrown hairs from upper 1/2 grafts; LF: regrown hairs from lower 1/2 grafts.
B: Longitudinal section of a regenerated follicle from an upper 1/2 graft, 2 years after grafting (magnification x10).
C: Light micrograph of the sebaceous gland regenerated from a lower 1/2 graft, 2 years after grafting (magnification x100)

dermal papilla showed a pyramidal shape. Lower half follicle implant reconstituted the complete hair follicle. The sebaceous gland was not regenerated, but there was an outgrowth in the sebaceous gland region.

Two years after grafting, the histological examination of the regenerated bulb from the upper half implant showed that the shape of dermal papilla was the same as control dermal papilla (Fig. 1b). The regenerated follicle from the lower half implant showed that the sebaceous gland was completely regenerated (Fig. 1c).

Discussion

Location of stem cells in human hair follicle

Recent evidence indicates that most stem cells may actually reside in the bulge which, when given the proper stimulus, generates the new inferior, cycling portion of the follicle.

First, a population of slow cycling label-retaining cells is localized in the bulge, when mouse follicular cells are labeled with ^{3}H-thymidine *in vivo* [4].

Second, over 95% of the keratinocyte colony-forming cells isolated from rat vibrissa are located in the bulge and the remainder are mainly present in the bulb [6]. Yang *et al.* [7] reported that the upper human hair follicle contains keratinocytes with superior *in vitro* proliferative potential, supporting the hypothesis that, as in rodents, the stem cells reside in the bulge.

However, bulge location of follicular stem cells posed problems for interpreting our transection experiments which showed that the lower half follicle implants (below the bulge-equivalent region) regenerated the hair follicle. Since we could not identify a well-defined bulge in most dissected follicles, we localized the site of insertion of the arrector pili muscle by immunostaining of smooth muscle-alpha-actin [10], and found that in adult human, it was always located in the upper half follicle.

Recently, Rochat *et al.* [8] demonstrated that most keratinocyte colony-forming cells are located below the midpoint of the human hair follicle, at a significant distance from the sebaceous gland, the bulge region, and the site of insertion of arrector pili muscle on one hand, and from the hair bulb on the other. However, our experiment showed that while 40% of the implanted upper half follicle regenerated, only 27% of the grafted lower half follicle regenerated. This indicated that more stem cells are located in the upper portion of the middle one-third.

It is possible that the bulge contains most of the stem cells in rodent hair follicle, but in human hair follicle, the stem cells are widely distributed in the middle one-third of the follicle.

Regeneration of pilo-sebaceous unit

Our experiments demonstrate that a papilla and outer root sheath in middle one-third of the follicle must be present if the hair is to grow and that perifollicular sheath cells which surround the transient portion of the follicle are the source of the new papillae.

Thus when the hair follicle is cut below the lower one-third, only the upper follicle can regenerate the hair follicle. In the upper follicle implant, the remaining perifollicular sheath cells are reorganized to form a new papilla. Then, the remaining keratinocytes in concert with the regenerated dermal papilla can form a complete follicle. In the lower follicle implant, the hair shaft of the lower portion is pushed up by subsequent regression of the lower portion, but a new hair follicle cannot regenerate in the next hair cycle because of the absence of hair follicular stem cells which are located in the middle one-third of the hair follicle. The finding contrasts with the results obtained with implants of vibrissa bulbs which always provide hair fibres [11]. When the hair follicle is cut near the middle portion where follicular epithelial stem cells and perifollicular sheath cells overlap, both the upper and the lower follicle implants can regenerate the hair follicle. In the upper follicle implant case, the remaining perifollicular sheath cells migrate to form the new papilla which is small and associated with the production of a fine hair. In the lower follicle implant, the lower portion undergoes catagen and telogen by programmed cell death. Then the hair shaft is shed 2 weeks after implantation. The remaining follicular stem cells regenerate a new epithelial column and make a new hair follicle through interaction with the dermal papilla. The diameter of the regenerated hair is the same as the original hair. When cutting the upper two-thirds, only the lower follicle implant can form a hair follicle. Because there are no perifollicular sheath cells in the upper portion, the upper follicle implant cannot form a new follicle.

Our data also indicate that the sebaceous gland can be regenerated even in the lower half follicle implant; this raises the possibility that the follicular stem cells ascend through the isthmus, giving rise to sebaceous glands. Our present observation argues against the possibility that the sebaceous gland may itself contain stem cells [12].

Melanocyte reservoir in human hair follicle

Active melanocytes located in the matrix of hair follicles synthesize melanin and produce pigmented fiber [13]. Our results show that surgical removal of the lower half including the matrix, containing active melanocytes, cannot prevent the regeneration of new black hair follicles. Thus, the melanocytes in the bulbs of regenerated hair follicles might come from the proliferation and migration of inactive melanocytes in the outer root sheaths of middle one-third of the follicle.

We have grafted the lower two-thirds of the scalp hair follicle onto the vitiligo skin and found that the grafted hair follicle induced the repigmentation of vitiligo (unpublished data). This observation also indicated that there was a melanocyte reservoir in human hair follicles and the repigmentation of vitiligo began with reproduction of melanocytes in the middle part of the hair follicles. Thus, amelanotic melanocytes which are located in the middle portion of the hair follicle may migrate upwards or downwards to become active melanocytes in epidermis or in matrix.

Acknowledgements

This work was supported by a grant from Kakinuma Medical and Omiya Skin Clinic in Japan.

References

1   Chase HB. Physiol Rev. 1954; 34: 112-126
2   Bishop GH. Am J Anat. 1945; 76: 153-181
3   Limat A, Breitkreutz D, Hunziker T, *et al*. Expt Cell Res. 1991; 194: 218-227
4   Cotsarelis G, Sun T-T, Lavker RM. Cell. 1990; 61: 1329-1337
5   Oliver RF. J Embryol Exp Morph. 1966; 15: 331-347
6   Kobayashi K, Rochat A, Barrandon Y. Proc Natl Acad Sci. USA. 1993; 90: 7391-7395
7   Yang J-S, Lavker RM, Sun T-T. J Invest Dermatol. 1993; 101: 652-659
8   Rochat A, Kobayashi K, Barrandon Y. Cell. 1994; 76: 1063-1073
9   Choi YC, Kim JC. J Dermatol Surg Oncol. 1992; 18: 945-948.
10 Jahoda CA, Reynolds AJ, Chaponnier C, *et al*. J Cell Sci. 1991; 99: 627-636
11 Cohen J. J Embryol Exp Morph. 1961; 9: 117-127
12 Doran TI, Baff R, Jacoba P, Pacia E. J Invest Dermatol. 1991; 96: 341-348
13 Staricco RG. J Invest Dermatol. 1960; 35: 185-194

Colour plate XI

Histological examination of human hair follicles grafted onto severe combined immunodeficient (SCID) mice

T. Hashimoto[1], T. Kazama[1], M. Ito[1], K. Urano[3], Y. Katakai[2, 3] and Y. Ueyama[2, 3, 4]

[1]Department of Dermatology, Niigata University, School of Medicine 1-Ashahimachidori, Niigata, 951, Japan
[2]Kanagawa Academy of Science and Technology Laboratory 3-2-1 Sakado, Takatsu-ku, Kawasaki, Kanagawa, 213, Japan
[3]Central Institute for Experimental Animals 1430 Nogawa, Miyamae-ku, Kawasaki, Kanagawa, 213, Japan
[4]Department of Pathology, Tokai University, School of Medicine Bohseidai Isehara, Kanagawa, 259-11, Japan

Introduction

An *in vivo* model of human hair follicles seems very important to investigate human hair biology and human hair follicles grafted on experimental animals seem to be the most useful. Normally, a piece of hairy human skin has been grafted onto mice [1-3]. However, in our experience, the follicles in such a scalp skin graft tend to bend in random directions, probably due to shrinkage of its dermal connective tissue, leading to difficulty in obtaining longitudinal sections of the follicles for histological study. Such skin grafts also require a large skin specimen to prepare adequate numbers of model mice. To overcome these problems, we have isolated human scalp hair follicles prior to transplantation so that a single hair follicle with a minimal amount of connective tissue was grafted into mouse skin and could be examined histologically, immunohistochemically and electron microscopically.

Materials and methods

Animal

C.B-17-*SCID* mice aged 4 to 8 weeks were used as recipients. The SCID mice have no functional T and B lymphocytes.

Isolation of hair follicles

Human anagen hair follicles were isolated mechanically from surgically obtained scalp skin specimens with scalpels, scissors and forceps under a dissecting microscope. Each grafted specimen always contained a single follicle. The infundibular epithelium partly remained at the upper end of the follicle but the sebaceous glands and arrector pili muscle were mostly removed. A little amount of the dermal tissue probably corresponding to connective tissue sheath remained around the follicle. Only anagen hair follicles were selected and grafted.

Transplantation

Under general anaesthesia, the back skin of each mouse was shaved with a razor and bored with a number 18 injection needle. An isolated hair follicle was inserted through the skin pore into the subcutaneous space of the mouse to adjust its upper end to the level of the mouse epidermis. The hair shaft was left on the skin surface and fixed with a surgical adhesive and a film. Ninety seven follicles were grafted onto 28 recipient mice with two to four follicles per mouse.

Preparation of specimens

Mouse back skin containing a grafted follicle was biopsied on days 7, 20, 25, 40, 45, 50, 55, 60, 70, 100, and 150 after transplantation. Specimens were fixed in 10% neutralized buffered formalin or 70% ethanol and embedded in paraffin. Deparaffinized sections were examined histologically with hematoxylin-eosin staining and immunohistochemically using a streptavidin-biotin-peroxidase system with a monoclonal antibody for proliferating cell nuclear antigen (PCNA). Some specimens were further examined ultrastructurally by transmission electron microscopy. The hair shafts obtained on day 100 were examined by scanning electron microscopy.

Results

Forty four (45%) out of 97 follicles were shown to be successfully engrafted by histology. The hair bulb and lower portion of the follicle were located in the subcutaneous space and its infundibular epithelium had a smooth connection to the epidermis of the mouse. In some instances, a follicle was entirely engulfed in the subcutaneous space with no connection to the mouse epidermis.

On day 7, the hair matrix cells and melanocytes decreased in number, resulting in atrophy of the hair bulb. The differentiation of the hair cortex and the inner root sheath (IRS) was observed to be disturbed. The vitreous membrane around the lower part of the follicle was thickened and corrugated. A few mononuclear cells were seen in the thickened connective tissue sheath (Fig. 1). These findings are consistent with those of the normal early catagen follicles. On day 20, the atrophy of the follicles was more advanced; there were no hair bulbs at the lower end of the follicles and no hair cortex or inner root sheath. The outline of the lower portion of the follicles was irregularly shaped. The lower end of the remaining hair shafts was usually observed to be tapered and the clubbed hair root, which is usually observed in telogen follicles, was seldom formed. On day 40, many small epithelial projections toward the connective tissue were seen in the lower half of the follicles. The dermal papilla cells were still present adjacent to the lower end of the follicles. The connective tissue sheath and the thickened vitreous membrane were left in the area where the lower follicle disappeared by shrinkage (Fig. 2). This feature of the follicles nearly resembles that seen in the mid-catagen phase of the normal hair cycle. Many PCNA-positive cells were seen mainly in the outer parts of the lower follicle by immunohistochemistry, but no PCNA-positive cells were observed in the central part of the follicle (Fig. 3). Many apoptotic cells still existed in the central part as demonstrated by electron microscopy (Fig. 4).

After day 45, grafted follicles had reconstructed anagen hair structures which were histologically identical with normal anagen hair follicles. The reconstruction seemed to have started on days ranging from day 45 to 60. After day 70, follicles always showed anagen phase. The anagen phase continued even to day 150 (Figs. 7 and 8). A new hair shaft was formed in the follicles and grew out of the mouse skin surface (Fig. 5). By scanning electron microscopy, normal imbricated hair cuticles were seen on the surface of the hair shaft (Fig. 6).

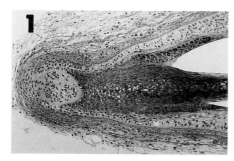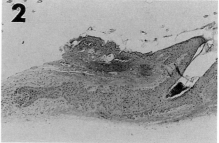

Figure 1. Day 7. H and E staining. The hair bulb shows atrophic changes
Figure 2. Day 40. H and E staining. The lower portion of the grafted follicle has regressed. The hair shaft is tapered in shape and the outline of the lower follicle is irregular. The dermal papilla cells exist adjacent to the end of the follicle

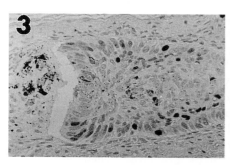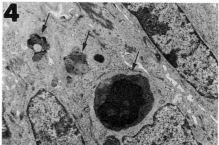

Figure 3. Day 40. Immunohistochemistry. Many PCNA positive-cells reside in the outer parts of the lower end of the shrunk follicle
Figure 4. Day 45. Ultrastructural study. The arrows indicate apoptotic fragments engulfed in still living keratinocytes in the central part of the lower follicle

144

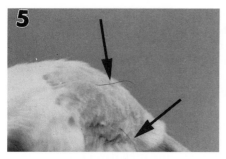
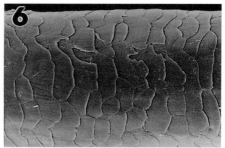

Figure 5. Day 120. The arrows indicate the hair shafts growing out of the skin surface
Figure 6. Day 100. SEM study. The regrown hair shaft shows a normal hair structure
with well imbricated hair cuticles

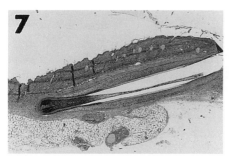
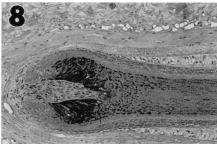

Figures 7, 8. Day 150. H and E staining. The hair follicle is almost straight in shape
and exhibits a well developed anagen state.

Discussion

In this model the grafted follicles reconstruct and maintain almost their original shapes, so that longitudinal sections can be easily obtained. In addition, the grafted human hair follicles maintain an anagen phase, growing a hair shaft for at least 90 days, starting about 70 days after transplantation. This means that this sytem has great advantages over the previous models. Furthermore, the grafted anagen follicles regress transiently and reconstruct a new anagen follicle. Human scalp skin grafted onto nude mice has been reported to shed hairs after transplantation and then grow new hairs, too. Although this phenomenon resembles the normal hair cycle, the shedding mechanism has not been clarified.

In the present study, some histological differences were seen during the regression phase compared to the normal catagen phase. These included a tapered, not clubbed, end of the shed hair shaft; dermal papilla cells apparently always existed adjacent to the lower end of the follicles; PCNA positive cells were present in the lower part of the regressing follicles and the upward shrinkage (regression) of the lower follicle seemed incomplete.

According to the bulge activation hypothesis [4], the catagen follicles may loose almost all keratinocytes in the lower follicle, perhaps by exhaustion of the proliferative potential of the hair matrix cells, and consequently the dermal papilla comes close to the bulge area. Stem cells, which may reside in the bulge area, are believed to supply new keratinocytes to regenerate a new hair bulb when stimulated by the dermal papilla cells. On the other hand, in the present model, it is not likely that the reconstructed hair bulb may be derived from such bulge stem cells, because the hair bulb regenerated from the lower end of the regressing follicle in a mid-catagen-like phase. Indeed, dermal papilla cells were adjacent to the lower end of the follicle where PCNA-positive cells were seen. The dermal papilla cells never reach the bulge area and should be unable to stimulate the bulge stem cells. Therefore, the anagen follicles in this model appear to be reconstructed by the keratinocytes which may survive in the lower follicles, but not by the newly provided ones from the bulge stem cells. The causes of this incomplete regression of the follicle are currently unclear, although some speculations are possible. Transplantation may lead to the temporary arrest of the follicular blood supply, mechanical damage to the bulb during the isolation of the follicles or, possibly, some growth factors in the fetal calf serum supplement or the culture medium in which the biopsies were maintained may affect the proliferative activity of the hair bulb.

Although the reconstructed anagen hair follicles undergo a natural hair cycle, it is unclear whether the present SCID mouse model can be used for the investigation of such a natural human hair cycle because of the shorter life span of the mice than that of human hairs. Some encouraging data showing modulation of the human hair cycle after transplantation of balding human scalp in another model i.e. testosterone conditioned nude mice have already been presented in this volume (Van Neste *et al.*) and support monitoring of hair cycles as a potentially relevant signal.

Furthermore, since the SCID mouse model of human hair follicles just after transplantation reveals morphological changes closely imitating those seen in human hair cycle *in vivo*, it may be useful as a model for early stages of the hair cycle. Moreover, since the reconstructed anagen hair follicles continue to grow hairs for a long term over several months, the present model could be used for some biological assays of human anagen hair follicles.

References

1   Gilhar A, Pillar T, Etzioni A. Br J Dermatol. 1988; 119: 767-770
2   Van Neste DJJ, Gillespie JM, Marshall RC, Taieb A *et al.* Br J Dermatol. 1993; 128: 384-387
3   Masui S, Matsumoto K, Yokoyama Y, Suzuki M. Jpn J Dermatol. 1994; 104: 681-684
4   Cotsarelis G, Sun TT, Lavker RM. Cell. 1990; 61: 1329-1337

Structure and function

Microvascular and collagen fibrillar architecture of whisker by scanning electron microscopy

S. Sakita[1], O. Ohtani[2] and M. Morohashi[1]

[1]Departments of Dermatology and [2]Anatomy, Toyama Medical and Pharmaceutical University, 2630 Sugitani, Toyama 930-01, Japan

Introduction

The whiskers, which are located on the upper lip of rats, cats, *etc.* are also called sinus hairs morphologically and tactile hairs functionally. The whisker is characteristically accompanied by the blood sinus. The whiskers have commonly been used for various hair researches for a long time. Recently, the three-dimensional (3-D) microvascular architecture of cat sinus hair has been observed by scanning electron microscopy (SEM) of vascular corrosion casts [1]. However, it failed to reach full representation of the 3-D microvascular organization of the whisker, especially of the whisker dermal papilla. Therefore, in this study, we have demonstrated the three-dimensional microvascular and collagen fibrillar architecture of the whisker by SEM of vascular corrosion casts and after cell-maceration to make good use of various kinds of hair researches in the future and we mention the functional significance of the microvascular and collagen fibrillar architecture of the whisker.

Materials and methods

Wistar adult rats were used. To study the 3-D microvascular architecture, SEM of vascular corrosion casts was made according to the usual method [2]. To study the 3-D collagen fibrillar architecture, SEM after cell-maceration was performed according to Ohtani [3].

Results

Scanning electron microscopy of vascular corrosion casts

The whisker was surrounded by two blood sinuses: a superficial ring sinus and a deeper cavernous sinus. Inside the cavernous sinus, there was a basket-like capillary network which surrounded the hair root. The network was denser at its lower part. Inside the ring sinus, there were only a few capillaries (Fig. 1a-c). The whisker dermal papilla had a developed capillary network which was connected

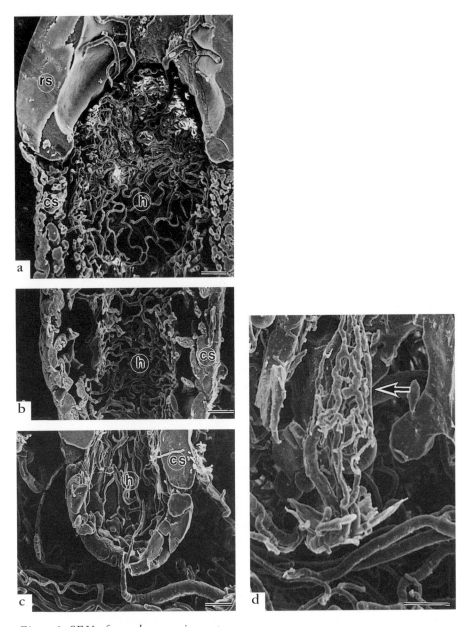

Figure 1. SEM of vascular corrosion casts
a-c: The whisker has a basket-like capillary network (h) which is dense inside the
cavernous sinus (cs) and sparse inside the ring sinus (rs)
d: The whisker dermal papilla has a developed capillary network (arrow).
Scale bar, 50μm.

with the dermal microcirculation (Fig. 1d).

Scanning electron microscopy after cell-maceration

In the external connective tissue capsule, thick collagen fibers were densely packed and formed a thick wall. The collagen fibers of the internal connective tissue capsule formed a thin cylindrical sheath which surrounded the hair root. Within the cavernous sinus, there was a 3-D network of collagen fibers. On the other hand, few collagen fibers were observed in the ring sinus (Fig. 2a). The dermal papilla also had a network of collagen fibers which was connected with the internal connective tissue capsule (Fig. 2b). The network of collagen fibers within the dermal papilla consisted of many thin collagen fibers and only a few thick ones (Fig. 2c).

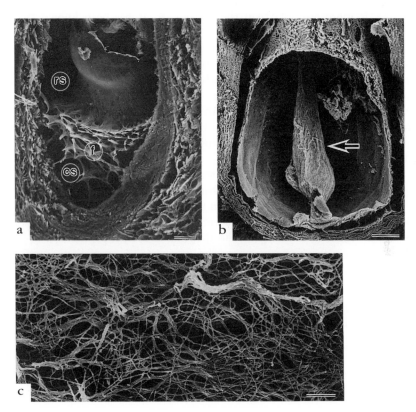

Figure 2. SEM after cell-maceration
a: The network of collagen fibers (f) exists within the cavernous sinus (cs) but not within ring sinus (rs). Scale bar, 50µm; b: Within the dermal papilla, there was a fine network of collagen fibers (arrow). Scale bar, 50µm: c: The network of collagen fibers within the dermal papilla consists of many thin collagen fibers and a few thick ones. Scale bar, 1µm.

152

Discussion

Our present study revealed that the whisker had a dense capillary network inside of the cavernous sinus while only a few capillaries inside of the ring sinus. This microvascular organization would facilitate an abundant supply of blood to the lower part of the hair root which is the most important area for hair growth.

Our SEM after cell-maceration also revealed that whisker had a 3-D architecture of the collagen fibers within the cavernous sinus. It should be noted that many of the collagen fibers are spun between the internal and external connective tissue capsule. Such an organization of collagen fibers would serve to anchor the lower part of the hair root and thereby, to protect the hair root from external forces. On the other hand, there is no network of collagen fibers within the ring sinus. This indicates that the upper part of the hair root surrounded by the ring sinus is more movable than the lower part. It has been known that Merkel cells and nerve terminals are condensed around this part of the hair root [4]. For this reason, the ring sinus, which has no network of collagen fibers, would facilitate the detection of forces upon the hair. On the other hand, the large cavernous sinus would serve as a shock absorber to diminish excessive vibration.

In our previous report, rat dorsal hair, which is much smaller than the whisker, had no visible capillary network within the dermal papilla [5]. However, in the present study, we have demonstrated a developed capillary network within the whisker dermal papilla. Using histochemical methods, Montagna et al. have previously reported that the terminal hair of human scalp had developed capillary network whereas the vellus hair of human scalp had poorly developed capillary network [6]. These observations indicate that the development of the capillary network within the dermal papilla may be in proportion to the size of the dermal papilla because the larger dermal papilla seems to need more abundant supply of blood including nutrients and oxygen than the smaller dermal papilla.

References

1 Ikeda M, Okada S. Okajimas Folia Anat Jpn. 1990; 67: 365-380
2 Murakami T. Arch Histol Jpn. 1971; 32: 445-454
3 Ohtani O. Arch Histol Cytol. 1987; 50: 557-566
4 Patrizi G, Munger BL. J Comp Neurol. 1966; 126: 423-436
5 Sakita S, Ohtani O, Morohashi M. Med Electron Microsc. 1994; 27: 95-98
6 Montagna W, Ellis RA. J Nat Cancer Inst. 1957; 19: 451-463

The changes in microvascular architecture of hair follicle by scanning electron microscopy

S. Sakita[1], O. Ohtani[2] and M. Morohashi[1]

[1]Department of Dermatology and [2]Anatomy, Toyama Medical and Pharmaceutical University, 2630 Sugitani, Toyama 930-01, Japan

Introduction

Although we have previously demonstrated the three-dimensional (3-D) microvasculature of rat anagen hair follicle [1], there is no literature describing the 3-D changes in the microvasculature of the hair follicle during the hair cycle. Therefore, we have examined the 3-D microvascular organization of the rat hair follicle during the hair cycle by scanning electron microscopy (SEM) of vascular corrosion casts and of alkali-collagenase-treated tissues. In addition, we have also performed transmission electron microscopy (TEM) to study the ultrastructural changes of the follicular capillaries during the hair cycle.

Materials and methods

Six Wistar rats were used. Three of them were 50-day-old and the remaining three were 70-day-old. In each group, one rat was used for SEM of vascular corrosion casts, one for SEM of alkali-collagenase-treated tissues, and one for TEM and light microscopy. Routine histological examinations showed that the hair follicles of the dorsal skin of the 50-day-old rat were mostly in the telogen phase and those of the 70-day-old rat were mostly in the anagen phase. The vascular corrosion casts were made by original method [2]. TEM was done according to the routine method. SEM of alkali-collagenase-treated tissues was performed by our original method with minor modifications [3]. In summary, we predigested tissue using 1% collagenase solution prior to the original method.

Results

70-day-old rats

SEM of vascular corrosion casts showed many basket-like capillary networks surrounding the hair follicles. The bottom of the capillary network reached the subcutaneous vascular plexus (Fig. 1a). SEM of alkali-collagenase-treated-tissues also showed the capillary network around the hair follicle, which

154

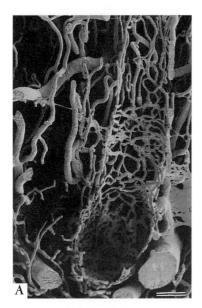
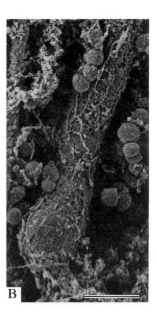

Figure 1. **A**: *SEM of vascular corrosion casts shows an anagen basket-like capillary network.* **B**: *SEM of alkali-collagenase-treated tissues shows an anagen hair follicle and its associated capillary network. Scale bar=100 μm.*

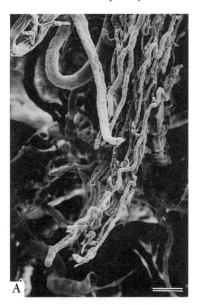
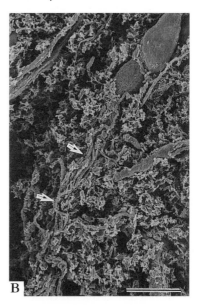

figure 2. **A**: *SEM of vascular corrosion casts shows a collapsed telogen capillary network.* **B**: *SEM of alkali-collagenase-treated tissues shows a telogen hair follicle and its associated capillary network (arrows). Scale bar=100 μm.*

corresponded to that revealed by SEM of vascular corrosion casts (Fig. 1b).

50-day-old rats

SEM of vascular corrosion casts showed many capillary networks that were arranged into the collapsed basket-like structures which gave the appearance of vascular strands (Fig. 2a). SEM of alkali-collagenase-treated-tissues also showed the collapsed capillary network below the tip of telogen hair follicle, which corresponded to that revealed by SEM of vascular corrosion casts (Fig. 2b).

Transmission electron microscopy

The capillaries around the anagen hair bulb possessed many fenestrations (Fig. 3a), while those of the collapsed capillary network located below the tip of the telogen follicle had virtually no fenestration (Fig. 3b).

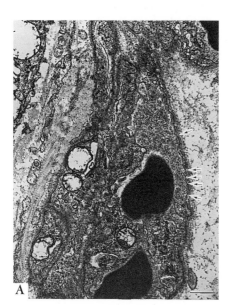
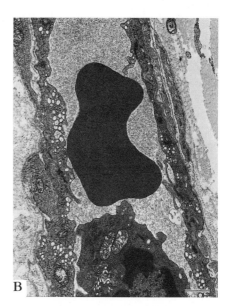

*Figure 3. **A**: Many fenestrations (arrows) were observed on capillary wall around the anagen hair bulb. **B**: No fenestration was observed on capillary wall within the telogen collapsed capillary network. Scale bar = 1 μm.*

Discussion

We have demonstrated the changes of microvascular organization around the hair follicle during the hair cycle. SEM of vascular corrosion casts has revealed the 3-D microvascular architecture associated with the follicle, but did not show the spatial relationship to the cellular elements. This disadvantage has been overcome by SEM of alkali-collagenase-treated tissues. This method can remove most of the collagen fibers, thus exposing the 3-D organization of cellular elements of the skin. As the skin contains abundant collagen and elastic fibers, it is imperative to incubate fresh skin in the collagenase solution prior to the original method [3].

Our previous study by SEM of vascular corrosion casts showed the basket-like capillary network of the anagen hair follicle, but the relationship of the capillary network to the hair follicle during the hair cycle remained to be studied. The present study has demonstrated that the anagen hair follicle is surrounded by a basket-like capillary network whereas the telogen follicle has a collapsed basket-like capillary network below its tapered tip. This indicates that the follicular capillary network collapses with the involution of the hair follicle during telogen and in turn develops with a new follicular downgrowth into the pre-existing collapsed capillary network to form the basket-like capillary network of the anagen follicle. The present study has also shown that the capillaries around the anagen hair follicle possess many fenestrations, while those of the telogen one possess virtually no fenestration. It is widely accepted that the fenestration of capillary endothelium is formed by the simultaneous opening of a pinocytic vesicle on both luminal and basal surfaces of the endothelial cell [4]. This indicates that substances required for the follicular growth during anagen are richly transported through the endothelial cells to the follicle cells, and that, as no follicle cell exists within the collapsed telogen capillary network, trans-endothelial transport across the capillaries occurs much less during telogen, thus resulting in no fenestration of the capillaries.

References

1   Sakita S, Ohtani O, Morohashi M. Med Electron Microsc. 1994; 27: 95-98
2   Murakami T. Arch Histol Jpn. 1971; 32: 445-454
3   Miller BG, Woods RI, Bohlen HG, Evan AP. Anat Rec. 1982; 203: 493-503
4   Kobayashi S. J Electron Microsc. 1968; 17: 322-326

157

Morphological and histochemical characterization of the human vellus hair follicle

K. Krüger, U. Blume-Peytavi and C.E. Orfanos

Department of Dermatology, University Medical Center Benjamin Franklin, The Free University of Berlin, Berlin, Germany

Introduction

The human vellus hair follicle (VHF) plays an important role in various physiological and pathological processes of the skin. Different endogenous and exogenous factors are involved in biological and biochemical regulation and differentiation processes of the human hair follicle. In androgen sensitive areas, for example at puberty, a vellus hair follicle can turn into a terminal hair follicle whereas in androgenetic alopecia a fully developed terminal hair follicle (THF) can involute to a follicle of the vellus hair type. In order to further elucidate responsible mechanisms it is necessary to investigate morphological and functional characteristics of the VHF, which have, in contrast to the human terminal hair follicle, not been in the center of interest until now. The aim of the present study was:

1. to establish morphological criteria marking the vellus hair follicle of human facial skin,
2. to investigate the expression of epithelial cytokeratins and trichohyaline,
3. to examine the lectin binding capacity in the several layers of the vellus hair follicle.

Materials and methods

The morphology of the human vellus hair follicle in facial skin of 17 patients was examined in paraffin and cryostat sections by means of light microscopy in comparison to human terminal scalp hair follicles. The histochemical characterization was performed using a panel of monoclonal antibodies (Moabs) against epithelial cytokeratins and trichohyaline (alkaline phosphatase anti-alkaline phosphatase technique [1]) and six different lectins detecting special glycoconjugates in cell membranes (avidin-biotin technique [2]). Sections were evaluated by light microscopy.

Results

Histomorphology (Fig. 1)

In the thin and non-medullated vellus hair follicle of human facial skin all different cell layers characterizing the human terminal hair follicle could be distinguished. However, in the VHF the inner root sheath (IRS) contains ≥ 3 cell layers (including Huxley's layer with ≥ 2 layers and Henle's layer consisting of a single cell layer) and the outer root sheath (ORS) often consists of a single cell layer only, especially in the suprabulbar region. In the presumed bulge region the ORS is pronounced and contains up to 4 cell layers. At the level of the sebaceous gland the VHF often shows a skirt- or apron-like configuration of the epithelial hood. The sebaceous gland itself is disproportionally large.

Histochemistry

Immunohistochemical investigations of the suprabulbar region of VHF reveal positive staining with the cytokeratins CK 5+8, CK 14 and CK 19 (Fig. 2) in the ORS, whereas cytokeratin CK 13, trichohyaline (Fig. 3, staining more prominent in Huxley's layer) and CK 18 (staining more prominent in Huxley's layer) labeled the IRS. The keratogenous zone of the IRS (Huxley's layer) showed constant labeling with CK 4. Intense staining of the cuticle was observed using CK 7 (Fig. 4) and CK 13. Lectin binding capacity: Constant positive staining in

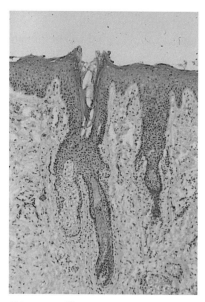

Figure 1. Characteristic histomorphology of the human vellus hair follicle (x 100)

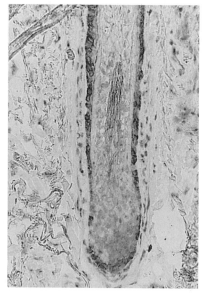

Figure 2. Positive staining of the outer root sheath with CK 19 (x 300)

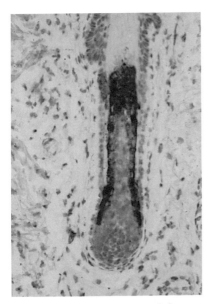

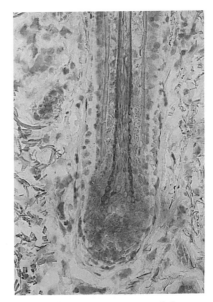

Figure 3. Positive staining of the inner root sheath with trichohyaline (x 250)

Figure 4. Positive staining of the cuticle with CK 7 (x 300)

the ORS could be observed using the lectins DBA, PNA, CON A and WGA. As for the IRS, we found intensive labeling with UEA-1, SBA, PNA and WGA. The cuticle showed positive staining with SBA, PNA and WGA. Labeling of the cortex could be observed neither with cytokeratins nor with lectins.

Conclusions

In the present study we could demonstrate characteristic morphological and histochemical features of the human vellus hair follicle. Our results indicate that the human vellus hair follicle (VHF) resembles a miniaturized terminal hair follicle presenting the same cell layers and compartments as the terminal hair follicle. In contrast to the terminal hair follicle (THF) as characterized by Forslind *et al.* [3] the main morphological characteristics of the VHF are a pronounced inner root sheath with more than 2 cell layers in Huxley's layer, a disproportional size of the sebaceous gland and a relatively small dermal papilla. At the level of the sebaceous gland we could observe a skirt- or apron-like configuration of the epithelial hood which was first described by Narisawa *et al.* [4]. Interestingly, in the VHF the bulge region is rather pronounced.

To further understand morphological and functional characteristics of the VHF we established the cytokeratin labeling pattern and the lectin binding pattern of the VHF. Using a wide panel of cytokeratins and trichohyaline as well as different lectins we could observe similar staining patterns in human terminal and vellus hair follicles. However we found characteristic differences: a homogenous expression of cytokeratin 19 (CK 19) in the outer root sheath and a constant expression of cytokeratin 4 (CK 4) in the keratogenous zone of the inner root sheath in the vellus hair follicle. In contrast in the THF we could observe a mosaic-like staining pattern with CK 19 in the ORS and a variable expression of CK 4 in the inner root sheath. As to CK 19, investigation of transversal sections of VHF by Narisawa et al. [5] demonstrated, in contrast to our findings, expression of CK 19 only in the bulge region. An intense, but heterogeneous basal cell staining in the deep outer root sheath, which was maximal just below the isthmus and dependent on body site and hair cycle, was described by Lane et al. [6] in VHF of different body sites. The expression of CK 4, in our study always detectable in well developed facial VHF in anagen, showed two different patterns: first a continuous staining of Huxley's layer and second a localized staining pattern in the keratogenous zone in Huxley's layer. To our knowledge, until now CK 4 has only been observed in the sebaceous gland of the pilosebaceous unit.

In conclusion the VHF presents a characteristic histomorphology and histochemistry different from the THF. However, further investigation concerning functional significance of these findings is in progress.

References

1   Cordell JL, Falini B, Erber WN, Ghosh AK, Abdulatiz Z, Macdonald S, Pulford KAF, Stein H, Mason Dy. J Histochem Cytochem. 1984; 32: 219-229
2   Bourne JA. Dako Corporation, Carpinteria, California. 1983; 1-36
3   Forslind B. In: Orfanos CE, Happle R (eds): Hair and hair diseases. Springer-Verlag Berlin Heidelberg New York. 1990; 73-97
4   Narisawa Y, Hashimoto K, Kohda H. Arch Dermatol Res. 1993; 285: 269-277
5   Narisawa Y, Hashimoto K, Kohda H. J Invest Dermatol. 1994; 103: 191-195
6   Lane EB, Wilson CA, Hughes BR, Leigh IM. Ann NY Acad Sci. 1991; 642: 197-213

Hair research for the next millenium
D.J.J. Van Neste and V.A. Randall (Eds)

Recognition of cellular differentiation in the human hair follicle at the light microscope level using SACPIC staining

M. Nutbrown and V.A. Randall

Department of Biomedical Sciences, University of Bradford, Bradford BD7 1DP, United Kingdom

Introduction

It is often important to identify the precise cell layers and growth stages of the human hair follicle when carrying out investigations into abnormal follicles or when using immunostaining. Although this is normally rather difficult at the light microscope level SACPIC staining has been used successfully to distinguish the layers in transverse wax sections of animal follicles [1, 2]. We have applied this method to human skin to investigate whether SACPIC staining would discriminate the various cellular layers and stages of differentiation in longitudinal wax and frozen sections of human hair follicles.

Materials and methods

Small samples of human skin taken from scalp, axilla and breast were either fixed for 18-24 hours in 10% neutral buffered formaldehyde and processed routinely into paraffin wax or snap frozen in OCT (Agar Scientific Ltd., Stansted UK) and stored at -80°C. Longitudinal serial sections of tissues containing follicles were cut at 5-8 μm; frozen sections were air dried for 2 hours and fixed in Bouin's solution for 15 minutes. All sections were stained with SACPIC or with Harris's haematoxylin and aqueous eosin (H & E) [3] and examined under the light microscope.

Sections were dewaxed and rehydrated where necessary. SACPIC sections were stained in celestine blue for five minutes and rinsed gently in running tap water. Following this sections were stained for five minutes in Gill's haematoxylin, rinsed in tap water and blued for between two and five minutes in Scott's tap water. The next stain was 2% safranin for five minutes followed by dehydration in 70% and 95% ethanol. The sections were then differentiated in picric acid/ethanol solution, rehydrated in 95% and 70% ethanol and quickly rinsed in running tap water. Final staining was in picro-indigo carmine for one minute. After rinsing in tap water, sections were dehydrated through a graded series of ethanol/water mixes, cleared in Histoclear and mounted under glass coverslips with DPX (Agar Scientific Ltd., Stansted UK).

H & E sections were stained with Harris's haematoxylin for 10 minutes and blued in running tap water for four or five minutes. Five to ten seconds differentiation in 1% acid alcohol was followed by a second blueing in tap water, and, after staining for 10 minutes in eosin, sections were washed for five minutes, dehydrated, cleared and mounted.

Results

Hair follicles stained with H & E were clearly distinguished from the surrounding dermis, but the various follicular layers were not readily identified. The cytoplasm of the outer root sheath cells was virtually unstained whereas the cell nuclei were stained intense blue with black inclusions. Henle's and Huxley's layers and inner root sheaths were stained uniformly pink with dark pink stained trichohyalin granules. Cells of dermal papillae stained dark blue, but the extracellular matrixes were virtually unstained whereas other connective tissues were also stained blue and the collagenous connective tissue stained very pale pink.

SACPIC staining produced multicolored sections in which the various parts of the hair follicle could be readily distinguished in both wax (Fig. 1a) and frozen

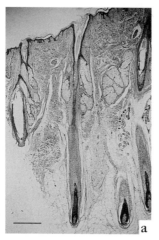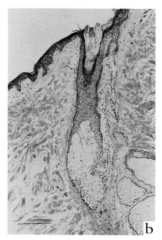

Figure 1a. Human scalp skin in wax stained with SACPIC
Keratinized parts of hair fibres (yellow) are easily distinguished. Collagen and the outer root sheath clearly stain a different blue from non-keratinizing epithelial cells of sebaceous glands and hair fibre. Scale bar: 600 µm
Figure 1b. Section of frozen human scalp skin stained with SACPIC
Collagen is stained an intense blue. Dark blue/black nuclei surrounded by purple cytoplasm are seen in the non-keratinizing portions of the epithelial tissues. Keratinized epithelium shows strong red staining. Scale bar: 200 µm

(Fig. 1b) sections of human scalp skin. Sections from frozen human scalp skin stained similarly to wax sections except that the intensity of the staining was greater than in wax sections. Collagen and outer root sheaths stained pale blue which was clearly different from the dark blues of non-keratinizing epithelial cells of sebaceous glands and hair fibre. Keratinized epithelium/epidermis showed strong red staining.

Individual human anagen hair follicles stained with SACPIC (Fig. 2a) showed remarkable diversity of staining color and intensity. Keratinized parts of hair fibres were easily identified as they stained bright yellow. The individual layers

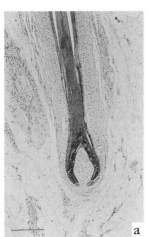 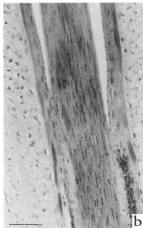 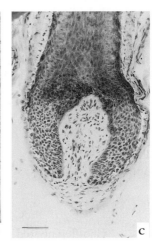

Figure 2a. Human anagen hair follicle; wax section stained with SACPIC
The individual layers of Henle, Huxley and the cuticle of the inner root sheath (all shades of red) are easily discerned. Differentiation of these layers is also distinguished by the changes in staining intensity and hue. Non-keratinizing epithelial cells all display dark blue nuclei with a purple/dark pink cytoplasm. Scale bar: 200 μm
Figure 2b. High power view of anagen follicle; wax section stained with SACPIC
This view shows the Henle and Huxley layers and inner root sheath at about three times dermal papilla height. Keratinizing cells of Henle's layer can be distinguished from non-keratinizing cells by the increased intensity of staining. Trichohyalin granules (orange/brown) can be seen in Huxley's layer in the lower part of the micrograph. Several changes can be seen in the staining pattern of the hair fibre, from the lower region of pre-keratinization (pink/blue) to higher portions of the fibre (yellow) which are fully keratinized. Scale bar: 50 μm
Figure 2c. Bulb of anagen hair follicle from frozen section of human scalp skin (SACPIC)
The extracellular matrix of the dermal papilla stains pale blue whereas the dermal papilla cells themselves are an intense blue with darker nuclei. The epithelial cells of the germinative layers and undifferentiated matrix have blue/purple nuclei with paler cytoplasm which contrasts with the brown/black deposits of melanin in the cells of the adjacent presumptive cortical region. Scale bar: 60 μm

of Henle, Huxley and the cuticle of the inner root sheath (all shades of red) were easily discerned. The progressive differentiation of these layers was also distinguished by the changes in staining intensity and hue. Non-keratinized epithelial tissues all displayed cells with dark blue nuclei in a purple/dark pink cytoplasm. At high power magnification (Fig. 2b) keratinizing cells of Henle's layer could be distinguished from non-keratinizing cells by the increased intensity of staining. Orange/brown trichohyalin granules could be seen in Huxley's layer. Several changes could be seen in the staining pattern of the hair fibres, from pink/blue of the lower regions of pre-keratinization through pink/red to yellow in higher parts of the fibre which are fully keratinized.

Detailed examination of bulbs of anagen hair follicles: from frozen sections of human scalp skin (Fig. 2c) also showed the extracellular matrixes of the dermal papillae stained pale blue and dermal papilla cells themselves stained an intense blue black. The epithelial cells of the germinative layers and undifferentiated matrix were blue/purple with clear extracellular matrixes which contrasted with the brown/black deposits of melanosomes in the adjacent presumptive cortical region.

Table 1.
Appearance of SACPIC stained sections

Collagen	blue
Smooth muscle	green
Undifferentiated keratinocytes	blue/pink
Keratinizing inner root sheath	red
Pre-keratinizing inner root sheath	blue/grey
Trichohyalin granules	orange/brown
Outer root sheath	blue
Connective tissue sheath	pale blue
Keratinizing hair fibre	yellow
Pre-keratinizing hair fibre	pink
Dermal papilla extracellular matrix	pale blue
Dermal papilla cells	blue/black
Outer borders of brush ends of catagen/telogen hair fibre	orange/yellow
Stratum corneum	dark red
Nuclei	dark blue/grey

When hair follicles at the end of catagen or in telogen were examined (Fig. 3a) the keratinized hair fibres were stained mostly yellow with red tinges at the brush end of the club hair. The collapsing sacs of connective tissue sheaths, which extended below the end of the hair fibre were stained pale blue. At higher

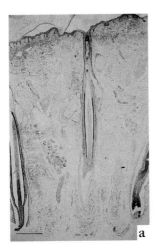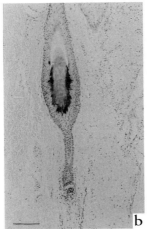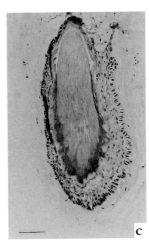

Figure 3a. Wax section of hair follicle at the end of catagen or in early telogen (SACPIC)
The keratinized hair fibre is stained mostly yellow with red tinges at the brush end of the club hair. The collapsing sac of the connective tissue sheath (pale blue) extends below the end of the hair fibre. Scale bar: 500 μm

Figure 3b. Late catagen/telogen follicle, oblique wax section (SACPIC)
The epithelial tissue including the epithelial stalk with the ball of the dermal papilla at its end are stained blue. Differential staining of the keratinized (yellow) and partly keratinized (red) hair fibres is evident. Scale bar: 120 μm

Figure 3c. Detail of brush end of hair fibre in telogen follicle from a frozen section of human scalp skin (SACPIC)
Distinction can easily be made between the fully keratinized hair fibre (yellow) and the brush border (red) of the end of the club hair. The non-keratinizing epithelial cells (blue) are clearly distinguished from the pale blue of the connective tissue sheath. Scale bar: 60 μ

magnifications (Figs. 3b and 3c) distinction could easily be made in late catagen/telogen between yellow staining of fully keratinized hair fibre and the red of the brush border of the end of club hairs. Blue of non-keratinizing epithelial cells was clearly distinguished from the much paler blue of the connective tissue sheaths.

Discussion

H & E staining discriminated between epithelial and connective tissues and to some extent distinguished between different stages of keratinizing tissues. However in none of the follicles examined was the ability to assess differentiation of follicular components or stages of the hair cycle as marked as with SACPIC staining.

SACPIC successfully stained both wax and frozen longitudinal sections of human hair follicles. Multicolored sections were produced giving ready definition of hair follicle structure (see Table 1). Although there were slight differences in degree or intensity of staining no significant differences in stain colors were seen between wax and frozen sections.

SACPIC staining allows ready identification of the stages of differentiation of the cellular layers in hair follicles and also between the stages of the hair growth cycle. There were no differences in staining patterns between human follicles and those of other mammals as reported previously by Auber [1] and Nixon [2].

In summary, SACPIC staining provides clear and useful information about the different layers and states of differentiation in the human hair follicle in both wax and frozen sections at the light microscope level. It is straightforward to apply and should be particularly useful for human studies where only limited amounts of material are available and sections may not be in an optimal plane.

References

1   Auber L. Trans Roy Soc Edin. 1952; 62: 191-254 + plates
2   Nixon AJ. Biotechnic & Histochemistry. 1993; 68: 316-325
3   Bancroft JD, Stevens A, eds. Theory and Practice of Histological Techniques. London: Churchill Livingstone. 1977; 85-94

Colour plates VII-IX

©1996 Elsevier Science B.V. All rights reserved.
Hair research for the next millenium
D.J.J. Van Neste and V.A. Randall (Eds)

Characterization of LHTric-1, a new monospecific monoclonal antibody to the trichocyte keratin Ha1

G.E. Westgate[1], D. de Berker[2], M.A. Blount[1], M.P. Philpott[1], N. Tidman[3] and I.M. Leigh[3]

[1]Unilever Research, Colworth House, Sharnbrook, Bedford, United Kingdom
[2]Department of Dermatology, Royal Victoria Infirmary, Newcastle, United Kingdom
[3]The London Hospital, Whitechapel, London, United Kingdom

Introduction

Epithelial keratins form a large multi-gene family of structural proteins, whose members can be detected by monospecific monoclonal antibodies. The complex patterns of epithelial differentiation in stratifying epithelia have been greatly elucidated by the use of these monoclonal antibodies [1]. The hair follicle is a heterogeneous tissue involving cells of both trichocyte and epithelial lineage; whilst the markers available for epithelial keratins can determine the distribution of these keratins in the outer and inner root sheath, fewer have been described for the trichocyte keratins found in hair fibre cortex and cuticle.

Results and discussion

We employed the proven strategy of raising monoclonal antibodies to a short synthetic peptide from the carboxy terminal sequence of the hair keratin Ha1, from the mouse sequence for Ha1 [2], (sequence used was CVPRPRCGPCNSFVR) and report here the successful production of a monospecific monoclonal antibody which we have called LH Tric-1.

We have characterized LH Tric-1 using standard immunostaining methods on rat and human tissues including embryonic and adult skin through the hair growth cycle, cultured human hair follicles, adult human tongue and human nail. We also established the specificity of the antibody by immunoblotting against a follicle extract.

Results of immunostaining showed that LH Tric-1 immunoreacted very specifically to the pre-cortical region of the hair follicle in early anagen and is specifically located in the cortical matrix in anagen (Fig. 1). There was no staining in the cuticle or root sheaths, demonstrating that the antibody was cortex specific. Telogen follicles did not react indicating that Ha1 is only expressed during fibre formation. The distribution of trichocyte keratins in nail

168

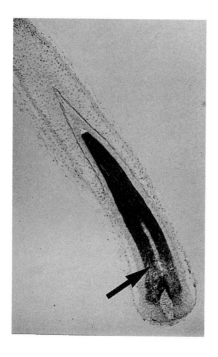

Figure 1. Anagen hair follicle isolated from human scalp, frozen without fixation and immunoreacted with LH Tric-1. Reaction detected using immunoperoxidase linked second antibody and diaminobenzidine as chromogen. Magnification x125. Earliest point of LH Tric-1 immunoreactivity in the cortex is indicated by an arrow.

and tongue was also confirmed by immunostaining with LH Tric-1, with reactivity restricted to the mid line above the connective tissue core in tongue and to the suprabasal layers of the nail matrix.

In immunoblotting, LH Tric-1 reacted with a single band of 44Kd, in contrast with the 2 bands seen when the monoclonal type antibody AE 13 [3] was used. This suggests that a single protein was recognized, although two dimensional blots would really confirm this.

We conclude that this antibody, by virtue of its known antigen sequence specificity, will be useful in research into the formation of hair and nail in normal and diseased states and for the examination of dual lineage pathways of differentiation in tissues containing trichocyte keratins.

References

1   Fuchs E, Tyner AL, Guidice GJ, Marchuk D, Chaudhury AR, Rosenburg M. The human keratin genes and their differential expression. In Current topics in developmental biology. 1987; 22: 5-34

2   Kaytes PS, McNab AR, Rea TR, Groppi V, Kawabe TT, Buhl AE, Bertolino AP, Hazenbuhler NT, Vogeli G. Hair Specific Keratins: characterization and expression of a mouse type I Keratin gene. J Invest Dermatol. 1991; 97: 835-842

3   Lynch MH, O'Guin WM, Hardy C, Mak L, Sun TT. Acidic and basic hair/nail («hard») keratins: their colocalization in upper cortical cells and cuticle cells of the human hair follicle and their relationship to «soft» keratins. J Cell Biol. 1986; 2593-2606

©1996 Elsevier Science B.V. All rights reserved.
Hair research for the next millenium
D.J.J. Van Neste and V.A. Randall (Eds)

Human trichohyalin

P. Steinert, E. Tarcsa, S.-C. Lee, S.-I. Jang, J. Andreoli and N. Markova

Skin Biology Branch, National Institute of Arthritis and Musculoskeletal and Skin Diseases, National Institute of Health, Bethesda, Maryland 20892-2755, U.S.A.

Introduction

Trichohyalin (THH) is a major structural protein of the inner root sheath layers of the hair follicle, the medulla of the hair fiber, and also of the epidermis, nail bed, hard palate, and filiform ridges of the tongue [1-4]. Isolated pig tongue THH is a highly insoluble largely α-helical protein [3, 4]. Established *in vivo* data have shown that THH is a major substrate for two types of post-translational modifications [5, 6]. These include conversion of many arginine residues to citrullines by the enzyme peptidylarginine deiminase (PAD), and crosslinking into an insoluble form by trans-glutaminases (TGases). We have recently cloned and sequenced human THH [4, 5]. It has a molecular weight of 250 kDa, consists of several subdomains characterized by irregular peptide repeats, and is likely to adopt the shape of an elongated rod at least 220 nm long of a largely single-stranded α-helical conformation. These physical properties are consistent with the possible function of THH as a keratin intermediate filament binding protein and/or a constituent of the cornified cell envelope of the tissues.

In an attempt to understand its function in tissues, we have now performed two different types of experiments. The first has been to better characterize *in vitro* the PAD and TGase substrate properties of THH. We have expressed in bacteria and used the largest domain of human THH, domain 8 (THH-8), since it is more soluble [7]. In a second series of experiments, we have explored the expression properties of the human *THH* gene in *in vitro* transfection assays and in transgenic mice.

PAD causes the unfolding of THH-8

The modification of arginines to citrullines in THH-8 by the type II PAD enzyme was monitored by amino acid analysis (Fig. 1). Up to 65% of the arginine residues in THH-8 could be modified to citrullines (~15% final citrulline content) using the highest enzyme: THH-8 ratio tested. By amino acid sequencing, virtually all arginines were modified >95% except those that were followed by a glutamic acid residue, which were not converted at all. By circular dichroism, the modification resulted in progressive loss of α-helicity (Fig. 2): 5%

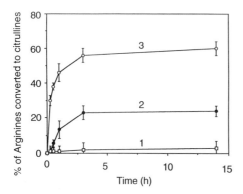

Figure 1. Kinetics of PAD modification of THH-8. The lines are enzyme: THH-8 ratios of: 1, 1:1000; 2, 1:100; 3, 10:1

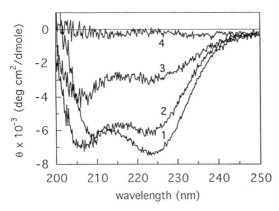

Figure 2. Circular dichroism of THH-8 modified by PAD. Line 0, before reaction, corresponding to ~100% α-helix. Lines 1-3: same as Figure 1

modification reduced the α-helical content to ~65% (line 2), ~25% modification to <25% (line 3), and 65% modification to disordered structure (line 4). The degree of denaturation resulting from 65% modification was equivalent to the effect of 5 M urea on THH-8 (data not shown). The citrulline side-chain is a substituted urea derivative. Thus we conclude that the net insertion of many citrullines interfers with H-bonding interactions in organized protein structures in a way similar to urea itself.

PAD-induced unfolding renders THH-8 a superior TGase substrate

Each of the epithelial tissues known to express THH also expresses the three TGase enzymes, TGase 1, TGase 2, TGase 3. By far the most abundant in terms of activity is TGase 3 enzyme, especially in the inner root sheath and medulla cell layers of the hair follicle [5]. We have found that THH-8 is a complete TGase substrate, in the sense that it provides both glutamines and lysines for crosslinking. Thus THH-8 is rapidly oligomerized by TGase 3 into species too large to enter an SDS gel (data not shown). On the other hand, by using the exogenous amine donor labeled putrescine, we measured the kinetic efficiency k_{cat}/K_M of the crosslinking reaction for THH-8 to be 12.8 $min^{-1}.\mu M^{-1}$. In maximally PAD modified THH-8, it was 36.9 $min^{-1}.\mu M^{-1}$. This means that THH-8 becomes a much better substrate for TGase cross-linking after deimination by PAD.

Together, the present data afford new insights on the role of THH in the skin. Intact THH is stored in insoluble granules, and based on histochemical staining, is largely unmodified by PAD [8]. Our data show that upon modification of many of its arginines to citrullines by PAD *in vivo* (up to 50% in the inner root sheath and 75% in the medulla, corresponding to citrulline contents of 11% and 17%, respectively) [9], the THH will be completely denatured. In this form it is likely to be a much more efficiently used substrate for the TGase 3 enzyme. Therefore, we predict that the specific purpose of PAD modification of THH is to permit its subsequent use as a major structural protein for the formation of highly crosslinked, rigid layers of cells in these tissues.

The regulation of expression of the human *THH* gene *in vitro*

In order to explore the regulation of the *THH* gene, we first sought a suitable cell culture assay system. By use of RT-PCR methods, we found that normal human epidermal keratinocytes express only very low levels of the THH mRNA [5]. However, both human and mouse hair follicle preparations [10] expressed the THH mRNA [5] and protein (data not shown) at much higher levels, which thus provides a more suitable assay system. Three constructs containing 0.1-3.8 kb of 5'-upstream sequences of the human *THH* gene were coupled to a β-galactosidase reporter gene and used for *in vitro* transient transfection experiments. Staining for enzyme activity showed that as few as the first 135 bp above the transcription start site were capable of driving the β-galactosidase gene in transfected mouse hair follicle preparations (Fig. 3B). The constructs containing 1.3 or 3.8 kb of upstream sequences were also expressed (Figs. 3C and 3D, respectively).

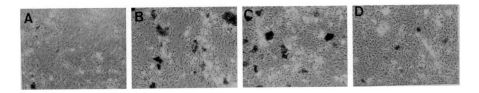

Figure 3. Staining for β-galactosidase enzyme activity in mouse hair follicle preparations transiently transfected with a promotorless β-galactosidase gene construct as a control (A), or this construct but containing the first 135 bp (B), 1.3 kb (C), or 3.8 kb (D) above the transcription start site of the human THH gene.

Expression of THH β-galactosidase constructs in transgenic mice

The 1.3 kb β-galactosidase construct was used to produce transgenic mice. Founder mice were assayed for the β-galactosidase gene by PCR from tail DNA preparations. The offspring of F1 generation transgenic siblings were analyzed for β-galactosidase expression. Using a whole-mount β-galactosidase enzymatic assay, the construct was expressed in the snout and palate in 0.5 day mice (data not shown). Immunostaining of 7 day old mice showed β-galactosidase staining only in the tongue filiform papilla (Fig. 4A) which co-localized with endogenous mouse THH (Fig. 4B), and palate (data not shown). However, immunostaining for β-galactosidase was not detected in the inner root sheath or medulla of hair follicles where endogenous THH is expresed (Figs. 4C and 4D). No β-galactosidase immunostaining was detected in nontransgenic siblings (data not shown).

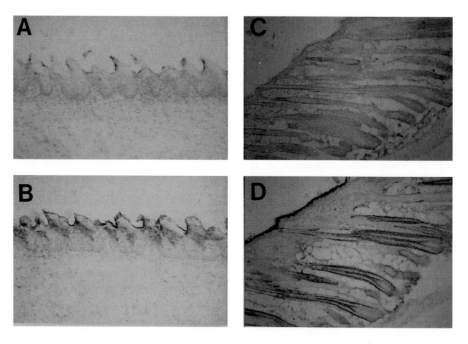

Figure 4. Immunolocalization of the expression of the 1.3 kb human THH β-galactosidase construct and of endogenous mouse THH in frozen sections in 7 day old transgenic mouse tongue (A,B) and skin (C,D). Serial sections were incubated with either a polyclonal antibody against β-galactosidase (A,C) or a polyclonal antibody against human THH (B,D). Primary antibodies were visualized following colorimetric detection of horseradish-peroxidase/streptavidin-biotin conjugated secondary antibodies.

Based on these results, we can conclude that as few as the first 135 bp above the transcription start site can drive *THH* gene expression in hair follicle cells *in vitro*, but at least 1.3 kb of sequences are required for proper *in vivo* expression in the tongue papilla and palate in transgenic mice. However, additional sequences are required to direct proper expression in the hair follicle. Further experiments using the 3.8 kb construct are in progress to see if they can regulate complete expression of the *THH* gene. In this way, we may be able to identify the specific regulatory sequences which direct *THH* gene expression to different tissues.

References

1 Rothnagel JA, Rogers GE. J Cell Biol. 1986; 102: 1419-1429
2 O'Guin WM, Sun TT, Manabe W. J Invest Dermatol. 1992; 98: 24-32
3 Hamilton EH, Sealock R, Wallace NR, O'Keefe EJ. J Invest Dermatol. 1992; 98: 881-889
4 O'Keefe EJ, Hamilton EH, Lee SC, Steinert PM. J Invest Dermatol. 1993; 101: 65S-71S
5 Lee SC, Kim IG, Marekov LN, O'Keefe EJ, Parry DAD, Steinert PM. J Biol Chem. 1993; 268: 12164-12176
6 Steinert PM. Biochemistry. 1988; 17: 5045-5052
7 Lee SC, Marekov LN, Steinert PM, Tarcsa E. J Invest Dermatol. 1995; 104: 576
8 Rogers GE. J Histochem Cytochem. 1962; 11: 700-706
9 Steinert PM, Harding HWJ, Rogers GE. Biochim Biophys Acta. 1969; 175: 1-9
10 Hennings H. In: Leigh I, Watt F, eds. Keratinocyte Methods. Cambridge University Press. 1994; 21-23

Hair research for the next millenium
D.J.J. Van Neste and V.A. Randall (Eds)

The Jackson Laboratory: repository for spontaneous and induced mouse mutations and information on the genetics and pathology of mice

J.P. Sundberg, B.A. Sundberg, R.S. Smith, J.S. Sharp, C. Blake, J.T. Eppig, T. Drake and M.T. Davisson

The Jackson Laboratory, 600 Main Street, Bar Harbor, ME 04609-1500, USA

Introduction

As the largest repository for transgenic, targeted, and spontaneous mouse mutations in the world, the Jackson Laboratory and its informational resources provides a unique resource for biomedical research scientists. The information is not limited to any one organ system, chromosome or cluster of genes, however, with several research groups at the Jackson Laboratory focusing on diseases of the skin and hair, information and training materials are available to support research in this area. The Jackson Laboratory has a number of programs, which are highlighted below. More information can be obtained through access to these programs *via* the World Wide Web. The URL address for The Jackson Laboratory is http://www.jax.org.

Mutant mouse resource

The Jackson Laboratory Mutant Mouse Resource (MMR), directed by Dr Kenneth R. Johnson and Dr Muriel Davisson identifies and characterizes new spontaneous mouse mutations for biomedical research, propagates new and established mouse mutations in useful stocks, publishes information on these mutations, and distributes mice carrying the mutations to scientists worldwide. The MMR arose out of early mutant mouse characterization studies done by Dr Elizabeth S. Russell and Dr George Dr Snell, in the 1930s and 1940s, and was established as a resource program by Dr Margaret Green in the late 1950s. The mission of the MMR is to (1) identify and analyze new mouse mutations, (2) publish information to describe new mutants to the scientific community, and (3) propagate and distribute mutant mice to scientific investigators. The resource focuses on mutations that arise spontaneously but also includes established mutations that were induced using radiation and mutagenic compounds such as ethylnitrosourea, as well as other classical approaches. Currently over 600 mouse mutations are available of which approximately 300 are maintained in small colonies, 300 as frozen embryos, and 30 in large production colonies [1, 2].

Not only are single gene mutations available as models for important groups of dermatological diseases, such as psoriasis, but groups of allelic mutations (new mutations with similar phenotypes that arise in the same gene) and those that are induced by mutations mapping to different *loci* are available. We now have such groups of mutations at The Jackson Laboratory for studying scaly skin diseases [3, 4], alopecia [4, 5], growth factors affecting hair development [4, 6-8], and for many other types of skin disorders [9].

Induced mutant resource

The Jackson Laboratory Induced Mutant Resource (IMR), directed by Dr John Sharp, was established in September 1992, in response to concerns from the scientific community. The IMR serves as a national clearing house for the collection and distribution of genetically engineered mice. The function of the IMR is to import, cryopreserve embryos, maintain, and distribute important transgenic, chemically induced, and targeted mutant strains of mice. Rederivation during importation rids mice of infectious diseases and cryopreservation of embryos provides backup in case of accidental loss or intentional elimination of breeding colonies due to reduced demand. The IMR also undertakes genetic development of stocks, such as transferring mutant genes or transgenes onto defined genetic backgrounds (congenic strains) and combining transgenes and/or targeted mutations to create new mouse models for research. The Pathology Program personnel work with IMR evaluating mutant mice to determine if the phenotype originally reported is maintained once they are rederived or put onto defined genetic backgrounds. Currently over 200 induced mutants have been accepted into the program and over 100 are being distributed [2,10], with an additional 30 strains expected to be available within the next 4 months. We are adding about 8 new strains/month and encourage investigators with new models to contact us.

Informatics program

The Jackson Laboratory Informatics Program, directed by Dr Janan T. Eppig, was formed in 1992. This effort evolved from previous successful informatics efforts including GBASE (*Genomic Database for the Mouse*), the first online database of mouse genomic information produced in the 1980s through the collaborative efforts of Dr Thomas H. Roderick and Dr Muriel T. Davisson. GBASE was merged into the new *Mouse Genome Database* (MGD) in 1994. *The Encyclopedia of the Mouse Genome* software, developed by Drs Joseph H. Nadeau, Lawrence E. Mobraaten, and Janan T. Eppig, is an interactive map display tool for mouse genetic data. First released in 1989, the Encyclopedia continues to be developed and improved. *The Encyclopedia* software uses data derived from Chromosome Committee maps, MIT Genome Center SSLP maps, and linkage information maps retrieved from MGD. MGD is a comprehensive database of information about the mouse genome, including genetic marker information, experimental genetic and physical mapping data, comparative mapping data for mouse, human beings, and 40 other mammals, probe, clone, and PCR primer information, genetic polymorphism data, phenotypic data including synoptic descriptions of genes (*Mouse Locus Catalog*) and inbred strain characteristics, and associated bibliographical references [11]. MGD can be used for browsing and as a source of data to be analyzed and graphically displayed in *the Encyclopedia of the Mouse Genome* or other display tools. The MGD is available to the scientific community *via* the World Wide Web (WWW) (http://www.informatics.jax.org), where it is complemented by links to external databases such as *Online Mendelian Inheritance in Man* (OMIM), *The Human Genome Database* (GDB), and GenBank. MGD is updated daily, providing a unique and valuable resource for scientists interested in animal models and biomedical tools. These tools are readily available «on-line» if researchers realize they exist, know how to access them, and know how to use them.

Pathology program

The Jackson Laboratory Pathology Program, directed by Dr John P. Sundberg, identifies and characterizes spontaneous diseases in inbred laboratory mice, evaluates mutations imported to the laboratory, and assists in characterization of new mutations [4, 12]. Based on the specialties of the three staff pathologists, work focuses on skin and hair, ocular, and neurological mutations in mice. The Pathology Program generates and distributes information on mouse mutations and diseases through publications [3, 4, 6, 7], on-line computer information *via* the WWW, and preparation of study sets consisting of glass microscope slides (four sets each containing nearly 400 slides are available for use at The Jackson Laboratory during meetings and a fifth set is on file at the Registry of Comparative Pathology, Armed Forces Institute of Pathology, Washington, D.C.). These are continually being expanded to include newly described mouse mutations.

The standardized nomenclature, repositories for mice, colonies for distribution of mice to researchers, and on-line, interactive information systems are some of the many important resources provided by The Jackson Laboratory to aid biomedical research using genetically defined, inbred laboratory mice.

Acknowledgements

This work was supported in part by National Cancer Institute grant number CA34196 (CORE) and National Institutes of Health grant number RR08911.

References

1   Davisson MT. Lab Animal. 1990; 19: 23-29
2   Sundberg JP, Sharp JS, Eppig JT, Davisson MT. Tox Pathol. (in press)
3   Sundberg JP, HogenEsch H, King Jr. LE. Dermatological Research Techniques. Maibach HI (ed.), Boca Raton, FL: CRC Press, Inc. 1995; 61-89

4   Sundberg JP. Handbook of mouse mutations with skin and hair abnormalities: animal models and biomedical tools. Boca Raton, FL: CRC Press, Inc. 1994
5   Sundberg JP, Shultz LD. J Invest Dermatol. 1991; 96: 95S
6   Sundberg JP, Smith RS, Hogan ME. Jax Notes. 1994; 459: 2-5
7   Sundberg JP, Hogan ME. Jax Notes. 1994; 460: 2-5
8   Herbert JM, Rosenquist T, Gotz J, Martin GR. Cell. 1994; 78: 1017-1025
9   Sundberg JP, King Jr LE. Progress in Dermatology, Moshel A (ed.), Bethesda, MD: NIH. 1994; 28: 1-12
10 Sharp JS, Davisson MT. Lab Animal. 1994; 23: 32-40
11 Nadeau JH, Grant PL, Mankala S, Reiner AH, *et al.* Nature. 1995; 373: 363-365
12 Sundberg JP. Comp Pathol Bull. 1989; 21: 1-4

Hair research for the next millenium
D.J.J. Van Neste and V.A. Randall (Eds)

Studies on biochemical indices in C3H mouse model as hair cycle markers

K. Hamada, K. Suzuki and I. Miyamoto

Cosmetics Laboratory, Kanebo Ltd, 3-28, 5-chome, kotobuki-cho, Odawara city, Kanagawa, 250 Japan

Introduction

Many animals possess hair follicle which is classified as a mammalian skin appendage and exhibit intrinsic hair cycle. The hair follicle passes through alternating periods of growth (anagen) and quiescence (telogen) producing successive generations of hairs. There is a brief involutionary phase between anagen and telogen called catagen. The relative duration of these phases varies with body sites, ages, nutritional status, hormone factors and other physiologic and pathologic factors. However, the regulatory mechanism of hair cycle is not fully understood.

In many mammals the cycles in adjacent hair follicles are coordinated, but in man they are generally asynchronous. Rabbits, mice, rats and stump-tailed macaques have been used for studying hair growth and its cycle, and many biochemical substances investigated pathologically. In the mice, after the first coat, waves of hair growth sweep posteriorly and dorsally from the throat region thus all the follicles in a particular area are in the growth phase at a given period [1]. C3H/HeNCrj mouse is thought to be useful as a model mouse for studying hair cycle, because it possesses wavy-typed hair cycle and its hair phase changes from telogen phase to anagen phase after depilation or epilation [2]. We have investigated the levels of biochemical indices while hair re-growth developed.

Materials and methods

Animals: C3H /HeNCrj male mice aged 7 weeks old were purchased from Charles River Ltd, Japan and kept at a temperature of $24 \pm 2°C$ in lighting for 12 hours (lights on 8:00 a.m. - 8:00 p.m.) with a humidity of $55 \pm 5\%$, and were freely given a cubed diet. In this conditions described above the mice were fed for one week before the experiment. After the prefeeding the dorsal areas (2 cm x 4 cm) of the mice were clipped with clipper and treated with the hair remover.

Administration of cyclosporin and minoxidil: The samples for administration were dissolved into 55% ethanol and 0.2ml of each sample was applied to each mouse twice a day.

Preparation of skin homogenates: dorsal skin of mice (n=3) was dissected out and trimmed according to the line of areas which were treated with clipper and the hair remover. After dissection, dorsal skin was minced in 9 times volume of phosphate buffered saline and homogenized for 15 seconds (twice) at 8,000 rpm with polytron-type homogenizer and centrifuged at 3,000 rpm for 10 min. The supernatant of each homogenate was used as the sample for each assay.

Assays for biochemical indices: Transglutaminase, sulfhydryl oxidase, cathepsin D, γ-glutamyltranspeptidase (GGT), alkaline phosphatase (AlP), acid phosphatase and tyrosinase (Tyr) activities and histamine content in the supernatant sample were assayed. The protein content was measured by the method of Lowry *et al.*

Results and discussion

The hair re-growth in C3H mouse was observed on 11 the days after depilation and completed during 18 days (Fig. 1). In this model the levels of eight biochemical indices were examined. The changes of transglutaminase, sulfhydryl oxidase, cathepsin D activities did not correlate with hair regrowth of C3H mice, but the increase of γ-glutamyltranspeptidase activity was relevant of

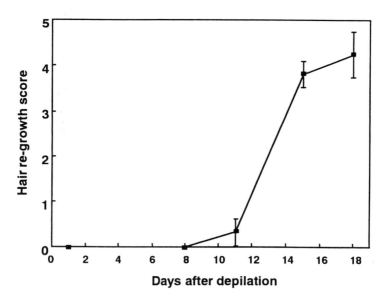

Figure 1. Hair re-growth score in dorsal skin of C3H mice after depilation. Results are the mean ± SD of ten animals scored individually.

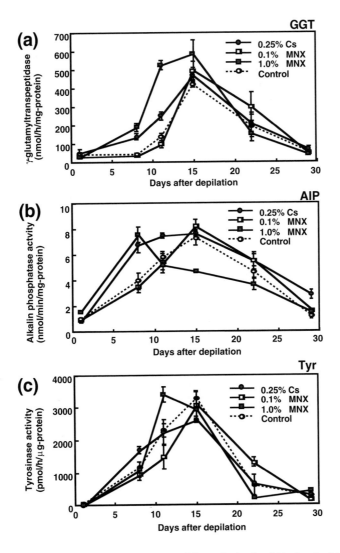

Figure 2. Effects of cyclosporin and minoxidil on the levels of biochemical indices in dorsal skin of C3H mice after depilation. Results are the mean ± SD of three samples each assayed individually.

(a) *γ-glutamyltranspeptidase (GGT)*

(b) *alkaline phosphatase (AlP)*

(c) *tyrosinase (Tyr).*

Enzyme activities are expressed as the following units; GGT: formation of p-nitroaniline per hour per mg-protein (nmol/h/mg-protein), AlP: formation of p-nitrophenol per mg-protein at pH 10.5 (nmol/mg-protein), Tyr: formation of L-3-(3,4-dihydroxy-phenol)-α alanine per mg (pmol/mg-protein).

the process of hair regrowth. Both the alkaline and acid phosphatase activities increased with hair regrowth, but the increasing rate of alkaline phosphatase activity was much higher than that of acid phosphatase activity. The change of tyrosinase activity was similar to those of γ-glutamyltranspeptidase, alkaline phosphatase activities, and well correlated with pigmentation of the clipped areas. The histamine content increased just after depilation treatment and returned to the normal level, compared with non-treated group.

As the results mentioned above the levels of γ-glutamyltranspeptidase, alkaline phosphatase and tyrosinase activities were monitored as hair cycle markers in order to evaluate the effects of cyclosporin and minoxidil on hair growth while hair regrowth is completed and hair cycle transformed into telogen phase (Fig. 2). The administration of 0.25% cyclosporin induced anagen phase much earlier than control group and prolonged its period. The administration of 1% minoxidil induced anagen phase earlier like cyclosporin, but 0.1% minoxidil did not. However, both the 0.1% and 1.0% minoxidil administration prolonged the anagen period.

In conclusion, the levels of γ-glutamyltranspeptidase, alkaline phosphatase and tyrosinase activities were parallel with the process of hair regrowth in C3H mouse model after depilation, but not others. Both the changes of alkaline phosphatase and tyrosinase activities in this period elevated a little earlier than that of γ-glutamyltranspeptidase activity. The administration of cyclosporin or minoxidil induced anagen phase earlier as compared with controls and prolonged this period.

All these results suggest that the markers examined in this C3H mouse model are useful for studying the distinctive hair regrowth, e.g. earlier induction of anagen phase and/or elongation of anagen period, and delay of catagen and telogen phase, by active substances.

References

1   Dry FW. J Genet. 1926; 16: 287-340
2   Silver AF, Chase HB, Aresenault CT. In: Advances in Biology of Skin. Hair growth. Montagna W (ed). 1969; 9: 265-286

Linear hair growth rate and diameter of hairs grown *in vitro*: a relevant correlation

C. Tételin and D. Van Neste

Skinterface, Skin Study Center, Tournai, Belgium

Introduction

It is known that linear hair growth rate (LHGR) and diameter are positively correlated: thick hairs, in situ [1, 2] or in scalp transplants onto nude mice [1], have been shown to grow faster than thin ones. The present trial was set up in order to look for such a correlation *in vitro*. Our data could help to validate this system model as a mimick of the *in vivo* situation.

Materials and methods

Isolation of human hair follicles

Human hair follicles were isolated according to previously published methods [3-5] by microdissection from human scalp skin taken from patients undergoing facelift surgery. The skin was firstly cut into strips not more than 5 mm wide. The epidermis and upper dermis were then separated from the underlying fat layer containing the hair follicle bulbs. The hair bulbs were isolated under a dissecting microscope, using fine watchmakers forceps, by gently gripping the outer root sheath of the follicles in the forceps and pulling the hair follicles out of the subcutaneous fat. This resulted in the isolation of intact, undamaged hair bulbs. Any adherent fat or collagen was removed using a fine scalpel blade.

Maintenance of hair follicles

Twenty-two isolated hair follicles were maintained free-floating in individual wells of 24-well plates containing 500 µl of culture medium described below. Follicles were incubated at 37°C in a humidified atmosphere of 5% CO_2/95% air, over 7 days.

Culture medium

Williams E medium was supplemented with L-glutamine (2 mM), penicillin (50 µg/ml), streptomycin (50 IU/ml), hydrocortisone (10 ng/ml) and bovine insulin (10 µg/ml). Williams E medium (minus L-glutamine), L-glutamine, penicillin and streptomycin were supplied by Gibco; other culture supplements were purchased from Sigma.

Assessment of hair follicle growth

Hair follicle growth was defined as the increase in length of the whole follicle with time in culture. Length and diameter of immersed hairs were measured using an inverted binocular microscope fitted with an eye-piece measuring graticule. The graticule measurements were converted to daily growth (linear hair growth rate, LHGR; mm/d) and diameter (μm).

With an accuracy in the order of 10 μm for the diameter measures, we chose to split the hair into thin (50 to 70 μm) and thick (70 to 90 μm) ones.

Statistical analysis

Linearity of continuous data (LHGR) distribution was checked. A two-way analysis of variance (ANOVA) was used to evaluate the variation of LHGR over time (day 2-3 (D2) vs day 6-7 (D7)) and co-variation according to the thickness of the hair. In order to minimize the noise vs signal ratio, differential LHGR of individual hair follicles were calculated as follows: $\delta LHGR = (LHGR$ at D2)-(LHGR at D7).

Variation of $\delta LHGR$ was studied with a one-way ANOVA against thickness of hair fibre. In case of significance ($p<0.05$), the profile of variation was analyzed with Scheffe-F test ($p<0.05$).

Results

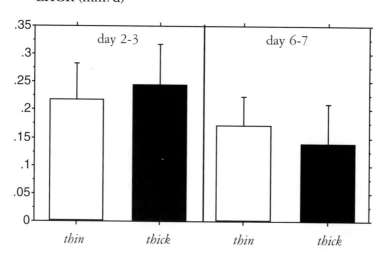

Figure 1. Variations of LHGR expressed as mm/day according to hair diameter (thin and thick: 50-70 μm and 70-90 μm respectively) and time spent in culture (2-3 days or 6-7 days)

From the data, it appeared that LHGR decreased with the time spent in culture: LHGR was higher at D2 (0.234 ± 0.069 mm/d) as compared with D7 (0.153 ± 0.065 mm/d).

A two-way ANOVA confirmed this observation and showed a significant decrease of LHGR over time (p = 0.0007). This evolution occurred for both thin (0.218 ± 0.065 mm/d at D2 vs 0.172 ± 0.051 mm/d at D7) and thick (0.245 ± 0.072 mm/d at D2 vs 0.139 ± 0.072 mm/d at D7) hair follicles.

Graphic display suggested that, at D2, LHGR of thick hair follicles was higher than LHGR of thin ones. Conversely, this trend was reversed at D7 when thin hair follicles seemed to grow faster than thick ones. Due to a high level of background, it was not possible to highlight a significant variation of LHGR against diameter of hair fibre (p = 0.8891), with the global ANOVA approach.

δLHGR reduced noise levels and thick hair follicles showed a more marked decrease of LHGR as compared with thin hair follicles (0.106 ± 0.027 mm/d and 0.045 ± 0.046 mm/d respectively; Scheffe-F test, p<0.05).

Discussion

Variation of LHGR over time

In vitro, the variation of LHGR over time presents two distinct stages. After a time of 4-5 days spent in culture, which coincides with an active period of hair fibre production, it appears that the trichocytes progressively de-differentiate. This involution leads to a progressive decline of LHGR.

Besides being in accordance with previously published data [3, 6, 7], our results specify that this profile of variation of LHGR occurs in both thin and thick hair follicles.

Correlation between LHGR and diameter

A positive correlation between LHGR and diameter seems to exist at early stages (D2) during *in vitro* culture of isolated human hair follicles, however our experimental data were not statistically significant. This may be due to:

- the small size of our study sample: 22 may be too small a number of hair follicles to highlight this correlation, compared to over 100 follicles from which this conclusion has been drawn [1];

- the lack of very thin vellus hairs: undamaged vellus hair follicles are indeed very difficult to extract with forceps, and our harvesting technique selects the roots of «deeply set» terminal type follicles.

At later stages (D7) of *in vitro* culture, the positive correlation between LHGR and diameter weakens and eventually tends to revert. Indeed, the productivity of thick hair follicles is significantly lower than that of thin hair follicles.

Analysis of paired δLHGR reveals that thick hair follicles have a more severe reduction in LHGR when compared to thin hair follicles. Several hypothesis could explain this differential fall in LHGR:

- the culture medium could be more rapidly exhausted for follicles having more demanding energetic needs;
- the proliferative compartment of follicles producing thick hair may be more sensitive to the surgery/isolation procedure and deteriorate more rapidly as compared to thin hair follicles.

Conclusion

This is the first time a study has been conducted on both LHGR and diameter of hairs grown *in vitro*. Our data highlight a relevant positive correlation between the above parameters at early stages of *in vitro* culture. As LHGR is the most common variable to test hair growth modulators *in vitro*, our data indicate that the hair diameter might be a significant factor of variation over time in the biologic response of isolated human scalp hair follicles maintained *in vitro*.

References

1   Van Neste D, de Brouwer B, Dumortier M. In: Stenn KS, Messenger AG, Baden HP, eds. Molecular and structural biology of hair. Annals New York Academy of Sciences. 1991; 642: 480-482
2   Hayashi S, Miyamoto I, Takeda K. Br J Dermatol. 1991; 125: 123-129
3   Philpott MP, Green MR, Kealey T. J Cell Science. 1990; 97: 463-471
4   Green MR, Clay CS, Gibson WT, Hughes TC, Smith CG, Westgate GE, White M, Kealey T. J Invest Dermatol. 1986; 87: 768-770
5   Westgate GE, Gibson WT, Kealey T, Philpott MP. Br J Dermatol 1993; 129: 372-379
6   Harmon CS, Nevins TD. Br J Dermatol. 1994; 130: 415-423
7   Jones LN, Fowler KJ, Marshall RC, Ackland ML. J Invest Dermatol. 1988; 90: 58-64

©1996 Elsevier Science B.V. All rights reserved.
Hair research for the next millenium
D.J.J. Van Neste and V.A. Randall (Eds)

The effects of removing the lower follicle bulb on human hair follicles maintained *in vitro*

M.P. Philpott, D.A. Sanders and T. Kealey

Department of Clinical Biochemistry, University of Cambridge, Addenbrooke's Hospital, Cambridge CB2 2QR, United Kingdom

Introduction

The mammalian hair follicle has a considerable capacity for regeneration [1-3]. Surgical removal of the entire follicle bulb *in vivo* results in the regeneration of a new bulb. The fibroblasts of the lower connective tissue sheath give rise to a new dermal papilla and the epidermal cells of the outer root sheath form a new population of germinative cells that give rise to a new hair fibre. The factors that control these regenerative processes are not known. We have previously reported on the isolation and *in vitro* growth of human hair follicles [4, 5] and have now used this model to study the effects of removing either the dermal papilla or the dermal papilla and hair follicle matrix on the *in vitro* patterns of growth of cultured human hair follicles.

Materials and methods

Isolation and maintenance of hair follicles

Human anagen hair follicles were isolated from scalp skin, taken from females undergoing facelift surgery, as previously described [4]. The DP was removed from hair follicles using watchmakers forceps and dissecting needles. DP and matrix cells were removed using a scalpel blade (No 15) to transect hair follicles at the apex of the DP. Isolated hair follicles were maintained in 500 µl of Williams E medium supplemented with 2 mM L-glutamine, 10 ng/ml hydrocortisone, 10 µg/ml insulin, 100 U/ml penicillin and 100 µg/ml streptomycin. Follicles were maintained at 37°C in an atmosphere of 5% CO_2 / 95% air. Hair follicle measurements were made using a Nikon Diaphot inverted microscope with eye piece measuring graticule.

Morphology and histology

The morphology of follicles in culture was examined using a Nikon Diaphot inverted microscope. Photographs were taken using Ilford FP4 film. Hair follicles were processed for histology by fixing overnight in 3.5% phosphate buffered formaldehyde and then mounted into 3% agar blocks, which facilitated the subsequent handling of the follicles during sectioning. Agar blocks, containing follicles, were then fixed overnight in 3.5% phosphate buffered formaldehyde and then embedded in wax. 5 µm sections were cut and stained using hematoxylin and eosin.

Autoradiography

Hair follicles were incubated for 6hr in Williams E medium supplemented with 5 µCi of (Methyl-^{3}H) thymidine (specific activity 3.3 µCi/nmole). Following incubation hair follicles were washed in PBS supplemented with cold thymidine and then fixed in phosphate buffered formaldehyde and processed for histology as described above. Autoradiography was carried out using Ilford K5 dipping emulsion.

Results

When the dermal papilla is removed, by micro dissection, from isolated human hair follicles, hair follicle elongation stopped. However, when the entire hair follicle bulbs containing the DP and matrix are removed hair follicles continued to elongate *in vitro*. However, this increase in hair follicle length was not due to hair fibre formation but appeared to be characterized by a marked expansion of undifferentiated cells from the ORS. Histology showed that following removal of the follicle bulb there was a marked expansion of undifferentiated ORS like cells from the site of amputation. Moreover, these cells, frequently formed a rounded bulb like structure and in some follicles aggregates of mesenchymal like cells, appeared at the base of these down growths. (^{3}H) thymidine autoradiography showed that following removal of the DP and matrix cells there appeared to be a marked increase in thymidine uptake in the basal cells of the ORS.

Conclusions

We have shown that, when the lower follicle bulb is removed from cultured human hair follicles, down growths of ORS cells from the site of amputation occur. These down growths are similar to those reported *in vivo* for both rat vibrissae [1, 2] and human hair follicles [3] following surgical removal of the follicle bulb and suggest that hair follicles *in vitro* also attempt follicular regeneration. Cultured hair follicles may therefore represent an excellent model for studying the early regenerative changes in hair follicles and for studying the role of cytokines in this process. However, the prospect of hair follicles fully regenerating *in vitro* may be limited by the fact that, at present, isolated follicles can only be maintained for up to 15 days *in vitro* before degenerating.

References

1   Oliver RF. J Embryol Exp Morphol. 1966; 16: 231-244
2   Jahoda CAB, Oliver RF, Forrester JC, Horne KA. J Invest Dermatol. 1989; 93: 452
3   Jahoda CAB, Horne KA, Mauger A, Bard S, Sengel P. Development. 1992; 114: 887-897
4   Philpott MP, Green MR, Kealey T. J Cell Sci. 1990; 97: 463-471
5   Westgate GE, Gibson WT, Kealey T, Philpott MP. Br J Dermatol. 1993; 129: 372-379

Reconstitution of hair follicles by rotation culture

A. Takeda, S. Matsuhashi, T. Nakamura, N. Shioya, E. Uchinuma and S. Ihara

Department of Plastic and Reconstructive Surgery, Kitasato University School of Medicine. Sagamihara, Japan

Introduction

The authors describe a method to test whether reconstruction of hair follicles is possible after complete dissociation of hair follicles into single cell suspensions followed by *in vitro* rotation culture.

Materials and methods

Skin samples and culture conditions

Dulbecco's modified Eagle medium (DMEM) and Ham's nutrient mixture F-12 (Ham's F12) were obtained in powdered form from Gibco/BRL Life Technologies, Inc. Each was supplemented with antibiotics, 20 mM HEPES and 10 mM sodium hydrogen carbonate. Fertile chicken eggs (Inoue Farm, Sagamihara, Japan) were incubated at 37°C and chick embryo extracts (diluted 1:1 in Tyrode's solution) were prepared from day-9 embryos. Nuclepore filters, 13 mm in diameter, 8.0 µm pore size (Nomura Micro Science Co., Ltd., Tokyo, Japan) were coated with collagen (Koken Co., Ltd., Tokyo, Japan) followed by air-drying and ultraviolet irradiation for 30 min.

Upper-lip fragments were taken from freshly excised Sprague-Dawley rat embryos. The day on which sperm appeared in the vagina was designated as fetal day 0. A total of 186 embryos from 15 pregnant rats was used for this study.

Dissociation of cells

Embryos were removed from the uterus of each mother rat killed by ether anaesthesia and the skin was dissected from the upper lip. Isolated fragments of skin were rinsed with DMEM and treated with 0.25% trypsin (DIFCO) in calcium and magnesium free Hanks' (CMF-Hanks'), pH 7.4, at 37°C for 30 min. Single cells were liberated by manually flushing the fragments with 10-30 gentle swirls with a pipette in the culture medium consisting of a 1:1 mixture of DMEM and Ham's F-12 (87%), fetal bovine serum (FBS) (10%) and chick-embryo extract (3%).

Culture procedure

Rotation: Each cell suspension was filtered through a sterile nylon mesh of 150 and 49 μm porosity followed by inoculation in 3 ml aliquots into plastic dishes (35 mm diameter x 12 mm high, Terumo Co., Tokyo, Japan) at a density of 1.5×10^6 cells per dish. This rotation [1] was based on the method of Moscona [2, 3]. The culture dishes were placed on a rotary shaker (Environmental Incubator Shaker, New Brunswick Scientific Co., Inc.), the rotation radius previously adjusted to 1 cm, and incubated for 20 hours at 37°C and 60 rpm.

Flotation: Cell aggregates obtained by rotation were placed on the collagen-coated Nuclepore membranes and cultured with flotation for 7 days on DMEM+Ham's F12 (1:1) supplemented with 10% FBS.

Grafting procedure

Silicone chambers were implanted in the backs of Sprague-Dawley rats with full thickness skin defect. The aggregates obtained by rotation culture or rotation and flotation culture were grafted on the panniculus carnosus beneath the chamber.

Histological study

On the 10th day after grafting, the tissue to be examined was excised along with surrounding connective tissue, fixed in 10% formalin and stained with hematoxylin-eosin for light microscopy.

Results

The reconstitution of hair follicles was confirmed by observation of hematoxylin-eosin specimens. Each specimen contained ordered structures, apparently consisting of a hair shaft, outer root sheath, inner root sheath, dermal papilla and dermal sheath. The structures were thus morphologically quite similar to hair follicles which develop normally in embryos. (Figs. 1 and 2).

Discussion

Tissue interactions in relation to hair follicle development in embryonic and adult skin have been extensively clarified. The dermal papilla and dermal sheath derive from aggregates of mesenchymal cells that form directly beneath epithelial hair germ at the start of follicular development. Appropriate sorting out of epithelial and mesenchymal cells, the rudiments of hair follicles, should thus occur prior to the interactions of these two cell types, that are requisite for histodifferentiation. Any experimental system for reconstruction of hair follicles should be such as to allow the progress of rudiment (re)formation and histodifferentiation even when starting with a single cell suspension.

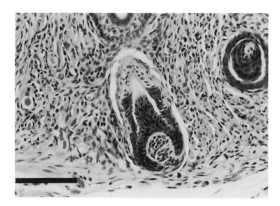

Figure 1. Reconstruction of hair follicles at 10 days after grafting of cell aggregates produced by rotation and flotation culture (H&E stains). Scale bar=100 μm

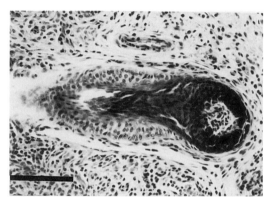

Figure 2. Reconstruction of hair follicles at 10 days after grafting of cell aggregates produced by rotation culture only (H&E stains). Scale bar=100 μm

We previously reconstructed hair follicles by *in vitro* procedures alone [1] with flotation culture to facilitate the histodifferentiation. This study was conducted to determine the possibility of grafting to adult skin as a means for greater differentiation of hair follicles. In one series of experiments, aggregates obtained by rotation only were used for grafting. In a second series, they were obtained by rotation and flotation culture and used for grafting. Well-differentiated hair follicles were reconstituted by either method. Tissue differentiation would thus appear to proceed as well during *in vivo* after grafting as during *in vitro* flotation.

References

1   Ihara S, Watanabe M, Nagao E, Shioya N. Cell and Tissue Research. 1991; 266: 65-73
2   Moscona A. Experimental Cell Research. 1961; 22: 455-475
3   Moscona M, Moscona A. Developmental Biology. 1965; 11: 402-423

Colour plate XIII

Alopecia areata

©1996 Elsevier Science B.V. All rights reserved.
Hair research for the next millenium
D.J.J. Van Neste and V.A. Randall (Eds)

Innervation and vasculature of the normal human and alopecia areata (AA) hair follicle: an immunohistochemical and laser scanning confocal microscopic study

M. Hordinsky, S. Lorimer, M. Ericson and S. Worel

Clinical Research Division, Department of Dermatology, University of Minnesota Health System, 420 Delaware Street SE, Minneapolis, Minnesota 55455-0392, USA

Introduction

The peripheral nervous system is now recognized to be an organized network which can deliver neuropeptides that modulate immunologic responses [1, 2]. Patients with AA experience itching, tingling or pain with their disease [3]. These sensations could be related to alterations in neuropeptide expression in cutaneous nerves or vessels. Although the occurrence and distribution of neuropeptides in human skin has been studied, very little information is available on their expression in the normal human scalp or that affected by AA [4, 5].

Materials and methods

Four mm scalp punch biopsies were obtained from three patients, 2 males and 1 female ages 45, 55, and 73, all of whom had extensive, untreated AA of the scalp (>75%). Control scalp biopsy samples were obtained from 2 males and 1 female, ages 24, 44, and 43 respectively. Each biopsy was placed in Zamboni's paraformaldehyde/picric acid fixative for 16 to 24 hours then transferred to a 20% sucrose phosphate-buffered saline solution (PBS) and refrigerated. Tissue samples were then mounted in O.C.T. (Miles, Elkhart, IN), frozen, and 70 to 110 µm sections were obtained with a freezing sliding microtome. Sections were treated with 5% normal goat serum (NGS) overnight (Quad Five, Ryegate, MT) in 0.1M PBS with 0.3% Triton X-100 to block nonspecific binding sites. The sections were incubated with primary antibody for a six hour period at 24°C, washed with PBS-0.3% Triton X and 1% NGS, and incubated with the secondary antibody for an additional six hours. Subsequently, all sections were incubated with *Ulex europaeus* agglutinin (UEA I) for 1 hour at 24°C (Table 1). Samples were dehydrated, cleared with methyl salicylate, and mounted in DPX mounting medium (Fluka, Ronkonkoma, NY). Sections were screened with an epifluorescent microscope and examined with a MRC-600 or MRC-1000 Confocal Imaging System (BioRad, Boston, MA). Images were collected in sequential 2 or 3 μm serial optical sections and integrated into single in-focus images. Montages of these images were created using the image processing Photoshop.

Table 1 Summary table of probes

Primary Antibodies	Secondary Antibodies
Protein Gene Related Peptide (PGP 9.5)[1] Ultraclone, Wellow, UK, 1:1000 (monoclonal antibody)	GAM Cyanine (Cy 3.18) Jackson ImmunoResearch West Grove, PA, 1:400
Substance P (SP)[2] Incstar, Stillwater, MN, 1:1000 (rabbit polyclonal)	GAR Cy 5.18 Jackson ImmunoResearch West Grove, PA, 1:400
Calcitonin Gene-Related Peptide (CGRP)[2] Amersham, Arlington Heights, IL, 1:1000 (rabbit polyclonal)	GAR Cy 5.18 Jackson ImmunoResearch West Grove, PA, 1:400

Lectin
Ulex europaeus agglutinin (UEA 1)[3] labeled with fluorescein isothiocyanate (1:200) Vector, Burlingame, CA, 1:200

[1]*PGP 9.5 is a cytoplasmic protein with characteristics of a general neuronal marker capable of identifying most cholinergic, adrenergic, and peptidergic neurons {6}.*
[2]*CGRP and SP are considered to be major neuropeptides involved in inflammation {4}.*
[3]*UEA 1 is a lectin that binds to α-L fucose which is present in the stratum granulosum and spinosum, infrainfundibular follicular keratinocytes and endothelial cells {7}.*

Results

In the AA patients as compared to the normal controls, CGRP expression was decreased in scalp epidermal nerves and in the subepidermal plexus. Both controls and patients expressed very little SP in their scalp skin. However, one patient showed prominent SP expression in the nerves surrounding her hair follicles. Both patients and controls expressed PGP 9.5 in epidermal nerves, the subepidermal plexus, arrector pili muscle, sweat glands, and blood vessels and on some infrainfundibular cells. In addition, a population of cells above the dermal papilla and in the hair follicle was highlighted with this antibody (Fig. 1A). PGP 9.5 was not expressed on the vascular plexus on the lower third of the hair follicle in both patients and controls. (Figs. 1A and 2A). In contrast to the controls, the

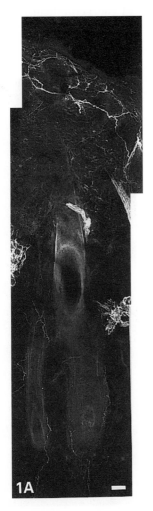 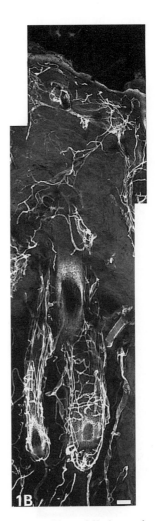

Figure 1. Montage of normal innervation and vasculature of hair follicles in the scalp of a 43- year-old white female (105μm). The montage is a projection of 35 optical sections taken at 3 μm intervals.
A. PGP 9.5. The subepidermal nerve plexus, arrector pili muscle, sweat glands, perifollicular nerves, and some hair follicle cells are immunoreactive with this antibody.
B. UEA 1. The stratum granulosum subepidermal vascular plexus, some hair follicle cells, and a prominent perifollicular vascular network stain with this lectin.
Scale bar = 100μm

200

longitudinal follicular nerves were not well demonstrated in the AA patients.

In the normal controls, UEA I prominently stained the subpapillary plexus, the perifollicular network and the stratum granulosum and spinosum. In contrast, patients demonstrated reduced staining of infrainfundibular keratinocytes, the subpapillary vascular plexus and the perifollicular vascular network, particularly around the hairbulb (Figs. 1B and 2B).

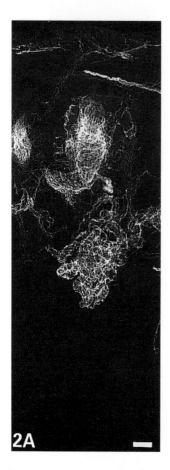 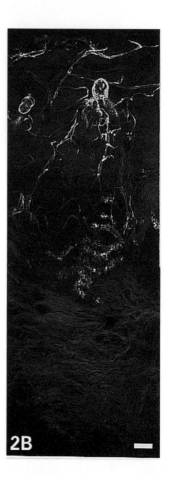

Figure 2. A montage of scalp AA follicles from a 73-year-old white female (100 μm). The montage is a projection of 33 optical sections taken at 3 μm intervals.
A. PGP 9.5. In contrast to the normal controls, the longitudinal follicular nerves are not well visualized and the nerves are clustered around the small follicles.
B. UEA 1. The subpapillary vascular plexus and perifollicular network are also not as prominent as in the normal controls. Scale bar = 100 μm.

Conclusions

Our study suggests that CGRP expression is reduced in scalp epidermal nerves and the subepidermal plexi of AA patients. To prove this observation, quantitative studies of neuropeptide expression would have to be done. The significance of the increased expression of SP in one patient is not known at this time. There is heterogeneity in neuropeptide expression in AA scalp skin but until additional patients and controls are studied, it is not clear whether this is related to the pathophysiology of AA or reflects normal variation. It also remains to be shown how these differences in neuropeptide expression relate to the scalp symptoms AA patients frequently experience. Both the normal and AA hair follicles express an epitope on infrainfundibular cells which reacts with PGP 9.5, a pan-neuronal marker. This observation may provide a link between the hair follicle and the nervous system.

Other noteworthy observations include reduced staining of the perifollicular vasculature and the subpapillary vascular plexus in the AA patients. The absence of PGP 9.5 expression on virtually all of the blood vessels in the lower portion of the hair follicle in both patients and controls was an unexpected finding and may be related to the involution this part of the hair follicle normally undergoes during hair differentiation.

References

1   Hosoi J, Murphy GF, Egan CL, Lerner EA, Grabbe S, Asahina A, Granstein RD. Regulation of Langerhans cell function by nerves containing calcitonin gene-related peptide. Nature. 1993; 363: 159-163

2   Ansel JC, Kaynard AH, Armstrong CA, Olerud J, Bunnett N, Payan D. Skin-nervous system interactions. Prog Dermatol. 1995; 29: 1-12

3   Ishizaki F, Sasaki K, Shimoda Y, Shimao S. EEG findings, rapid ACTH test and autonomic nervous symptoms in patients with alopecia areata. J Neural Transm. 1976; 39: 71-75

4   Eedy DJ. Neuropeptides in skin. Br J Dermatol. 1993; 128: 597-605

5   Hashimoto K, Ito M, Suzuki Y. Innervation and vasculature of the hair follicle. In : Orfanos CE, Happle R (eds) : Hair and Hair Diseases, Springer-Verlag, Berlin. 1990; 117-147

6   Karanth SS, Springgall DR, Kuhn DM, Levene MM, Polak JM. An immunocytochemical study of cutaneous innervation and the distribution of neuropeptides and protein gene product 9.5 in man and commonly employed laboratory animals. Am J Anatomy. 1991; 191: 369-383

7   Holthöfer H, Virtanen I, Kariniemi AL, Hormia M, Linder E, Miettinen A. Ulex europaeus 1 lectin as a marker for vascular endothelium in human tissue. Lab Invest. 1982; 47: 60-66

Hair research for the next millenium
D.J.J. Van Neste and V.A. Randall (Eds)

Ultrastructural and immunohistological changes of the follicular keratinocytes in alopecia areata: comparison from active lesion, stable lesion and non-lesional scalp

W.S. Lee

Department of Dermatology, Yonsei University Wonju Medical College, 162 Ilsan-Dong, Wonju, Kangwon-Do, 220-701, Korea

Introduction

The primary target injured during the immunologic mechanism of alopecia areata is not definitely established. Recently, particular interest has been focused on the follicular keratinocytes which show morphological and antigenic alterations in active lesions [1-7]. Another important point is the «subclinical state» concept. This is based upon the observation that the patterns of the T lymphocyte infiltration and the ultrastructural changes of dermal papilla cells are nearly identical in active lesions and in non-lesional areas of alopecia areata [8]. The aim of this study is to determine and to compare the ultrastructural and immunohistological changes of the follicular keratinocytes from active lesion, stable lesion and non-lesional scalp of alopecia areata.

Materials and methods

Scalp biopsies were taken from both lesional and non-lesional scalps (occipital) of six alopecia areata patients, four in an active stage and two in a stable stage of the disease, together with two normal controls. The active stage was defined by bald patches that were increasing in size at the time the biopsy was taken and from where numerous tapering hair shafts were removed by gentle pulling i.e. the hair pull technique. Stable stage was identified by patches that did not change dimension for at least 4 weeks before biopsy and showing no hairs with the hair pull technique. All subjects were without treatment for at least 4 weeks before the biopsy and only patients presenting alopecia areata for the first time were included. One half of each biopsy was immediately fixed and processed for routine transmission electron microscopy, while the cryostat sections of the other half were stained immunohistologically with HLA-DR, CD1 and ICAM-1 mouse monoclonal antibodies (DAKO) using a streptavidin system.

Results

The morphological changes seen in follicles from active lesions when compared to normal controls were also present in follicles from stable lesions and non-lesional areas. The follicular keratinocytes showed extensive degenerative changes. In addition, there were a few grouped or singly scattered apoptotic keratinocytes and dark cell transformations (Figs. 1 and 4). However, there were immunohistochemical differences between scalps with active lesions and those with stable lesions or normal controls. Active lesions and non-lesional areas from the same individuals were immunohistologically similar with CD1 antigen always expressed by lower bulb keratinocytes. HLA-DR and ICAM-1 antigen were also found in some lesions. None of these molecules were detected in stable lesions and their matched non-lesional areas nor in the normal controls (Tables 1 and 2).

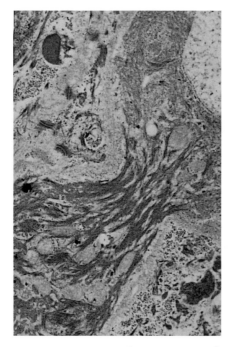

Figure 1. Apoptotic keratinocytes with tonofilament clumping. Active lesion, Case 1

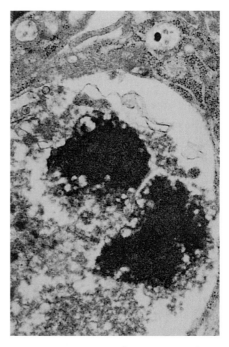

Figure 2. Apoptotic keratinocytes shows nuclear segregation and fragmentation. Non-lesional scalp from patient with active lesions (see fig. 1), Case 1

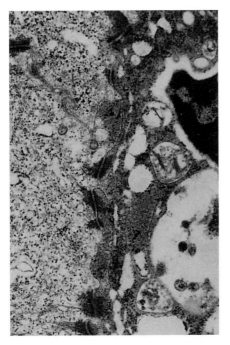

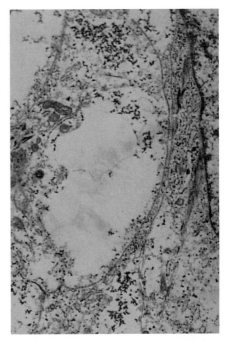

Figure 3. Dark cell shows cellular condensation and vacuolation. Active lesion, Case 2

Figure 4. Necrotic keratinocytes show severe cytoplasmic oedema. Non-lesional scalp, Case 6

Table 1.

The expression of antigens by follicular keratinocytes: comparison between lesional and non-lesional scalp of patients with alopecia areata

Antibodies	Lesion	Non-lesional scalp	Control
HLA-DR	1/6 (3/22)	1/6 (3/18)	0/2 (0/8)
CD1	4/6 (13/22)	4/6 (8/18)	0/2 (0/8)
ICAM-1	2/6 (7/22)	2/6 (4/18)	0/2 (0/8)

n/n (n/n) number of subjects positive/examined (number of follicles positive/examined)

Table 2.

Expression of antigens by follicular keratinocytes: comparison between active and stable scalp lesion of alopecia areata vs controls

| Antibodies | Active | | Stable | | Control |
	Lesion	Non-lesional	Lesion	Non-lesional	
HLA-DR	1/4 (3/16)	1/4 (3/12)	0/2 (0/6)	0/2 (0/6)	0/2 (0/8)
CD1	4/4 (13/16)	4/4 (8/12)	0/2 (0/6)	0/2 (0/6)	0/2 (0/8)
ICAM-1	2/4 (7/16)	2/4 (4/12)	0/2 (0/6)	0/2 (0/6)	0/2 (0/8)

n/n (n/n): number of positive subjects/examined (number of positive follicles/examined)

Discussion

Follicular keratinocytes in alopecia areata show morphological and antigenic alterations. Ectopic HLA-DR expression might be expected to enable them to function as antigen presenting cells and to activate MHC restricted T lymphocytes [1]. But, it is unclear whether this is a primary event [2] or a nonspecific result of the local diffusion of γ-interferon from the lymphoid infiltrate around hair follicle [3, 4]. Ectopic T6 antigen expression could signify an «activation state» of the bulbar keratinocytes, because this antigen was only found in an active stage [1]. Activated keratinocytes are able to release IL-1, the second signal for T cell activation, which could enhance and perpetuate the putative autoimmune response that might be operating in alopecia areata. Positive ICAM-1 expression by follicular epithelial cells in alopecia areata would permit the entry of monocyte/macrophages and T cells directly into the epithelial compartment of the hair follicle [5]. Electron microscopy revealed degenerative changes of upper bulb pre-cortical keratinocytes in regrowing white hairs [6]. It also found that keratinocytic degeneration may affect layers of matrix cells in alopecia areata, unlike the apoptosis of scattered outer root sheath cells in normal catagen [7].

Another important observation is the «subclinical state» of alopecia areata. It is based upon the observation that the «active» and «normal» areas of alopecia areata scalps are similar immunohistologically (number, distribution and ratio for T4 and T8 positive cells) and ultrastructurally (pleomorphic nature of the dermal papilla cells, critical changes in the dermoepithelial junction of the hair follicle bulb) [8].

In our study, we tried to determine and to compare the changes of the follicular keratinocytes according to disease activity. Our results indicate an active involvement of the follicular keratinocytes in alopecia areata and reconfirm the concept of a subclinical condition of the disease since changes were detected in non-lesional areas. These results also suggest that the morphological changes themselves do not mean disease activity, but the aberrant antigenic alterations, especially CD1 expression of the follicular keratinocytes are closely associated with active progress of alopecia areata lesions.

References

1   Lotti T, Knoepfel B. Int J Dermatol. 1992; 106: 103-106
2   Messenger AG, Bleehen SS. J Invest Dermatol. 1985; 85: 569-572
3   Broecker EB, Echternacht-Happle R, Hamm H, *et al.* J Invest Dermatol. 1987; 88: 564-568
4   Khoury EL, Price VH, Greenspan JS. J Invest Dermatol. 1988; 90: 193-200
5   Nickoloff BJ, Griffiths CEM. J Invest Dermatol. 1991; 96: 91S-92S
6   Messenger G, Bleehen SS. Br J Dermatol. 1984; 110: 155-162
7   Tobin DJ, Fenton DA, Kendall MD. Am J Dermatopathol. 1991; 13: 248-256
8   Macdonald Hull S, Nutbrown M, Pepall L, *et al.* J Invest Dermatol. 1991; 96: 673-681

Increased apoptosis in the perilesional hair follicles of active alopecia areata may not be mediated by Fas antigen

G.Y. Ahn, C.K. Hong, K.Y. Song[1] and B.I. Ro

Department of Dermatology and [1]Pathology, College of Medicine, Chung Ang University, Seoul, Korea
65-207, Hangang-ro, 3-ka, Yongsan-ku, Seoul, 140-757, Korea

Introduction

Apoptosis occurs in many cells and organs such as hematopoietic cells, epidermal cells and cycling hairs [1]. In the normal hair cycle, apoptosis is observed in the dermal papillae and outer root sheath cells of catagen hair. There is premature entry into catagen with CD4$^+$ T lymphocytic infiltration in the alopecia areata. Among the molecules involved in apoptotic signals, Fas antigen is the major target molecule of CD4$^+$ T lymphocyte [2] and it has been studied in the field of skin biology. In alopecia areata, CD4$^+$ T lymphocytic infiltration is predominant around the hair follicle [3]. Therefore we hypothesized that apoptosis is abnormally increased in the perilesional hair follicles of active alopecia areata and Fas antigen might be involved in the premature entry into catagen initiated by CD4$^+$ T lymphocyte attack and that the ensuing apoptotic process results in the development of alopecia areata.

Materials and methods

Scalp biopsies

Hair follicles were obtained from excisional biopsies of lesional and perilesional scalp of patients with actively progressing alopecia areata. Normal scalp of patients with hair transplantation served as a control. Specimens were preserved immediately at -70°C.

Isolation of hair bulb

Bulb portion includes the dermal papilla, matrix cells, outer root sheath cells and inner root sheath cells. They were carefully trimmed under the stereomicroscope on the ice-ridden Petri dish to minimize enzyme activation.

DNA elution

Genomic DNAs were eluted and isolated by using the proteinase K and Qia amp tissue kit (Qiagen, U.S.A.).

DNA electrophoresis

Extracted DNAs were run on the 2% agarose gel with 40 voltage current power for 6 hours.

In situ detection of apoptotic bodies

In situ detection of apoptotic bodies was performed in both alopecic and normal scalp using the ApoTag *in situ* apoptosis detection kit (Oncor, U.S.A.).

Immunohistochemical stain of Fas antigen

We stained the specimens with monoclonal human anti-Fas antigen antibody.

Results

DNA electrophoresis

The results of DNA electrophoresis are shown in Fig. 1.

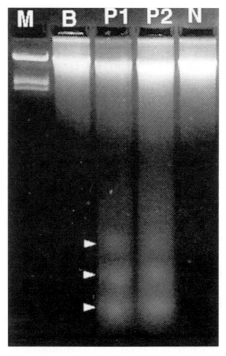

Figure 1. Characteristic ladder appearance in the lanes of perilesional scalp of active alopecia areata, but not in the lanes of bald area of alopecia or normal scalp. (M: marker, B: bald scalp,
P: perilesional scalp, N: normal scalp, DNA electrophoresis on 2% agarose gel)

In situ detection of apoptotic bodies

The results of *in situ* detection of apoptotic bodies are shown in Fig. 2.

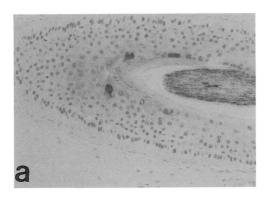

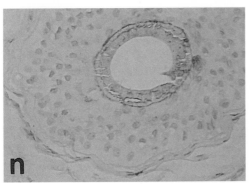

*Figure 2. Markedly increased apoptosis in the perilesional hair follicles of active alopecia areata (**a**: scalp of alopecia areata, **n**: normal scalp, TdT immunostain, x200)*

Immunohistochemical stain of Fas antigen

The results of our study are summarized in Table 1.

Table 1
Immunoreactivities of Fas antigen in alopecia and normal scalp

	Alopecia		Normal control
	Anagen	Telogen	Anagen
Inner root sheath cell	+ +	-	+ +
Outer root sheath cell	+	-	+ +
Dermal papillar cell	±	-	±

Discussion

These results suggest that increased apoptosis occurs in the perilesional hair follicles of active alopecia areata and it may be a major pathway of premature catagen entry during the development of alopecia areata. We think that Fas antigen may not be a major mediator of apoptotic signal in the development of alopecia areata.

References

1   Haake AR, Polakowska RR. J Invest Dermatol. 1993; 101: 107-112
2   Stalder T, Hahn S, Erb P. J Immunol. 1994; 152: 1127-1133
3   Taylor NT, Turner R, Wood GS, Stratte PT, et al. J Am Acad Dermatol. 1984; 11: 216-223

Hair research for the next millenium
D.J.J. Van Neste and V.A. Randall (Eds)

Evaluation of PCNA, cyclin B and bcl-2 protein in normal anagen hair follicles and hair follicles of alopecia areata

K. Ito, A. Nakamura and M. Ito

Department of Dermatology, Niigata University School of Medicine, 1 Asahimachidori, Niigata 951, Japan

Introduction

Proliferative and cyclic activities of hair follicle have not been fully understood. Analysis of cell proliferation has been performed by tritiated-thymidine uptake [1], BrdU uptake [2], Ki-67 (MIB 1) monoclonal antibody [3, 4], anti-DNA polymerase α antibody [5] and antibody to proliferating cell nuclear antigen (PCNA) [6]. In addition, recent studies have determined cyclins which regulate cell cycle. Among them, cyclin B, one of M cyclins, has been found mainly during G_2 and M phases of the cell cycle [7]. On the other hand, PCNA is present through G_1, S and G_2 phases.

Apoptosis is also associated with cell proliferation and is suppressed by bcl-2 protein. It is the product of *bcl-2* gene [8] and is expressed in basal cells of epidermis and dermal papilla cells and isthmus of hair follicles in human fetal skin [9, 10].

In the present study, expression of PCNA, cyclin B and bcl-2 protein was evaluated in order to investigate the proliferative and cyclic activity of hair follicles in the scalp skin of normal subjects and alopecia areata patients.

Materials and methods

Normal scalp skin materials were obtained from 8 normal subjects and 15 cases of alopecia areata including 9 cases with single or multiple lesions and 6 cases of alopecia totalis. Biopsy specimens were fixed and embedded in paraffin. Monoclonal antibodies to PCNA (PC10, DAKO, Glostrup, Denmark), cyclin B (GNSI, Santa Cruz Biotechnology, Santa Cruz, CA, U.S.A) and bcl-2 protein (124, DAKO, Glostrup, Denmark) were applied on paraffin sections after microwave antigen retrieval treatment with 10 mM citrate buffer, pH 6.0 [11]. Immunohistochemical procedure was performed using Streptavidin-biotin-peroxidase method. As a chromogen, 3, 3'-diaminobenzidine was used.

214

Results

In normal anagen hair follicles, PCNA and cyclin B were positive in several outer layers of outer root sheath cells and bulbar region. There were more PCNA positive cells than cyclin B positive cells (Figs. 1a, 1b, 1e and 1f). These reactions were reduced in the follicles of alopecia areata patients (Figs. 1c, 1d, 2a and 2b).

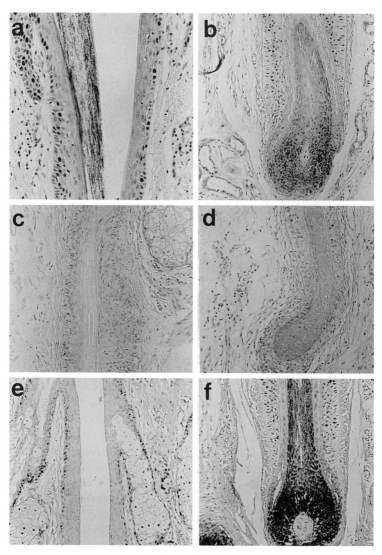

*Figure 1. PCNA expression in normal scalp hair follicles (**a**, **b**) and in alopecia areata (**c**, **d**) and cyclin B in normal scalp hair follicles (**e**, **f**)*

Bcl-2 protein was strongly expressed in outermost cell layer of outer root sheath at infundibular and bulge levels in normal anagen hair (Figs. 2c and 2d). This expression was diminished in alopecia areata (Fig. 2f). Dermal papilla cells in normal scalp were also positive for bcl-2 protein (Fig. 2e). In alopecia areata, dermal papilla cells were negative for bcl-2 protein (Fig. 2g).

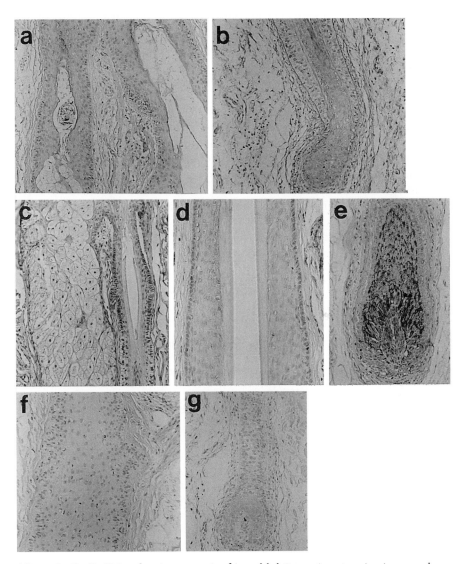

*Figure 2. Cyclin B in alopecia areata (**a**, **b**) and bcl-2 protein expression in normal scalp hair (**c**, **d**, **e**) and in alopecia areata (**f**, **g**)*

Discussion

Cyclin B is expressed at G_2 to M transition which is more restricted than the expression stages of PCNA. PCNA is expressed through G_1, S and G_2. Therefore cyclin B seems to be closely associated with mitosis [7]. From the present results, cyclin B is a better marker to detect proliferating cells in tissue sections than PCNA. Reduced expression of PCNA and cyclin B in the outer root sheath and bulbar areas in alopecia areata demonstrated that the proliferative activity of hair follicles is diminished in this disorder.

Bcl-2 protein is regarded to suppress apoptosis and has been found in the basal cells of epidermis and dermal papilla cells and isthmus of hair follicles of human fetal skin indicating that it is expressed in the potentially proliferative areas of the tissues [9, 10]. The expression of bcl-2 protein in outermost cell layer of outer root sheath at infundibular and bulge levels in normal adult specimens also suggested that these areas are associated with the proliferation of hair follicles. Recent studies hypothesize that the hair follicle stem cell is located at the bulge area [12]. Therefore, the presence of bcl-2 protein might be associated with the stem cells. Reduced expression in upper hair follicle might be related to the pathogenesis of alopecia areata. In addition, loss of bcl-2 protein expression in dermal papilla cells in alopecia areata suggests that dermal papilla cells are also involved in its pathogenesis.

Further studies on the proliferation and apoptotic process in the hair follicles in normal and alopecia areata patients are required from *in vitro* and molecular biological aspects.

References

1 Weinstein GD, Mason Mooney K. J Invest Dermatol. 1980; 74: 43-46
2 Gratzner HG. Science. 1982; 218: 474-475
3 Schlüter C, Duchrow M, Wohlenberg C, Becker MHG, *et al.* J Cell Biol. 1993; 123: 513-522
4 Tezuka M, Ito M, Ito K, Sato Y. J Dermatol Sci. 1990; 1: 335-346
5 Tanaka S, Hu S-Z, Wang, TS-F, Korn D. J Biol Chem. 1982; 257: 8386-8390
6 Hall PA, Levison DA, Woods AL, Yu C-W, *et al.* J Pathol. 1990; 162: 285-294
7 Galaktionov K, Beach D. Cell. 1991; 67: 1181-1194
8 Hockenbury DM, Zutter M, Hickey W, Nahm M, *et al.* Proc Natl Acad Sci USA. 1991; 88: 6961-6965
9 LeBrun DP, Warnke RA, Cleary ML. Am J Pathol. 1993; 142: 743-753
10 Lu QL, Poulsom R, Wong L, Hanby AM. J Pathol. 1993; 169: 431-437
11 Cattoretti G, Becker MHG, Key G, Duchrow M, *et al.* J Pathol. 1992; 168: 357-363
12 Lavker RM, Sun TT. J Invest Dermatol. 1995; 104s: 38s-39s

Hair research for the next millenium
D.J.J. Van Neste and V.A. Randall (Eds)

The clinical phase of alopecia areata is related to lymphocyte subsets

G. Orecchia, P.G. Malagoli and F. Borghini

Department of Dermatology, University of Pavia, Italy

Introduction

Alopecia areata (AA) is a common and sometimes disabling chronic inflammatory disorder of the hair and nails. Genetic factors, which we are beginning to identify, are undoubtedly important in determining susceptibility and disease severity but it seems unlikely that AA depends on a single gene defect. In common with other inflammatory diseases, environmental factors are probably important in initiating disease expression [1].

Investigations of cell-mediated immunity in AA have concentrated on findings in the peripheral blood. These, however, have failed to reveal a consistent pattern of abnormality and demographic differences between the groups studied are likely to be involved in the disparity.

The aim of this study was to examine lymphocyte subsets, in an attempt to correlate cellular immunity to the clinical phases of the disease.

Materials and methods

Fifty two patients affected by AA (21 in progressive stage, 16 in stationary and 15 in regressive), 29 females and 23 males aged 8 to 71 years (median 27) entered the investigation.

Twenty six patients suffered from patchy AA, 20 patients from alopecia totalis and 6 from alopecia universalis; 46 healthy age and sex matched individuals were used as controls.

They were studied for the determination of lymphocyte subsets in peripheral blood; the labelled cells were analyzed using a fluorescence-activated cell sorter (FACStar-1: Becton Dickinson Immunocytometry Systems).

Thus the distribution of T-cell subsets were related to the different stages of AA.

Results

Patients in the active phase showed a significant increase of CD3 HLA-DR +

(activated T lymphocytes) (p < 0.005), CD16 + CD56 (natural killers) (p < 0.01) and CD11aLFA1 (lymphocyte functional antigen) (p < 0.05); patients in the stationary phase evidenced a significant increase of CD11aLFA1. In the regressive stage we did not observed any significant difference from the healthy control subjects (Table 1).

Table 1.
Lymphocyte subsets and AA in different phases

Lymphocyte subsets	Active phase	Stationary phase	Regressive phase	Controls
CD3 HLA-DR +	662.4	234.3	216.5	283.3
CD16 + CD56	421.3	89.2	28.1	109
CD11aLFA1	2197.1	1823.1	1784.3	1206.3

Discussion

The populations of CD3 HLA-DR + cells, CD16 + CD56 cells and CD11aLFA1 cells are increased in the peripheral blood of patients affected by AA.

The increase of CD3 HLA-DR + and CD16 + CD56 cells suggests, according to other studies [2], that T cells and NK cells are activated and may play a role in the disease, through an increased release of γ-interferon by CD3 HLA-DR + cells that leads to a stimulation of the NK cells [3].

As regards the increase of CD11aLFA1, the detection of LFA1 molecules on lymphocytes in the peripheral blood may reflect their activation state. In fact, LFA1 expression is known to represent the mode of interaction between lymphocytes and follicular keratinocytes abnormally expressing, in the area of AA, the intercellular adhesion molecule-1 (ICAM-1) [4-9].

Even if not disease specific, high levels of CD3 HLA-DR + , CD16 + CD56 and CD11aLFA1 cells are related to a worsening of AA.

However we are aware that the relevance of cellular immune abnormality in the peripheral blood may be questionable since many cells participating in the specific inflammatory process of AA may be sequestrated in the perifollicular tissues.

In conclusion, our study seems to confirm a role for some lymphocyte populations in the mechanisms of the disease in relation to the different clinical stages, but further investigations are needed to better define the importance of the observed phenomena.

References

1 McDonagh AJG, Messenger AG. The aetiology and pathogenesis of alopecia areata. J Dermatol Sci. 1994; 7: 125-35

2 Imai R, Miura J, Numata K, Aikawa Y *et al*. Analysis of T cell, activated T cell and NK cell subsets in peripheral blood lymphocytes from patients with alopecia areata. In: Van Neste D, Lachapelle JM, Antoine JL, eds. Trends in Human Hair Growth and Alopecia Research. Dordrecht: Kluwer Academic Publishers. 1989; 299-304

3 Sayers TJ, Mason AT, Ortaldo JR: Regulation of human natural killer cell activity by interferon-γ: lack of a role in interleukin 2-mediated augmentation. Journal of immunology. 1986; 136: 2176-2180

4 Lucarini G, Offidani AM, Cellini A, Castaldini C *et al*. Abnormal immuno-morphological features of hair follicles in alopecia areata. A quantitative investigation. Investigative report Eur J Dermatol. 1994; 4: 232-237

5 Backer JNWN, Allen MH, MacDonald DM. The effect of in vivo interferon-gamma on the distribution of LFA-1 and ICAM-1 in normal human skin. J Invest Dermatol. 1989; 93: 439-442

6 Dustin ML, Springer TA. Role of lymphocyte adhesion receptors in transient interactions and cell locomotion. Ann Rev Immunol. 1991; 9: 27-66

7 Cagnoni ML, Ghersetich I, Campanile G, Lotti T. Caratterizzazione immunofenotipica dell'infiltrato e identificazione di alcune molecole di adesione (ICAM-1, ELAM-1, LFA-1) in 10 casi di alopecia areata. G It Dermatol Venereol. 1982; 127: 463-469

8 Springer TA. Adhesion receptors of the immune system. Nature. 1990; 346: 425-434

9 Nickoloff BJ, Griffiths CEM. Aberrant intercellular adhesion molecule-1 (ICAM-1) expression by hair follicle epithelial cells and endothelial leukocyte adhesion molecule-1 by vascular cells are important adhesion-molecule alteration in alopecia areata. J Invest Dermatol. 1991; 96: 91-92

©1996 Elsevier Science B.V. All rights reserved.
Hair research for the next millenium
D.J.J. Van Neste and V.A. Randall (Eds)

Expression of T-cell receptor Vβ-chains in alopecia areata

C. Arand, R. Happle and R. Hoffmann

Department of Dermatology, Philipp University, Deutschhausstrasse 9, 35033 Marburg, Germany

Introduction

The T-cell receptor (TCR) is a cell surface heterodimer, combining α and β chains. This receptor is used by approximately 95% of human T cells to recognize antigens in combination with molecules of the major histocompatibility complex (MHC). Both α and β chains have variable (V), junctional (J) and constant (C) regions. The β chain has, in addition, regions of diversity (D). The human $V\beta$ gene segments are organized in at least 24 families. Each T cell that expresses TCR Vβ chains on its cell surface has rearranged at least one of the available Vβ chains to generate the antigen receptor. The RNA transcripts for the TCR β chains are then spliced to yield a continuous V-D-J-C template for translation. Increasing evidence supports the view that antigen specific responses can be explained, at least in part, by the presence of antigenic epitopes sharing structural features. It has been shown that these epitopes are recognized by related TCR structures [1]. Therefore, analysis of rearrangement of TCR Vβ chains is important for establishing the clonality of antigen specific T cells present in inflammatory skin diseases [2], or clonality of malignant cells in lymphatic leukemia [3].

There is increasing evidence that immune/inflammatory cells such as T cells participate in the pathophysiology of various types of alopecia [4]. In alopecia areata (AA), the onset of hair loss is accompanied by a peri-and intrafollicular lymphocytic infiltrate consisting primarily of CD 4+ T lymphocytes [5]. However, the nature of the noxious signal and the specific target remains unknown, although it has been assumed that an autoimmune process is involved. Recently, melanocytes of affected hair follicles have been proposed to be the primary target of the lymphocytic attack and an antigen associated with this melanocytes has been hypothesized [6]. If this hypothesis holds true, antigen specific T cells should be present in lesional scalp and this should be reflected by a clonal rearrangement of the *TCR Vβ* gene families. Recent studies revealed a distinct TCR Vβ repertoire in normal skin as compared to blood lymphocytes and a clonal expansion within the skin was suggested [7]. A detailed knowledge of the TCR Vβ repertoire in AA is so far lacking. Characterization of AA specific T-cell clones would be needed for a better understanding of the immune response. To address this question, we examined the TCR Vβ repertoire in scalp biopsies and blood lymphocytes from patients with AA by reverse-transcriptase polymerase chain reaction. RT-PCR analysis using Vβ-region specific primers has become an important tool to study T cells responding to a variety of antigens and to discriminate monoclonal from polyclonal T cell responses [8].

Materials and methods

Patients

With informed consent, excisional scalp biopsies were taken from 20 patients (25-55 years, mean 36 years) with alopecia areata of the totalis type. Venous blood was drawn into preservative-free heparin and the mononuclear fraction was separated by sedimentation on a Ficoll-Hypaque gradient. Collected peripheral blood lymphocytes (PBLC) were immediately stored in liquid nitrogen.

Chemicals

Guanidinium thiocyanate, Tween 20, Tris-HCL, Tris-borate, glycerol, bromophenol blue, Tris-HCl, $NaClNa_2H_2$ ethylenediaminetetraacetic acid (EDTA), Ficoll, Denhardt's solution, sodium lauryl sulfate (SDS) and herring sperm DNA were purchased from Sigma (Deisenhofen, Germany) and phenol, isopropanol and chloroform from Merck (Darmstadt, Germany). The *taq* polymerase and the kit for reverse-transcription (RT kit) came from Pharmacia (Uppsala, Sweden). Ethidium bromide and the DNA-VIII molecular weight marker came from Boehringer Mannheim (Mannheim, Germany). Primers for PCR amplification of *TCR Vβ* and *Cα* gene segments and biotinylated Cβ oligonucleotide probes were bought from Clonetech (Palo Alto, USA). The primer and probe sequences are provided by Clonetech.

Extraction of total RNA and RT-PCR analysis of TCR Vβ and Cα mRNA

Total RNA from scalp skin and PBLC was isolated according to Chomczynski and Sacchi [9]. Standard curves for the amount of RNA, PCR cycle numbers and quantification by HPLC were established as described previously [10]. The specificity of the PCR products was demonstrated by southern blotting.

Results

Although the pattern of TCR Vβ expression varied slightly from one patient to another, a consistent pattern of TCR Vβ overexpression emerged. We detected steady state mRNA levels for all TCR Vβ families tested in scalp areas affected by AA (Fig. 1). The expression levels, however, varied. Some of the detected TCR Vβ families showed only little expression, whereas others were highly expressed. Predominantly used *TCR Vβ* gene segments were Vβ 4, Vβ 5.1 and Vβ 13. Using an identical technique we investigated the *TCR Vβ* gene expression in

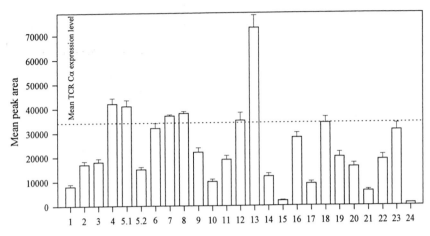

Figure 1. T cell receptor Vβ chain expression scalp biopsies affected by alopecia areata

PBLC from the same patients. TCR Vβ 4 and Vβ 5.1 were likewise highly expressed, whereas TCR Vβ 13 was low (data not shown). Therefore, in scalp biopsies from patients with AA we detected an preferential expression of TCR Vβ 13.

Discussion

The rationale of our study was the recent detection of abnormal antibodies to hair follicle melanocytes in AA [6]. When melanocytes are the principal target in AA, a resulting immune response ought to be reflected by a clonal rearrangement of specific T cells. Selective recruitment of T lymphocytes bearing a particular TCR Vβ region has so far not been demonstrated in alopecia areata. Despite the fact that all Vβ genes were detected by RT-PCR in tissue samples from patients with AA, a rather oligoclonal expression pattern emerged. The predominant TCR Vβ used was Vβ 13. This expression pattern differs from the recently reported pattern in normal skin [7] and supports the view of a selective immunological situation in scalp areas involved by AA. This result is suggestive of a selective clonal expansion of T cells within the scalp. The nature of the antigen(s) that trigger clonal proliferation of specific T cells is unknown. In other diseases such as psoriasis a role of superantigens have been postulated [2]. In this regard persistent streptococcal infection has been shown to trigger clonal expansion of TCR Vβ 2 and TCR Vβ 5.1 bearing T cells. In AA recent streptococcal infection is very uncommon and in our opinion not associated with the occurence or progression of hair loss. Our findings are more consistent with possible self-antigens located within affected hair bulbs. In this regard AA-

224

specific T cells from involved scalp areas have been cloned and shown to release factors that *in vitro* inhibit the proliferation of epithelial cells [11]. However, these T cells have not been characterized further. Future studies have to show what kind of *TCR Vβ* genes these T cells express.

Our results may prove to have therapeutic implications. At present topical immunotherapy appears to be the most effective approach for the induction of hair regrowth, even in long-standing AA [12,13]. This treatment is, however, difficult to handle and may be accompanied by undesired side effects. Studies on *TCR* gene expression in experimental allergic encephalomyelitis, a prototypic animal model for autoimmunity induced by T cells, have shown a major role of certain TCRα and β products in the immune response. Treatment of mice with monoclonal antibodies specific for the predominant TCR Vβ-region reverses the disease [14]. Additional approaches used immunization with synthetic peptides from the TCR Vβ-regions that are rearranged. Application of such treatment requires identification of disease-causing T cells and preferential *TCR Vβ* gene usage [15]. AA does not appear to be a disease severe enough to introduce such mode of treatment. However, animal models may help in the design of alternative therapeutic approaches.

Acknowledgements

This work was supported by a grant from the Deutsche Forschungsgemeinschaft (Ho 1598/1-1), Bonn, Germany.

References

1   Davis MM. T-cell receptor gene diversity 2nd selection. Annu Rev Biochem. 1990; 59: 475-96
2   Lewis HM, Baker BS, Bokth S, Powels AV, Garioch JJ, Valdimarsson HV, Fry L. Restricted T-cell receptor *Vβ* gene usage in the skin of patients with guttate and chronic plaque psoriasis. Br J Dermatol. 1993; 129: 514-20
3   Preesman AH, Hu HZ, Tilanus MGJ, Geus B, Schuurman HJ, Reitsma P, Wichen DF van, Vloten WA van, Weger RA de. T-cell receptor Vβ family usage in primary cutaneous and primary nodal T-cell non-Hodgkin's lymphomas. J Invest Dermatol. 1992; 99: 587-93
4   Bystryn JC. Immunologic aspects of hair loss. J Invest Dermatol. 1991; 96: 88S
5   Perret C, Wiesner-Menzel L, Happle R. Immunohistochemical analysis of T-cell subsets in the peribulbar and intrabulbar infiltrates of alopecia areata. Acta Dermatol Venereol (Stockh). 1984; 64: 26-30
6   Tobin DJ, Orentreich N, Fenton DA, Bystryn J-C. Antibodies to hair follicles in alopecia areata. J Invest Dermatol. 1994; 102: 721-724
7   Dunn AD, Gadenne AS, Simha S, Lerner EA, Bigby M, Bleicher PA. T-cell receptor Vβ expression in normal human skin. Proc Natl Acad Sci USA. 1993; 90: 1267
8   Kotzin J, Karuturi S, Chou YK, Lafferty J, Forrester RM, Better M, Nedwin GE, Offner H, Vandenbark AA. Preferential T-cell receptor β-chain variable gene use in myelin basic protein-reactive T-cell clones from patients with multiple sclerosis. Proc Natl Acad Sci USA. 1991; 88: 9161-9165

9 Chomczynski P, Sacchi N. Single-step method of RNA isolation by acid guanidinium thiocyanate-phenol-chloroform extraction. Anal Biochem. 1987; 162:156-159

10 Henninger HP, Hoffmann R, Grewe M, Schulze-Specking A, Decker K. Purification and quantitative analysis of nucleic acids by anion-exchange high-performance liquid chromatography. Biol Chem Hoppe-Seyler. 1994; 274: 625-634

11 Baadsgaard O. Potential immunological mechanisms in alopecia areata. Eur J Dermatol. 1994; 4: 261

12 Happle R, Kalveram KJ, Büchner U, Echternacht-Happle K, Göggelmann W, Summer KH. Contact allergy as a therapeutic tool for alopecia areata: application of squaric acid dibutylester. Dermatologica. 1980; 161: 289-297

13 Shapiro J, Tan J, Ho V, Abbott F, Tron V. Treatment of chronic severe alopecia areata with topical diphenylcyclopropenone and 5% minoxidil: a clinical and immunopathologic evaluation. J Am Acad Dermatol. 1993; 29: 729-735

14 Hanawa H, Kodama M, Inomata T, Izumi T, Shibata A, Tuchida M, Matsumoto Y, Abo. Anti-α β T-cell receptor antibodies prevents the progression of experimental autoimmune myocarditis. Clin Exp Immunol. 1994; 96: 470-475

15 Vandenbark AA, Chou YK, Bourdette R, Whitham RH, Hashim GA, Offner H. T-cell receptor peptide therapy for autoimmune diseases. J Autoimmun. 1992; 5: 83

Incidence and significance of single stranded DNA antibodies in alopecia areata

S. Alaiti[1], G. Ulyanov[1], M. Teodorescu[2], W. Lee[1], B. Kappogiannis[2] and V.C. Fiedler[1]

[1]Department of Dermatology, University of Illinois at Chicago, USA
[2]Department of Immunology, University of Illinois at Chicago, USA

Introduction

Alopecia areata (AA) is thought to be an autoimmune disease. It is occasionally associated with other autoimmune diseases especially thyroid disease and vitiligo [1, 2]. Various autoantibodies (gastric parietal cell, thyroid, smooth muscle, mitochondrial, reticulin, rheumatoid and antinuclear antibodies) have been reported in patients with AA [2]. No prior studies have reported on the incidence and significance of ssDNA antinuclear antibodies in AA patients.

Materials and methods

Serum Assays

Sera from patients and controls were tested for ssDNAabs by the ELISA method [4]. Normal maximum for ssDNAab was < 99 units/ml with 1000 units/ml being a high value.

Patients

Blood samples were obtained from sixty five alopecia areata patients attending the Alopecia Clinic at the University of Illinois Hospital (Table 1).

Controls

Blood samples were obtained from 52 volunteers who were seen at the University of Illinois Hospital Dermatology Clinic for various dermatologic problems. None of the controls had a personal history of autoimmune disease (Table 2).

Table 1.
Patients

	Females	Males
Number (N = 65)	39	26
Mean age (years)	35.3 ± 12.3	37.3 ± 10.4
Mean duration of current episode (years)	7.13 ± 6.3	4.9 ± 5.7
Mean age on onset (years)	24.3 ± 13.1	26.5 ± 15.3
Mean duration of AA (years)	11.6 ± 8.3	10.7 ± 10.8
Autoimmune disease:		
Patient	11 (28%)[1,2]	2 (8%)[1,3]
Family	19 (49%)[4]	9 (35%)[5]
Severity (> 75%)[6]	17 (44%)	10 (38%)
Atopy 34 (87%)	18 (69%)	
Responsiveness to treatment:		
Non cosmetic	18 (46%)	17 (65%)
Cosmetic	21 (54%)	9 (35%)

[1] *Female patients vs male patients; p < 0.05*
[2] *1 Vitiligo, 2 Graves', 1 DLE, 6 Hashimoto's, 2 Crohn's*
[3] *1 Hashimoto's, 1 RA*
[4] *SLE: one grandmother, one mother*
[5] *DLE: one daughter*
[6] *Previously we have shown that patients with ≥ 75% hair loss are less responsive to treatment [3]*

Table 2.
Controls

	Females	Males
Number (N = 52)	22	30
Mean age (years)	42.5 ± 13.9	33.8 ± 9.7
Autoimmune disease:		
Subject	0	0
Family	1 (5%)[1]	1 (3%)[2]
Atopy	12 (55%)	8 (27%)

[1] *RA: one grandmother*
[2] *DM: one aunt*

Results

ssDNAab positive patients vs controls

Twelve (18.4%) of 65 patients vs 2 (3.8%) of 52 controls were ssDNAab positive (p < 0.05). Nine (23%) of female patients vs 0 (0%) of female controls were ssDNAab positive (p < 0.05). Three (11.5%) of male patients vs 2 (6.6%) of male controls had positive ssDNAabs (p > 0.05).

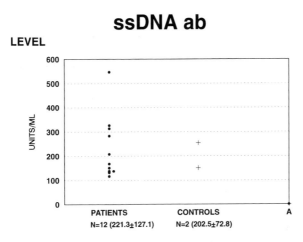

Figure 1. ssDNAab positive patients (mean = 221 units/ml) and controls (mean = 203 units/ml)

Correlation of ssDNAab with other clinical parameters

Six (46%) of 13 patients with autoimmune disease vs six (11%) of 52 patients without autoimmune disease were ssDNAab positive (p < 0.05). Five (45%) of 11 female patients with autoimmune disease vs 4 (14%) of 28 females without autoimmune disease were positive for ssDNAab (p < 0.05), and one (50%) of 2 male patients with autoimmune disease vs 2 (8%) of 24 males without autoimmune disease were ssDNAab positive (p = 0.07).

Only one of the ssDNAab positive patients had DLE; none had SLE. None of the ssDNAab negative patients or controls had a personal or family history of LE.

Eight (29%) of 28 patients with a positive family history of autoimmune disease vs 4 (11%) of 37 patients who did not have such a positive family history were ssDNAab positive (p = 0.06). Five (26%) of 19 female patients with a family history of autoimmune disease vs 4 (20%) of 20 females without such a family history were ssDNAab positive (p > 0.05); 3 (33%) of 9 male patients with family history of autoimmune disease vs 0 (0%) of 17 male patients without such a family history were ssDNAab positive (p < 0.05).

No significant associations were found between positive ssDNAab and atopy, severity of AA, treatment response of AA, or duration of the current episode of AA (Table 3). Similarly, total duration of AA showed no significant association with ssDNAab. ssDNAab positive patients had a mean total duration of AA of 6.3 ± 2.6 years vs 6.2 ± 0.8 years for patients who were ssDNAab negative ($p > 0.05$).

Table 3.
ssDNAab positive patients[2]

	All	Females	Males
Atopy:			
Present	10/52 (19%)	7/34 (21%)	3/18 (17%)
Absent	2/13 (15%)	2/5 (40%)	0/8 (0%)
Severity of AA:[1]			
≥ 75%	7/27 (26%)	5/17 (29%)	2/10 (20%)
< 75%	5/38 (13%)	4/22 (18%)	1/16 (6%)
Regrowth:			
Cosmetic	5/30 (17%)	4/21 (19%)	1/9 (11%)
Non cosmetic	7/35 (20%)	5/18 (28%)	3/17 (12%)
Duration current Episode AA:			
> 2 year	8/52 (15%)	7/34 (21%)	1/18 (6%)
< 2 year	4/13 (31%)	2/5 (40%)	2/8 (25%)

[1] *Severity of AA: ≥ 75% scalp hairloss vs < 75% scalp hairloss*
[2] *No significant associations between ssDNAab and clinical parameters listed in Table 3*

Discussion

Significantly more AA patients than controls were positive for ssDNA antinuclear antibodies as measured by the ELISA method. Only one of the ssDNAab positive patients had DLE; none had SLE. Patients with associated autoimmune disease were significantly more likely to be ssDNAab positive. No other clinical parameters measured were significantly associated with the presence of ssDNAabs. Many of the organ-specific autoimmune diseases occur in association with each other, and they also occur with increased frequency in patients with alopecia areata and their families [1]. Various autoantibodies are reported to be present in patients with AA [2] suggesting that they may have generalized B-cell stimulation. B cells capable of producing anti-DNAabs occur with high frequency in normal subjects as well as in patients with SLE. It is possible that anti-DNA B cells are preferentially expressed in settings of generalized B-cell stimulation [5]. Our data suggest that ssDNAab positive patients are not likely to develop LE. Anti-DNAabs from LE patients versus normal controls have been shown to have different cross-reactive antigen-binding properties which are thought to influence their capacity to produce clinical disease [6]. It is possible that AA patients may express ssDNAabs similar to those found in normal controls which would account for the apparent low frequency ($< 1\%$) of LE associated with AA [1].

Conclusion

There is an increased incidence of ssDNAabs found in AA patients compared with controls. AA patients with positive ssDNAabs are more likely to have an associated autoimmune disease, most commonly Hashimoto's thyroiditis. Positive ssDNAabs do not correlate with any other clinical parameters of AA.

References

1   Muller SA, Winkelmann RK. Alopecia areata. Arch Dermatol. 1963; 88: 290-297
2   Friedmann PS. Alopecia areata and autoimmunity. Br J Dermatol. 1981; 105: 153-157
3   Friedler-Weiss VC. Topical minoxidil solution (1% and 5%) in the treatment of alopecia areata. J Am Acad Dermatol. 1987; 16: 745-748
4   Fritzler MJ. Antinuclear antibodies in the investigation of rheumatic diseases. Bulletin on the Rheumatic Diseases. 1985; 35(6): 1-10
5   Pisetzky DS. The role of anti-DNA antibodies in systemic lupus erythematosus. Clinical Aspects of Autoimmunity. 1988; 2(6): 8-15
6   Sabbaga J, Panekewycz OG, Luffit V, et al. Cross reactivity distinguishes serum and nephritogenic anti-DNA antibodies in human lupus from their natural counterparts in normal serum. Journal of Autoimmunity. 1990; 3: 215-235

©1996 Elsevier Science B.V. All rights reserved.
Hair research for the next millenium
D.J.J. Van Neste and V.A. Randall (Eds)

Hair follicle structures targeted by antibodies in alopecia areata

J.-C. Bystryn, D.J. Tobin, S.-K. Hann[1] and M.-S. Song[1]

The Ronald O. Perelman Department of Dermatology, New York University Medical Center, 560 First Ave, New York, NY, 10016, USA
[1]Yonsei University College of Medicine, Seoul, Korea

Introduction

Although the cause of alopecia areata (AA) is not known, it is believed to result from an autoimmune reaction to hair follicles (HF) based on indirect observations that have been reviewed [1].

We have recently made several major observations that strongly and directly support this hypothesis. These are that

1) high levels of IgG antibodies to HF are present in most patients with AA, but are rare in persons without hair loss [2];

2) these antibodies are most commonly directed to HF antigens of 44, 47, 50 , 52, 57 and/or 62 kD, several of which are expressed only in HF [2] and

3) similar antibodies are present in a mouse model of AA. These observations provide the underlying framework necessary to explain the selective damage to HF that occurs in AA.

This study was conducted to identify the structures within the HF that are targeted by AA antibodies; to examine whether there are differences in the antigenic properties of HF in scalp of persons with and without the disease; and in those with the disease, between areas of scalp that are and are not involved with lesions.

Results

The sera of 10 patients with AA, 5 normal individuals, and 3 persons with unrelated autoimmune skin diseases were tested for circulating antibodies to HF in perilesional and uninvolved scalp obtained from 10 AA patients.

Antibodies (titer ≥ 50) to HF were detected in 60% of AA sera but in only 12% of controls and were specifically directed to HF as they did not react with autologous adjacent epidermis or dermis in the same scalp specimen.

Hair follicle structures targeted by AA antibodies

The most common HF structure targeted by AA antibodies was the outer root sheath (Fig. 1) followed by the hair shaft, inner root sheath, and matrix.

234

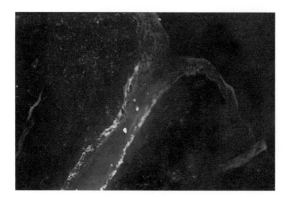

Figure 1. Indirect immunofluorescence photomicrograph of serum from an AA patient reacted with AA scalp tissue. Antibodies react to keratinocytes of the outer root sheath of HF.

Antibodies to these structures were present in 40%, 20%, 20%, and 10% of AA patients respectively (using scalp from AA patient #4 as target) but in only 12%, 0%, 0%, and 0% of control individuals. None of these sera reacted with the follicular papilla.

Different patients developed different patterns of antibodies to different HF structures. These differences were not due to differences in antigen expression, as the same scalp specimen was used for these studies.

Heterogeneity of AA-reactive antigens within the same HF structure

Some AA sera reacted to antigens present in some scalp specimens but not in others. Indication of multiple antigens within the same HF structure is illustrated in Figure 2. Here antibodies in the serum reacted with an antigen(s) expressed throughout the outer root sheath in one specimen (Fig. 2a), whereas antibodies in the same AA serum reacted to an antigen(s) distributed in the innermost cells of the same structure in a different specimen (Fig. 2b). As the

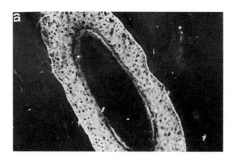
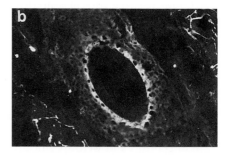

Figure 2. Heterogeneity of antigens within the same HF structure. Serum from an AA patient was incubated with scalp of two AA patients. a) The serum reacted to antigens in the first specimen that were distributed evenly throughout the entire outer root sheath but b) reacted to an antigen(s) distributed only in the innermost cell layer of the same structure in the second scalp specimen.

same serum was used in both cases, this difference indicates the existence of two or more antigens/epitopes in this HF structure.

Antigen expression in perilesional and uninvolved scalp of AA patients

To determine whether the differences in antigen expression between different areas of the scalp could account for the localization of AA lesions, the panel of 10 AA sera were tested for reactivity to HF obtained from perilesional and uninvolved scalp of 10 patients with active AA. Most sera reacted similarly with HF obtained from either perilesional or uninvolved AA scalp, indicating that there is no gross difference in the distribution of HF antigens between areas of scalp involved and spared by the disease.

Variation in antigenic properties of HF between patients with AA and normal individuals

To examine whether the development of AA is related to differences in antigen expression between persons with and without the disease, a panel of 10 AA sera was tested for reactivity against uninvolved scalp of 10 patients with active AA and against scalp of 5 normal persons without hair abnormality.

Antibodies to HF in one of the AA patients reacted to an antigen(s) that was present in 8 (80%) of scalp specimens obtained from 10 patients with AA, but in none of 5 scalp specimens obtained from normal individuals. The antibodies in another patient with AA reacted to an antigen(s) that was present in 40% of the AA patients but in none of the normal individuals (Table 1).

Table 1.
Variation in antigenic properties of HF in AA and normal scalp[a]

AA patient	% scalp specimens reactive with HF antibodies	
	AA scalp (pts =10)	Normal Scalp (pts=5)
AA 1	80%	0%
AA 2	40%	0%

[a]*Sera were reacted with uninvolved scalp from ten AA patients and with scalp from five normal individuals.*

Discussion

The most important findings of this study are that the antibodies to HF that are present in most individuals with AA target multiple structures in HF, that this antibody response is heterogeneous, and that it is directed in part to antigens expressed to a greater extent in patients with the disease than in normal individuals.

This study confirms, using a different assay system, that high levels of antibodies to HF occur in most patients with AA [2]. These antibodies are unrelated to «natural» cytoplasmic and keratin antibodies present in normal individuals, as they do not react to adjacent scalp tissues. The HF structure most commonly targeted by AA antibodies was the outer root sheath, followed by the inner root sheath, hair shaft, and matrix. Each of these HF structures contained several immunologically distinct AA-reactive antigens and/or epitopes, and patients with AA develop various combinations of antibodies to one or more of these antigens.

The factors responsible for the appearance of lesions of AA in some areas of scalp, but nor others, and more fundamentally, for the development of the disease itself, remain unknown. But in other autoimmune skin diseases (eg. pemphigus vulgaris), the distribution of skin lesions is related to the amount of autoantigen expressed in the skin. By contrast, in AA we did not find any difference in HF antigen expression between areas of scalp involved with hair loss and areas away from it. This suggests that factors other than antigen concentration are responsible for the location of areas of hair loss in the scalp of patients with AA.

An intriguing finding was that the expression of some AA antigens was increased in scalp of patients with the disease compared to normal individuals. This suggests that the development of AA may be related to the amount of certain antigens expressed in HF, ie. high antigen expressors may be more likely to develop an autoimmune response to HF and thus to develop AA. It suggests that antigen expressed may relate to extent and severity of the disease.

The role of antibodies to HF in the pathogenesis of AA remains to be defined. It is unlikely that they are produced non-specifically as they are not seen in normal individuals despite the constant release of HF antigens that occurs as a result of up to 70% of the anagen HF being destroyed during the transition from anagen to telogen during the normal hair growth cycle. Nor do they appear to be related to «natural» cytoplasmic or keratin antibody as they do not react with these antigens in adjacent epidermis. Thus, the production of antibodies to HF-specific antigens in AA may be a primary event and as such a possible cause rather than a result of the disease process.

Acknowledgements

This study was supported in part by the National Alopecia Areata Foundation.

References

1   Bystryn J-C, Tamesis J. J Invest Dermatol. 1991; 96: 88S-89S
2   Tobin DJ, Orentreich N, Fenton DA, Bystryn J-C. J Invest Dermatol. 1994; 102: 721-724

©1996 Elsevier Science B.V. All rights reserved.
Hair research for the next millenium
D.J.J. Van Neste and V.A. Randall (Eds)

Alopecia areata is associated with antibodies to hair follicle-specific antigens located predominantly in the proliferative region of hair follicles

D.J. Tobin and J.-C. Bystryn

The Ronald O. Perelman Department of Dermatology, New York University Medical Center, 560 First Ave, New York, NY, 10016, USA

Introduction

The cause of alopecia areata (AA) is not known. The favored hypothesis is that it is an autoimmune disease of hair follicles (HF) based on several indirect observations which have been reviewed [1]. The major problem with this hypothesis is that, until recently, there was no direct evidence of an abnormal immune response directed specifically to HF in AA.

We have made three basic observations that strongly and directly support this hypothesis. One is that HF express unique antigens that can stimulate autoimmune responses [2]. Another is that AA in humans is associated with antibodies to HF-specific antigens [3]. The third is that similar antibodies to HF are present in a mouse model of this disease. The presence of tissue-specific autoantigens in HF, and of an abnormal antibody response to some of these antigens in AA, provides the underlying framework necessary to explain the selective damage to HF that occurs in AA; and is the strongest evidence to date that AA is an autoimmune disease. Another clue to the pathogenesis of AA is that the inflammatory infiltrate around HF is predominantly present around anagen HF and spares telogen HF. This suggests that the autoimmune responses that may be present in this disease target antigens which are preferentially expressed in anagen HF, either because they are differentiation-associated antigens, or because they are preferentially expressed in proliferative areas of HF.

Here we review these findings, and present data on the nature of HF antigens targeted by AA antibodies, their anatomical location within the HF, and their preferential expression in the proliferative areas of the HF. These findings provide an explanation for the selective destruction of anagen HF in this disease.

Results

Presence of unique antigens in hair follicles

Using selected human sera as probes, we found that HF express what appear to be unique antigens [2]. Several features of these antigens are of note;

1) they react with individual's own antibodies, indicating they are autoantigens,

2) several of these antigens are expressed in HF but cannot be detected in similarly prepared extracts of autologous adjacent scalp epidermis and dermis,

3) low level (titer ≤20) of antibodies to some of these antigens can be present in some normal individuals.

These results indicate that HF express unique antigens that may provide the targets necessary to explain selective damage to HF by an autoimmune process.

Antibodies to hair follicles in alopecia areata

We have recently found that AA is associated with an abnormal antibody response to HF [3]. This is the first demonstration of this fundamental abnormality. We tested sera of 39 patients with active AA and 29 control individuals for antibodies to antigens in 6M urea extracts of normal anagen HF by immunoblotting. The results are illustrated in Figure 1 and summarized in Table 1.

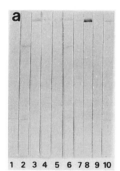 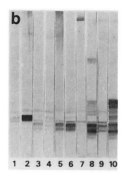

Figure 1. Immunoblot analysis of HF antigens reacted with control (a) or AA (b) sera. 20 μg protein per lane. Serum dilution 1:80

Table 1.
Antibodies to HF in patients with AA

HF antigen	HF antibodies				
	Control (n=29)		AA (n=39)		P**
	%	level*	%	level*	
60 kD	0	0	12	20.0	< 0.0005
57 kD	11	3.1	67	34.3	< 0.0005
52 kD	33	5.3	46	22.5	< 0.005
50 kD	19	7.8	46	38.5	< 0.005
47 kD	11	2.4	67	34.3	< 0.005
44 kD	19	2.1	36	28.3	< 0.005

average level measured by computer assisted densitometry.
** *significance of difference in antibody level between AA & controls*

High titer (≥ 80) of antibodies to one or more HF antigens of 62, 57, 52, 47, 44 kD were detected in most AA patients, but only in few control individuals. The difference between AA and control individuals was particularly striking for antibodies to 47 kD and 57 kD antigens, antibodies which were present in 67% of patients with AA but in only 11% of control persons. The titer of antibodies to HF was much greater (up to 14 times greater for some antigens) in patients with AA than in control individuals.

Several features of the HF antibodies associated with AA are of note. Such antibodies are more common and present in higher levels in AA than in control persons. They are directed most commonly to antigens of 44-62 kD. They do not appear to be secondary to the autoimmune process or to HF damage, as initial experiments indicate their incidence is not increased in patients with unrelated autoimmune (pemphigus or bullous pemphigoid) or inflammatory diseases of HF such as lichen planopilaris.

They are predominantly of the IgG type (present in all 15 patients). IgM antibodies are relatively rare (present in 3 of 15 patients). This suggests that the antibodies may be pathogenic since «natural» autoantibodies present in normal persons are usually IgM, whereas those associated with autoimmune are normally IgG.

Several of the antigens defined by AA antibodies (those ranging from 44-52 kD) are selectively expressed in HF. They are not detected in extracts prepared similarly from adjacent, freshly excised, autologous scalp tissues, or in cultured follicular papilla or melanoma cells [3]. Some HF antigens defined by AA antibodies are expressed to a much greater extent in scalp of AA, as compared with normal individuals (see elsewhere in this volume).

Anatomical location of alopecia areata antigens within hair follicles

Antibodies to the 44, 62 and 105 kD HF antigens, in a patient with active AA, were individually affinity-purified by elution from immunoblots and used to probe cryostat-cut sections of scalp biopsies by indirect immunofluorescence. The location of some of these antigens is illustrated below (Fig. 2) and is summarized in Table 2. The antigens, reactive with AA antibodies, were present in the lower HF and hair shaft apart from the follicular papilla and inner root sheath. All AA antigens were HF-specific, as they were not detected in adjacent scalp epidermis or dermis.

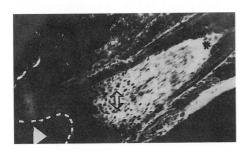

Figure 2. Staining of anagen HF by affinity-purified antibody to a 44 kD antigen

Table 2.
Expression of antigens defined by AA antibodies in the lower HF

Site of antigen expression	Antigen		
	44 kD	62 kD	105 kD
Outer root sheath	+	+	–
Inner root sheath	–	–	–
Hair shaft	+	+	+
Matrix	–	–	–
Pre-cortex	+ +	+	+ +

HF antigens defined by AA antibodies were expressed predominantly in the lower part of the growing anagen HF and in particular, close to or at the proliferative region. Furthermore, the expression of the antigen(s), as denoted by fluorescence intensity, was higher in these regions. For example, cells of the pre-cortex , located just above the follicular papilla, reacted most strongly with AA antibodies. Although AA antibodies also reacted with the non viable hair shaft, these antibodies are unlikely to be involved in pathogenesis.

Relation of antigens defined by alopecia areata antibodies with hair follicle-specific keratins

Antigens defined by AA antibodies were characterized by

1) their co-location in the anagen HF with monoclonal antibodies (moab) to HF proteins by indirect immuno fluorescence,

2) co-migration in SDS-PAGE with HF-specific keratins and

3) immunoprecipitation of antigens by AA antibodies with anti-keratin moabs.

A 44 kD HF antigen, defined by AA antibody, co-located in the anagen HF with 44/46 kD specific keratins defined by the monoclonal antibody AE13. Both antibodies reacted strongly with the pre-cortex but not the bulbar matrix. Further, all (100%) of 17 AA sera contained antibodies that precipitated the 46 kD hair-specific keratins, while 64% precipitated the 44 kD hair-specific keratin. By contrast, none of 22 control sera reacted with the 44 kD hair-specific keratin and only 18% of control sera reacted with the 46 kD hair-specific keratin. This also contrasts to «natural» antibodies to the 56-60 kD type II basic keratins which are not HF-specific, antibodies which were present in all individuals with or without AA.

Discussion

The results of these studies show that abnormalities in circulating antibodies to HF antigens are present in individuals with AA and provide direct evidence of an abnormal immune response to HF in this disease.

We have previously shown that HF express unique antigens not detected in adjacent scalp epidermis or dermis, that low levels of IgM and IgG antibodies to these antigens are common in normal individuals [2], and that high titers of predominantly IgG antibodies to HF are present in all AA patients but are rare in control persons. These antibodies do not appear to be secondary to the autoimmune process, as incidence does not increase in individuals with unrelated autoimmune disease of the scalp such as pemphigus or bullous pemphigoid.

In this study we examined the anatomical location of individual antigens defined by AA antibodies within the HF by indirect immunofluorescence study of cryostat-cut sections of normal human scalp incubated with affinity-purified antibodies directed to three antigens (ie. 44, 62, and 105 kD). These antibodies were eluted from HF antigens resolved by SDS-PAGE and transferred to PVDF membrane. All the affinity-purified antibodies tested were HF-specific. One of these antigens (ie. of 44 kD) appears to be identical to the 44 kD HF-specific keratin and all three antigens were expressed predominantly in the lower HF in or close to the proliferative region. None of these antigens could be detected in telogen HF.

The biologic relevance of antibodies to HF-specific antigens in AA remains to be determined. The findings that many of these antibodies are directed to antigens that are expressed in or close to the proliferative region of anagen HF, but cannot be detected in telogen HF, provides an explanation for why anagen HF are targeted in AA, and for the termination of hair growth.

Acknowledgements

This study was supported in part by the National Alopecia Areata Foundation.

References

1 Bystryn J-C, Tamesis J. J Invest Dermatol. 1991; 96: 88S-89S
2 Tobin DJ, Orentreich N, Bystryn J-C. Arch Dermatol. 1994; 30: 395-397
3 Tobin DJ, Orentreich N, Fenton DA, Bystryn J-C. J Invest Dermatol. 1994; 102: 721-724

Cytokines characteristic of alopecia areata regulate the expression of ICAM-1 and MHC class I and II molecules in cultured dermal papilla cells

A. König, R. Happle and R. Hoffmann

Department of Dermatology, Philipp University, Marburg, Germany

Introduction

Alopecia areata (AA) is associated with an aberrant lesional expression of IFN-γ, IL-2 and IL-1β [1, 2] and an overexpression of ICAM-1 and MHC molecules on hair follicle keratinocytes and dermal papilla cells [3-7]. Interestingly, after successful treatment with the potent contact allergen diphenylcyclopropenone (DCP) the expression of adhesion molecules on the surface of dermal papilla cells is reduced despite an augmented inflammation. Cytokines are very likely to be involved in this process, and recently reduced levels of IFN-γ, IL1-β and an increased lesional expression of IL-8, IL-10, TGF-β1 and TNF-α were detected in scalp biopsies after DCP treatment [1, 2]. The mechanism by which DCP-therapy is beneficial in AA is unknown. However, the idea is advanced, that cytokines such as IL-10 or TGF-β1 are involved, probably by inhibition of adhesion molecule expression. Furthermore, cyclooxygenase-products might play a role in this process. We therefore decided to study the effects of various cytokines and prostaglandins on the formation and regulation of ICAM-1, HLA-DR and HLA-ABC in cultured dermal papilla cells obtained from healthy donors, thus imitating the situation of AA *in vitro*.

Materials and methods

Full thickness biopsies were obtained from the occipital scalp region of healthy volunteers. Hair follicles were isolated under the dissecting microscope. For this purpose the upper half of the dermis was removed and intact anagen hair follicles were isolated by gentle traction using watchmakers' forceps. The dermal papilla was then teased out by means of fine needles. Intact dermal papillas were transferred into a 24-well culture plate containing Amniomax medium. After outgrowth the dermal papilla cells were removed by trypsinization and transferred into tissue flasks. Only subconfluent monolayers of the second and third passage were used for the experiments.

The cells were incubated for 33 or 43 hours with IFN-γ, IL-1β, TNF-α, TGF-β1, IL-10 and with PGE2, Alprostadil, Iloprost and Diclofenac. A neutralizing anti-IL-1β-antibody was used to study the effects of endogenous IL-1β. Furthermore, co-incubations with IFN-γ and the mentioned mediators were performed. To detect and quantitate the surface molecules expressed on dermal papilla cells, we used FITC-conjugated monoclonal mouse anti-human antibodies directed towards HLA-DR, HLA-ABC and ICAM-1. All antibodies belonged to the IgG1-kappa isotype, and isotype-controls were performed using a FITC-conjugated mouse monoclonal IgG1 antibody directed towards Aspergillus niger glucose oxidase. Cells were incubated on ice following the supplier's instructions. Fluorescence intensity was determined by FACScan analysis.

Chemicals

Antibodies directed towards HLA-DR as well as isotype-control antibodies were obtained from Dako, Denmark, those directed towards HLA-ABC from Pharmingen, USA, and anti-ICAM-1 antibodies from Immunotech, France. IL-1β, IL-10, TNF-α were obtained from Biosource, USA, TGF-β1 from Serva, and PGE2 from Sigma, Germany. IFN-γ was bought from Stratagene, USA. A neutralizing monoclonal mouse anti-human IL-1β-antibody was purchased from Genzyme, USA. Commercially available solutions of Diclofenac (Voltaren®, Geigy), Iloprost (Ilomedin®, Schering) and Alprostadil (Prostavasin®, Schwarz Pharma) were used. Amniomax medium came from Gibco, Germany.

Results

In untreated cells we noted a relatively high constitutive expression of HLA-ABC and a lower expression of ICAM-1 and HLA-DR (data not shown). Incubation with IFN-γ (100 ng/ml) led to a time-dependent upregulation of the studied surface molecules. IL-1β (4 ng/ml) and TNF-α (100 ng/ml) were found to have a potent and synergistic effect on the upregulation of ICAM-1 (Fig. 1, Table 1) but they did not induce MHC molecules (Table 1). However, both cytokines significantly reduced the IFN-γ-induced HLA-DR expression (Fig. 2, Table 1). IL-10 (60 ng/ml) and TGF-β1 (10 ng/ml) did not affect the basal or agonist-induced expression of surface molecules. Neither preincubation of cells with the cyclooxygenase-inhibitor Diclofenac (10 µM), nor any of the studied prostanoids (PGE1 and PGE2) inhibited IFN-γ-elicited ICAM1 or HLA-DR expression, or had any endogenous effect on the studied surface molecules. Treatment of cells with a neutralizing anti-IL-1β-antibody did not cause changes in TNF-α-induced effects, although TNF-α was shown to stimulate endogenous IL-1β-release (own unpublished data).

Table 1.

Change in Mean Fluorescence Intensity (%)

	IFN-γ	IL-1β	TNF-α	IFN-γ + IL-1β	IFN-γ + TNF-α
ICAM-1 (33h)	54 ± 3	51 ± 9	78 ± 9	130 ± 24	142 ± 13
ICAM-1 (43h)	109 ± 10	74 ± 14	139 ± 14	162 ± 11	214 ± 15
HLA-DR (43h)	121 ± 16	7 ± 2	3 ± 3	74 ± 14**	97 ± 21*

ICAM-1 is synergistically upregulated by IFN-γ (100 ng/ml), IL-1β (4 ng/ml) and TNF-α (100 ng/ml) in a time-dependent manner. HLA-DR-expression is stimulated by IFN-γ but this effect is significantly reduced by IL-1β and TNF-α. Neither IL-1β nor TNF-α had any effects on the basal expression of HLA-DR. Values are Mean ± Std. Dev. n=6. Change in MFI is calculated by the formula

$$\frac{\text{(MFI of cells treated with cytokine)} - \text{(MFI of cells treated with medium only)}}{\text{(MFI of cells treated with medium only)}} \times 100$$

*$p<0.05$; ** $p<0.005$ compared to the IFN-γ effect (Student t-test performed on raw data)*

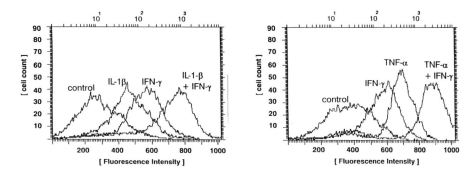

Figure 1. Single registrations of a typical experiment showing the effect of IFN-γ, IL-1β (a) and TNF-α (b) on the expression of ICAM-1. Similar results were obtained in 5 other experiments.

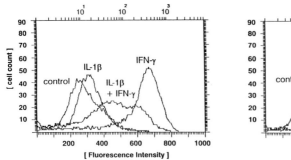
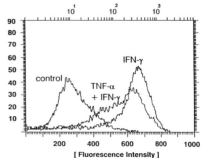

Figure 2. Single registrations of a typical experiment showing the effect of IFN-γ, IL-1β (a) and TNF-α (b) on the expression of HLA-DR. Similar results were obtained in 5 other experiments.

Discussion

We conclude that, with regard to the studied surface molecules, we can imitate the *in vivo* situation of AA *in vitro*. Cytokines found in AA are able to induce ICAM-1 and MHC molecules on cultured dermal papilla cells the same way as *in vivo*. After successful DCP-therapy, reduced ICAM-1 and HLA-DR molecule expression on dermal papilla cells has been described *in vivo* [3, 7]. Cytokines of the late contact allergy may mediate this effect and in this way the beneficial effect of contact sensitization in AA. IL-10 and TGF-β1 are likely candidates for such an action, because they have been repeatedly shown to modulate/suppress immune responses [8]. From our results, however, we have no evidence that these mediators are important; both cytokines were ineffective to reduce IFN-γ-elicited ICAM-1 or MHC molecules *in vitro*. Although IL-1β and TNF-α proved to be potent inductors of ICAM-1-expression, they have, on the other hand, a capacity to reduce MHC class II molecules on IFN-γ-stimulated dermal papilla cells. Most remarkably, we found increased lesional levels for TNF-α after successful DCP-therapy [1]. TNF-α is able to modulate immune responses by limiting antigen-presentation [9]. Theoretically this may happen in DCP-treated AA and as a consequence of this, activation and recruitment of AA-specific T-cells would be diminished. As a result of a reduced immune response around the hair follicles hair regrowth would occur. It remains to be shown, whether our hypothesis holds true, but prolonged expression of TNF-α might be one effector of the therapeutic response achieved by DCP-treatment in AA.

Acknowledgements

This study was supported by a grant from the «Stiftung für therapeutische Forschung» (Sandoz)

References

1 Hoffmann R, Wenzel E, Huth A, Henninger HP, Steen P, Schäufele M, Happle R. Cytokine mRNA levels in alopecia areata before and after treatment with the contact allergen diphenylcyclopropenone. J Invest Dermatol. 1994; 103: 530-533

2 Hoffmann R, Wenzel E, Huth A, Steen P, Schäufele M, Happle R. Diphenylcyclopropenone (DCP) therapy of alopecia areata is reflected by increased expression of TGF-β1 mRNA. Exp Dermatol. 1994; 3: 121

3 Bröcker EB, Echternacht-Happle K, Hamm H, Happle R. Abnormal expression of class I and class II major histocompatibility antigens in alopecia areata: modulation by topical immunotherapy. J Invest Dermatol. 1987; 88: 564-568

4 Hamm H, Klemmer S, Kreuzer I, Steijlen PM, Happle R, Bröcker E. HLA-DR and HLA-DQ antigen expression of anagen and telogen hair bulbs in long-standing alopecia areata. Arch Dermatol Res. 1988; 280: 179-181

5 Khoury EL, Price VH, Greenspann JS. HLA-DR expression by hair follicle keratinocytes in alopecia areata: evidence that it is secondary to the lymphoid infiltration. J Invest Dermatol. 1988; 90: 193-200

6 Nickoloff BJ, Griffiths CEM. Aberrant intercellular adhesion molecules-1 (ICAM-1) expression by hair follicle epithelial cells and endothelial leukocyte adhesion molecule-1 (ELAM-1) by vascular cells are important adhesion-molecule alterations in alopecia areata. J Invest Dermatol. 1991; 96: 91S-92S

7 Shapiro J, Tan J, Ho V, Abbott F, Tron V. Treatment of chronic severe alopecia areata with topical diphenylcyclopropenone and 5% minoxidil: a clinical and immunopathologic evaluation. J Am Acad Dermatol. 1993; 29: 729-735

8 Beissert S, Hosoi j, Grabbe S, Asahina A, Granstein RD. IL-10 inhibits tumor antigen presentation by epidermal antigen-presenting cells. J Immunol. 1995; 154: 1280-1286

9 Rivas JM, Ullrich SE. The role of IL-4, IL-10 and TNF-α in the immune suppression induced by ultraviolet radiation. J Leukocyte Biol. 1994; 56: 769-775

Interleukin 1β stimulation of interleukin-6 production by cultured dermal papilla cells in alopecia areata

A.J.G. McDonagh, K.R. Elliott and A.G. Messenger

Department of Dermatology, Royal Hallamshire Hospital, Glossop Road, Sheffield, S10 2JF, U.K.

Introduction

The dermal papilla of the hair follicle (DP) is crucial in inducing epithelial differentiation in the hair bulb and may be involved in regulating the hair growth cycle [1]. Several studies have suggested that DP function may be disturbed in alopecia areata (AA) and we have previously found evidence that DP cells cultured from perilesional sites in AA produce interleukin-6 (IL-6) and factors capable of stimulating lymphocyte proliferation *in vitro* [2]. This study was designed to investigate the possibility that regulation of IL-6 production in the hair follicle may be abnormal in AA principally by investigating the behavior of cells cultured from non-lesional sites in individuals with AA (NLAA) in comparison with normal controls.

Materials and methods

Scalp biopsies were obtained from AA patients (n=7). Three were from the margins of expanding hairless patches (perilesional); 4 from clinically uninvolved scalp (NLAA). Normal scalp tissue for controls was obtained from patients having removal of benign tumours/naevi or cosmetic surgery (n=6). DP cells and interfollicular fibroblasts (DFs) were cultured from tissue isolated by microdissection. Cultures were established in 25cm^2 flasks with an initial population of 2 x 10^5 cells in 4 ml Dulbecco's modified Eagle's medium (DMEM), 2 mM L-glutamine, 10% heat-inactivated pooled human serum (PHS), penicillin 50 IU/ml, streptomycin 50 μg/ml and amphotericin B 2.5 μg/ml. Cells were used between 2nd-4th passages and cell-free supernatants prepared from confluent cultures by passing conditioned media through a 0.22 μm filter. A 4 hour pulse with IL-1β 0.5 U/ml was applied to confluent cultures at the start of experiments. Cells were washed (x3) with PBS on medium change. IL-6 was measured at baseline then daily for 7 days after the IL-1β pulse. For the collagen gel cultures, rat tail collagen was used with glucose, PHS, glutamine and antibiotics as above. Sodium bicarbonate was added to achieve neutral pH. 200 000 cells (in 100 μl DMEM) were added to 900 μl collagen mixture in the wells of a 24 well plate. 1 ml culture medium was added to each well (with 0.5 U/ml IL-1β where appropriate). Cells were washed (x3) with PBS on medium change. IL-6 in filtered supernatant was measured at baseline, 4, 24, 48 and 72 hrs. Immunoreactive IL-6 was measured by ELISA (Cistron Biotechnology/ Laboratory Impex, UK).

Results

There was wide variation between cell lines in levels of IL-6 production in both normal and NLAA cell cultures (not illustrated). The effect of IL-1β stimulation on IL-6 levels in the culture supernatants was variable and generally small in comparison with the variation between cell lines. Similar responses to IL-1β were observed with supernatants derived from both DP and DF cell lines. In collagen gelcultures, variability between cell lines was much less than in monolayer cultures and there was a trend towards higher peak levels of IL-6 in the response of NLAA cell lines in comparison with normal and perilesional lines but this difference was not statistically significant (Fig. 1). A similar profile of IL-6 response to IL-1β was observed in normal controls, NLAA and perilesional cell lines.

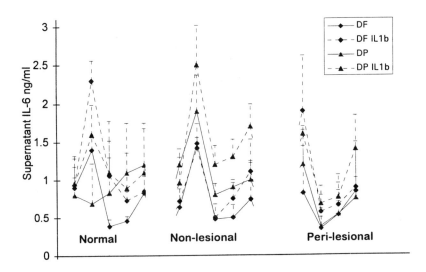

Figure 1. IL-6 response to IL-1β in collagen gels. Each point represents the mean + SEM for 3 or 4 cell lines

Discussion

In monolayer cultures, starting cell numbers and cell confluency state were critical influences on IL-6 production which showed wide variability between cell lines that outweighed differences between cell lines derived from AA/normal tissues. Using collagen gel cultures, the variability between cell lines found using monolayer cultures was reduced and there was a trend towards a larger IL-6 response to IL-1β production by NLAA cells rather than perilesional or normal cells. Such a finding could fit well with the genetic polymorphism of IL-1 receptor antagonist that has been identified as a severity association with AA [3]. However, further studies are required to confirm the significance of these findings.

Acknowledgements

This work was supported by a grant from the National Alopecia Areata Foundation.

References

1   McDonagh AJG, Messenger AG. The aetiology and pathogenesis of alopecia areata. J Dermatol Sci. 1994; 7: S125-135
2   McDonagh AJG, Al'Abadie MSK, Symons JA, Duff GW, Messenger AG. Cytokine production by dermal papilla cell cultures in alopecia areata. J Invest Dermatol. 1993; 100: 569
3   Tarlow JK, Clay FE, Cork MJ, Blakemore AIF, McDonagh AJG, Messenger AG, Duff GW. Alopecia areata is associated with a polymorphism in the interleukin-1 receptor antagonist gene. J Invest Dermatol. 1994; 103: 387-390

Hair research for the next millenium
D.J.J. Van Neste and V.A. Randall (Eds)

Hair follicle specific autoantibodies associated with alopecia areata in sera from the DEBR rat model and humans

K.J. McElwee, S. Drummond and R.F. Oliver

Department of Biological Sciences, University of Dundee, Dundee, Scotland, United Kingdom

Introduction

The psychologically devastating hair loss disease alopecia areata (AA) is widely believed to be the result of autoimmune action against hair follicles [1]. In other autoimmune diseases autoantibodies can play an active role in disease pathogenesis but despite many studies on autoantibodies in AA the results are confusing. Attempts to detect autoantibodies against hair follicle components in sera from AA patients have largely failed [2]. However, recent reports from two research groups do provide supporting evidence [3, 4].

Using the DEBR rat model for AA, we previously developed a refined indirect immunofluorescent technique to examine the sera from individual rats for presence of autoantibodies to the hair follicle and other tissues [5, 6]. In this study, we examined the staining properties of sera derived from DEBR rats and humans with AA when applied to cryostat sections of human and rat hair follicles.

The DEBR rat is an impressive model of AA showing hair loss in association with a mononuclear cell infiltrate in and around hair follicles [7]. Although the two substrains, one black hooded, the other brown hooded, are isogenic in nature, the extent of the hair loss lesion can vary between each individual rat-even littermates. The genetic contribution to the AA lesion can be described as dominant with incomplete penetrance. Hair loss expression can range from loss of vibrissae or small, isolated bald patches on the head through to total hair loss.

Materials and methods

The blood samples used were obtained from 30 DEBR rats with an age range of 1 to 19 months. Control blood samples for comparison were obtained from 15 normal PVG/Ola hooded rats with an age range of 2 to 14 months. 13 AA affected humans with an age range of 20 to 52 years donated blood samples and 5 control blood samples were obtained from normal, healthy humans with an age range of 25 to 51 years. 6 μm tissue sections of rat vibrissae, attached pelage follicles and epidermis were taken from PVG/Ola rats and sections were cut in the same way from normal, human skin biopsies.

The refined indirect immunofluorescence method employed has been described elsewhere in more detail [6]. Briefly, partially purified rat and human sera, diluted 1: 80 in tris-phosphate buffered saline, were applied to frozen tissue sections of normal rat or human hair follicles for 72 hours at 4°C . After incubation with FITC conjugated mouse anti-rat or anti-human antibodies, diluted 1:100 for 1 hour at 4°C , slides were mounted and analyzed for intensity and specificity of staining.

Results

Individual rat and human sera revealed detailed differences in specificity for hair follicle structures. Target tissues for DEBR rat sera were defined as hair cortex and cuticle, and the inner root sheath Henle, Huxley and/or cuticle layers using both rat and human tissue (Figs. 1 and 2). Generally, each rat had similar staining patterns with both tissue types. Human sera also showed variable

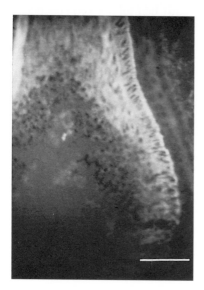

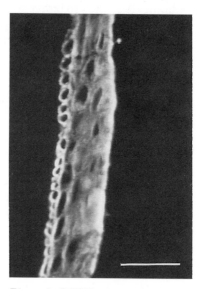

Figure 1. DEBR rat serum on normal rat vibrissae bulb tissue. Specific, positive staining for the hair cortex and cuticle. Bar = 200 μm

Figure 2. DEBR rat serum, different from that used in Fig. 1, on normal human tissue. Positive staining for the inner root sheath Henle, Huxley and cuticle layers. Other, adjacent components of the hair follicle are present but not stained. Bar = 100 μm

staining for the same epidermal structures (Figs. 3 and 4) but there was a less exact correlation between each sera's staining pattern in rat, compared to human tissue. Some human sera also expressed specific staining for the outer root sheath, sebaceous glands and epidermis. In addition some human sera also stained nerve fibres and blood vessel endothelium in rat, but not human tissue.

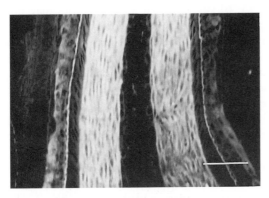

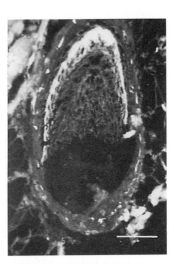

Figure 3. Human serum on rat vibrissae tissue. Intense, positive staining for the hair cortex and inner root sheath cuticle with light staining for the Henle layer. Bar = 200 μm

Figure 4. Human serum, different from that used in Figure 3, on normal human tissue. Intense, positive staining for the inner root sheath. Bar = 200 μm

Non-specific staining was seen in all rat sera whether from control PVG/Ola or DEBR rats for the dermal papilla, dermal sheath, blood sinus and the collagen capsule and with human sera all showed a light non-specific, uniform stain for the dermis. These observations aside, it was clear that 1 of the 15 control sera from PVG rats showed specific positive staining for the inner root sheath Henle layer and 1 of the 5 human control sera may have shown faint staining also for the inner root sheath Henle layer.

Discussion

Previous studies using sera from DEBR rats on normal and lesional rat hair follicles had revealed hair follicle specific IgG autoantibodies which in some cases could be titrated to over 1:1280 and still maintain staining intensity [5, 6]

[S. Drummond-unpublished observations]. Here we attempted to compare and contrast the staining properties of DEBR rat derived autoantibodies and autoantibodies isolated from sera of human AA sufferers. Sera from both DEBR rats and human AA sufferers were able to variably stain hair follicle structures but intriguingly sera from humans contained autoantibodies specific for a wider range of targets compared to sera from DEBR rats.

It is clear that the lesional DEBR rats and humans with AA were able to mount a humoral immune response against hair follicle specific antigens. However, there was apparently no consistent target of attack and the autoantibodies targeted normally expressed hair follicle antigens. This in conjunction with previous studies [5, 6] suggests that autoantibodies may not play a fundamental role in the pathogenesis of AA. In autoimmune diseases where autoantibodies are the primary cause of the disease, such as myasthenia gravis, there is a dominant target of attack found in the majority of sufferers, in this case muscle cell acetyl choline receptors. Autoantibodies may be variably present against other targets which may or may not aid tissue destruction but they can be described as secondary, not necessary for progression of the disease. We are inclined to believe that the hair follicle specific autoantibodies revealed in our studies are secondary to a more important, probably cell mediated insult in AA.

Autoantibodies may arise as a result of a prior, cell mediated attack leading to release of antigenic debris. B cells are not found in significantly elevated numbers around hair follicles [7] and so these antigens are most likely presented to B cells in the lymphoid organs in the usual way to stimulate production of autoantibodies. These autoantibodies are clearly released into the blood stream and as they target normal hair follicle tissue they could potentially have a systemic effect. If the autoantibodies were capable of inducing hair loss independently of mononuclear cells by precipitation of the complement cascade we might then expect the lesion would be relatively uniform over the entire body. It is notable however that the sera used in this study was predominantly derived from rats and humans with limited, distinct patches of AA. Consequently, if the autoantibodies are capable of adversely affecting hair follicles they must require the support of other factors localized at the site of the lesion-the clear candidates being the mononuclear infiltrate cells localized in lesional areas but relatively absent from non-lesional areas. Autoantibodies may accentuate cell mediated tissue disruption by permitting binding of mononuclear cells via their Fc receptors. Alternatively, these autoantibodies may be largely ineffective and their activity only observed at the subclinical level. Another option is that the autoantibodies do not promote hair follicle disruption rather they act as opsonins encouraging phagocytic removal of antigenic particles released into the blood stream as a result of cell mediated activity.

It is notable that autoantibodies targeting the inner root sheath Henle layer could be found at a titration of 1:80 in one control rat serum and one control human serum but that the donors were clinically unaffected with no obvious adverse activity. This would suggest that even in so called normal individuals low levels of circulating hair follicle specific autoantibodies can be produced as part of the normal functioning of the immune system. The function of these autoantibodies is unknown but they apparently do not have a significant clinical effect.

In conclusion, in this study we have shown that hair follicle specific autoantibodies can be found in the sera of human AA sufferers and that they can be revealed using a refined indirect immunofluorescent technique. The autoantibodies are able to target the same tissues as DEBR rat autoantibodies including the hair cortex and cuticle, and the inner root sheath. In addition human sera also targeted the outer root sheath, sebaceous glands and epidermis. The inconsistent staining patterns observed with different sera suggest that these autoantibodies probably arise as a result of antigen exposure from a prior cell mediated attack on hair follicles. We suggest that autoantibodies may play a minor role in accentuating cell mediated activity but are not necessary for the initiation or progression of alopecia areata.

References

1   Editorial. Lancet. 1984; i: 1335-1336
2   Friedmann PS. Br J Dermatol. 1981; 105: 153-157
3   Calver NS, MacDonald Hull S, Parkin SM et al. Br J Dermatol. 1992; 127: 432
4   Tobin DJ, Orentreich N, Fenton DA, Bystryn J-C. J Invest Dermatol. 1994; 102: 721-724
5   McElwee KJ, Pickett P, Oliver RF. J Invest Dermatol. 1995; 104 (Suppl.): 34s-35s
6   McElwee KJ, Pickett P, Oliver RF. Br J Dermatol. 1996; 134: 55-63
7   Zhang JG, Oliver RF. Br J Dermatol. 1994; 130: 405-414

Effects of potent immunotherapies, oral cyclosporin A and topical FK506 in the DEBR rat model for alopecia areata

K.J. McElwee[1], J.G. Lowe[2] and R.F. Oliver[1]

[1]Department of Biomedical Sciences, University of Dundee, Scotland,
[2]Department of Dermatology/Photobiology, Ninewells Hospital, Dundee, Scotland, United Kingdom

Introduction

For the last ten years the Dundee Experimental Bald Rat (DEBR) has been developed as an animal model for alopecia areata (AA) at the University of Dundee. The colony exists as two isogenic substrains, one black hooded, the other brown hooded [1]. All DEBR rats grow a normal coat of hair from birth up to four and a half months of age. However with time up to 30% of males and 80% of females will exhibit clear macroscopic signs of AA and present a mononuclear cell infiltrate in and around hair follicles with a perifollicular $CD4^+ : CD8^+$ T cell ratio of 2 / 1 [2]. In the affected rats the AA lesion can exist as small distinct patches of hair loss through to total body hair loss.

As well as having significant value for use in analyzing the pathogenesis of the lesion, it shows promise as a suitable model for development and evaluation of new and existing therapies for AA. A wide range of treatments are available for AA but none are consistent in their efficacy and many have unwanted side effects.

A considerable volume of work on the effects of therapies on the AA lesion in DEBR rats has been developed in our laboratories [3, 4] including work on several specific immune cell inhibitors. Cyclosporin A (CyA) and FK506 are potent immunosuppressive agents which selectively inhibit $CD4^+$ T lymphocyte activation and proliferation. Here we compare two separate investigations into hair growth responses to oral cyclosporin A and topical FK506 application in the DEBR rat model for AA.

Materials and methods

Cyclosporin A was administered orally as a 10% solution in olive oil to 6 established lesional rats (10 mg/kg 5 days/week for 7 weeks). 6 equivalent control rats received olive oil vehicle alone. FK506 was applied topically as a 0.1% solution in a polyethylene glycol vehicle to 2 cm^2 patches marked on one bald flank of 6 established lesional rats (0.125 μg/mm^2 5 days/week for 8 weeks). A 2 cm^2 patch marked on the opposite flank of each rat received polyethylene glycol vehicle alone. The external appearance of each rat was regularly recorded and a macrophotographic record was taken on days 0, 35 and 56 of treatment. Hair growth continued to be monitored after completion of the therapy course until day 100. To confirm macroscopic observations, sequential skin biopsies taken throughout the duration of treatment were analyzed by histological examination for changes in hair follicle morphology and mononuclear cell infiltrate variations.

Results

Pretreatment, all the rats had large bald flank areas and partial hair loss was also evident on the head and shoulders with vibrissae absent or aberrant (Figs. 1 and 3). Both drugs induced a hair growth response visible as an even regrowth within 19 days from the start of therapy in all treated rats. Systemic CyA induced a whole body response and FK506 induced hair growth within the site of application. By 5 weeks hair growth with both drugs appeared to be nearly equal to a normal pelage coat. This condition was maintained for the duration, and sometimes after completion, of therapy but eventually gradual reinstatement of the AA lesion was observed. Control rats or control regions of skin did not respond with hair growth.

For CyA treated rats hair growth was first seen after 14 days and there was simultaneous regrowth of hair over the whole body. Initial growth existed as a dense fuzz. By day 35 the pelage coat of all rats was fully rehaired with a smooth, soft pelage (Fig. 2). This condition was maintained for the duration of the therapy. From around 80 days there was no further regrowth and eventually hair loss was initiated in all rats.

Analysis of sequential biopsies revealed reduction of the cellular infiltrate associated with conversion of dystrophic anagen follicles to normal, hair-producing follicles for both immunomodulatory drugs.

For our FK506 study hair growth was first seen in three rats fifteen days after the first application and all six rats showed hair production by day 19. Initial growth existed as a dense fuzz limited to the 2 cm^2 site of FK506 application on the right flank. Further hair growth was rapid and by day 35 the pelage coat within the drug application site had apparently reached their respective maximum densities (Fig. 4). By day 56, the final day of drug application for surviving rats, hair growth on the right flanks of 2 rats was good but not as dense as would be expected in a normal coat of hair. The other three rats showed a near perfect pelage coat. Beyond day 56, hair growth continued in all rats until around day 70. From day 77 onwards the hair produced was maintained but no new growth was observed. By day 100 hair loss from the drug site was apparent but the regions could still be clearly distinguished from surrounding skin by the presence of hair.

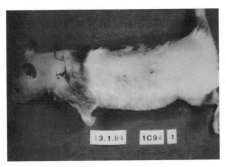

Figure 1. A lesional female DEBR rat aged 12 months at the start of CyA therapy. Complete loss of hair on the shoulders and flanks with extensive hair loss on the head. The hairless hooded area is blue/grey indicating the presence of pigmented anagen bulbs.

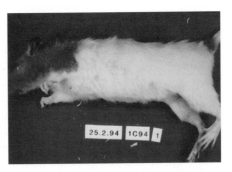

Figure 2. Same rat as figuge 1 after 35 days of orally administered CyA therapy now fully rehaired with a smooth, soft pelage.

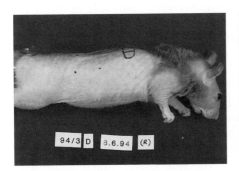

Figure 3. A lesional female DEBR rat aged 12 months at the start of FK506 therapy. Complete loss of hair on the flanks and extensive hair loss on the head. Note total absence of hair in the marked 2 cm² area on the flank.

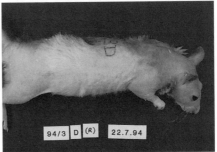

Figure 4. Same rat as figure 3 after 35 days of topically applied FK506 therapy to the 2 cm² patch. The area of drug application is fully rehaired. Note hair loss has continued on the head and shoulders.

Discussion

The antibiotic macrolide FK506 (Prograf ®), like CyA (Sandimmun®), is a specific immune cell inhibitor and although its molecular structure is distinct from CyA, it is known to have similar effects on the immune system [5]. Unlike CyA, systemic FK506, in experimental use, to suppress graft rejection does not have the side effect of hypertrichosis and does not induce hair growth when administered to lesional DEBR rats [6]. Recently however, comparison of topical activity of FK506 and CyA indicated FK506 may have significant potential for treating human skin diseases. Studies on topical application of FK506 to mice have shown its ability to induce anagen in catagen/telogen pelage hair follicles and prolongation of the hair follicles in the anagen growth phase [7]. CyA is known to be not effective when topically applied to the skin of AA patients or DEBR rats. Lack of effect with topical CyA could be a result of poor skin penetrance due to its high molecular weight (MW 1202) [8]. But it does induce hirsutism in non AA patients and hair regrowth in AA sufferers when taken orally [9] and is known to prolong the anagen phase of normal hair follicles *in vitro* [10].

The activity of AA is localized to epidermal appendages and thus it is not necessary nor desirable to immunosuppress an individual's entire immune system. Such blanket immune system disruption using CyA may release AA affected hair follicles from their dystrophic state but it can potentially leave patients partially exposed to infection and side effects including neurotoxicity and impairment of renal function. If the immunomodulation could be limited to specific areas of the skin most if not all adverse drug activity may be avoided. Therefore, topical application of an effective immunomodulatory drug with penetrance limited to the immediate area of application would be an ideal therapy method.

Topical application of FK506 to the 2 cm^2 region coincided with hair growth within that area. This would suggest that FK506 has a localized effect and is not taken up systemically. Indeed, as hair grew at the application site, hair elsewhere on the rats continued to be lost (Figs. 3, 4). Such localized effect bodes well for use in humans while reducing/avoiding the side effects which occur with systemic application. The ability of FK506 to act topically is a significant advantage over systemic use of CyA. In addition FK506 is a superior anti-lymphocytic agent. When used systemically in transplant patients FK506 can be used at concentrations 100 fold lower than CyA concentrations and still have the same immunosuppressive ability.

Our findings in this pilot study show FK506 to have promising potential as a potent topical application for people with AA. Further work should identify threshold dose levels without reducing its ability to promote hair growth. The DEBR model has, and will continue to be vital in analyzing and evaluating therapies for the combat of AA.

References

1   Michie HJ, Jahoda CAB, Oliver RF, Johnson BE. Br J Dermatol. 1991; 125: 94-100
2   Zhang JG, Oliver RF. Br J Dermatol. 1994; 130: 405-414
3   Sundberg JP, Oliver RF, McElwee KJ, King Jr LE. J Invest Dermatol. 1995; 104: 33s-34s
4   Oliver RF, Lowe JG. Clin Exp Dermatol. 1995; 20: 127-131
5   Thomson AW, Carroll PB, McCauley J *et al*. Springer Semin Immunopathol. 1993; 14: 323-344
6   Sainsbury TSL, Duncan JI, Whiting PH *et al*. Transplant Proc. 1991; 23: 3332-3334
7   Jiang H, Yamamoto S, Kato R. J Invest Dermatol. 1995; 104: 523-525
8   Meingassner JG, Stutz A. J Invest Dermatol. 1992; 98: 851-855
9   Gupta AK, Ellis IN, Cooper KD *et al*. J Am Acad Dermatol. 1990; 22: 242-250
10   Taylor M, Ashcroft ATT, Messenger AG. J Invest Dermatol. 1993; 100: 237-239

1996 Elsevier Science B.V.
Hair research for the next millenium
D.J.J. Van Neste and V.A. Randall (Eds)

Hair growth in the skin grafts from alopecia areata (AA) grafted onto severe combined immunodeficient (SCID) nude mice

H. Tsuboi, T. Fujimura and K. Katsuoka

Department of Dermatology, Kitasato University School of Medicine, 1-15-1 Kitasato, Sagamihara, Kanagawa 228, Japan

Introduction

It is known that CD4 positive T lymphocytes are infiltrating around the hair bulbs in the skin lesion of alopecia areata (AA), but the immunological brief mechanisms of T lymphocytes remain unclear. Recently, in our experiments using severe combined immunodeficient (SCID) nude mice, we successfully observed normal hair growth in the grafted AA skin lesion. SCID nude mice are capable of maintaining and proliferating human T cells in the grafted human specimens. We have studied the immunological effects of lymphocytes on the hair growth in the skin grafted onto SCID nude mice.

Materials and methods

Male and female BALB/cA-SCID nu/nu mice were used at ages of 6 to 8 weeks. Mice were obtained from Central Research Laboratory of experimental animals. SCID nude mice were grafted with 6 mm punch skin samples obtained from 3 patients with alopecia areata and 11 with alopecia universalis (AU) (Table 1).

13 of the 14 grafts were successfully accepted in mice and normal hair growth was observed in 12 cases for less than 3 months.

When the hair growth was observed, the mice were sacrificed and the graft areas were taken for HE staining and immunoperoxidase technique. Anti-human CD4 (MT310) and anti-human CD8 (DK25) MoAb were purchased from Dako (Denmark). Anti-human HLA-DR MoAb was obtained from the culture supernatant of mouse hybridoma L243. Immunohistological study was performed both in pre- and post-graft skins obtained from 5 cases.

Table 1.
Patients with alopecia areata

Case No	Age (year)	Sex	Duration (months)	Clinical type
1	20	M	117	Alopecia universalis
2	45	F	17	Alopecia universalis
3	23	F	156	Alopecia universalis
4	30	M	123	Alopecia universalis
5	27	F	240	Alopecia universalis
6	14	M	108	Alopecia universalis
7	60	M	37	Alopecia universalis
8	25	M	24	Alopecia universalis
9	22	M	60	Alopecia universalis
10	18	M	14	Alopecia universalis
11	52	F	18	Alopecia areata
12	43	F	6	Alopecia areata
13	20	F	14	Alopecia areata
14	31	M	72	Alopecia universalis

Results

As shown in figures 1a and 1b, telogen follicles turned to change to anagen in the specimens after grafting, and the cell infiltrates around the bulb area disappeared. In addition, 90 days after grafting, the number of lymphocytes was significantly increased around the upper portion containing the stem cell zone of the follicle (Fig. 1c). Immunohistochemical findings in 5 cases are shown in

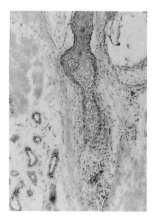

Figure 1a. HE staining, before grafting, x100

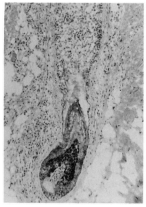

Figure 1b. HE staining, after grafting, x100

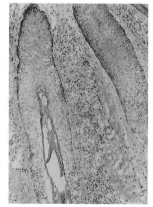

Figure 1c. HE staining, after grafting, x100

Table 2. CD4 positive human T cells were infiltrating around the bulb before grafting (Fig. 2a). After grafting, infiltrates of CD4 positive T cells were present around the upper portion including the stem cell zone of follicles (Fig. 2b). CD8 positive T cells existed around the bulb before grafting, but disappeared after grafting. These infiltrated lymphocytes did not react against anti-mouse H-2Dd. HLA-DR molecules were strongly expressed both in the follicular keratinocytes and infiltrated lymphocytes after grafting (Fig. 2c).

Table 2.
Phenotype and location of infiltrated T cells and HLA-DR expression in follicular keratinocytes

	CD4				CD8				HLA-DR			
	peri-bulb area		peri-bulge area		peri-bulb area		peri-bulge area		keratinocyte of bulb area		keratinocyte of bulge area	
	Before	After	Before	After	Before	After	Before	After	Before	After	Before	After
Patient 1	4+	-	+	4+	2+	+	-	-	+	+	+	2+
Patient 2	2+	-	+	2+	+	-	-	-	+	-	+	2+
Patient 3	4+	+	+	2+	+	-	-	-	+	-	+	2+
Patient 5	2+	-	+	+	+	-	-	-	+	-	+	+
Patient 6	2+	-	+	+	+	-	-	-	+	-	+	+

Number of positive T cells in follicle:

0 : -
0-10 : +
10-50 : 2+
50-100 : 3+
>100 : 4+

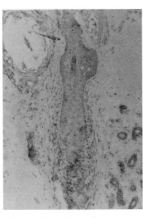

Figure 2a. Anti human CD4 staining, before grafting, x100

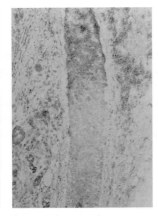

Figure 2b. Anti human CD4 staining, after grafting, x100

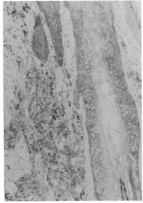

Figure 2c. Anti HLA-DR molecule staining, after grafting, x100

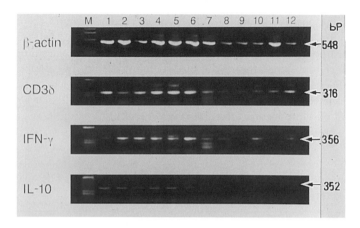

Figure 3. Expression of IFN-γ and IL-10 mRNAs in the specimens from the AA lesions and from the grafted lesions with normal hair growth
Lane 1: Case 1, before grafting   Lane 2: Case 1, after grafting
Lane 3: Case 2, before grafting   Lane 4: Case 2, after grafting
Lane 5: Case 3, before grafting   Lane 6: Case 3, after grafting
Lane 7: Case 4, before grafting   Lane 8: Case 4, after grafting
Lane 9: Case 5, before grafting   Lane 10: Case 5, after grafting
Lane 11: Case 6, before grafting   Lane 12: Case 6, after grafting
M: Molecular weight marker, CD3δ: T-cell marker

We also examined IFN-γ and IL-10 mRNA expression in these specimens before and after grafting using RT-PCR method (Fig. 3). The CD3δ PCR product was detected in all samples. Expression of IFN-γ mRNA was detected in all the samples after grafting. On the other hand, IL-10 was not necessarily expressed in the same samples.

SADBE, one of the contact allergens, is well known to cause hair growth in the patients with AA. For control study, we also investigated the specimens obtained from AA patients before and after treatment with SADBE. Similarly, many lymphocytes were infiltrating around the upper portion of follicles including the stem cell zone. The expression pattern of the cytokine messages showed to be the same as those in the experiments using SCID nude mice (Fig. 4).

Discussion

Th1 type cells have been considered to take important parts in the pathogenesis of AA. Gollnick H. *et al.* showed the expression of the messages of IFN-γ in the skin of AA patients [1] and R. Hoffmann *et al.* demonstrated the

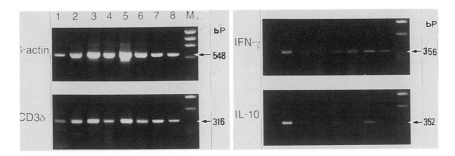

Figure 4. Detection of IFN-γ and IL-10 mRNAs in the specimens obtained from patients with AA before and after treatment with SADBE. M: Molecular weight marker.
Lanes 1, 3, 5, 7: before treatment. Lanes 2, 4, 6, 8: after treatment.

possible involvement of IL-10 in hair regrowth by suppressing IFN-γ [2]. In our studies, the correlation of IL-10 and IFN-γ was not demonstrable. The expression of IFN-γ mRNA was detected in all specimens with hair growth. Only in the specimens with hair regrowth, the histological findings demonstrated the infiltrates of CD4 positive T cells around the upper portion of hair follicles, where the bulge exists. The bulge contains the stem cells which are important in hair growth [3, 4]. Therefore, we considered that the infiltrates of lymphocytes could affect the bulge and result in hair growth in the alopecic skin.

References

1   Gollnick H, Orfanos CE. In: Orfanos CE, Happle R, eds. Hair and Hair Diseases. Berlin: Springer-Verlag, 1990; 529-569
2   Hoffmann R, Wenzel E, Huth A, Steen P van der, *et al.* J Invest Dermatol. 1994; 103: 530-533
3   Lavker RM, Miller S, Wilson C, Cotsarelis G, *et al.* J Invest Dermatol. 1993; 101: 16-26
4   Yang J-S, Lavker RM, Sun T-T. J Invest Dermatol. 1993; 101: 652-659

1996 Elsevier Science B.V.
Hair research for the next millenium
D.J.J. Van Neste and V.A. Randall (Eds)

Genetics and mechanisms of alopecia areata: a mouse model

L.E. King Jr.[1], J.-C. Bystryn[2], D.J. Tobin[2], D. Norris[3], X. Montagutelli,[4, 5] and J.P. Sundberg[5]

[1]Vanderbilt University and Department of Veterans Affairs Medical Center, Nashville, TN, USA
[2]NYU Medical Center, New York, NY, USA
[3]University of Colorado, Denver, CO, USA
[4]The Institut Pasteur, Paris, France
[5]The Jackson Laboratory, Bar Harbor, ME, USA

Human alopecia areata is a relatively common disease characterized by alopecia of acute onset that is focal, diffuse, or combinations of the two. Microscopically, this non-scarring human alopecia consists of dystrophic anagen or telogen hair follicles accompanied by a mononuclear cell infiltrate in and around hair follicles [1, 2]. Comparable diseases have been sporadically reported in domestic animals and some non-human primate species [3]. A spontaneous mutation occurred in the rat which has been developed as an animal model for alopecia areata, designated the Dundee Experimental Bald Rat (DEBR) [4].

A large number of spontaneous and induced mutations with alopecia as a major part of their phenotype are described and most are available through national repositories, such as the one at The Jackson Laboratory [2, 3, 5-7]. Although initial review of the literature and case materials failed to identify a mouse model for alopecia areata, in 1991 a single C3H/HeJ female mouse from a large production colony was diagnosed with what appeared to be alopecia areata. Subsequent investigations have confirmed that alopecia areata occurs spontaneously as an aging disease of very low frequency in this strain. The disease occurs most commonly in females 6 months of age and older and in males that are 12 months and more of age [1]. Crosses set up between affected male and female C3H/HeJ mice have not resulted in a significant increase in incidence. Crosses between affected C3H/HeJ and strains known to not developed alopecia areata that are related (C3HFeB/OuJ) and unrelated (C57BL6J) yielded mice in the F1 generation with alopecia areata indicating that this disease is controlled by at least one dominant or semi-dominant gene with reduced penetrance.

Affected C3H/HeJ mice can be first recognized by a diffuse ventral alopecia that starts on the medial aspects of the proximal portion of the rear legs [1]. Alopecia of the dorsal trunk develops as circular foci that can be solitary or multifocal. These foci wax and wane. Approximately 17% progress to generalized alopecia [1]. Therefore, mice can present a variety of lesions ranging from focal alopecia, large areas of alopecia that appear to involve hair cycle waves, a generalized thinning of the hair coat, to diffuse alopecia [2].

Microscopically, all hair follicle types [2] are affected. Only follicles in anagen are found with a severe mixed inflammatory cell (predominantly lymphocytic) infiltrate in and around the follicles. The isthmus and to a lesser degree the bulb regions are primarily involved. Intrafollicular migration of lymphocytes is associated with disruption of the follicular sheaths, focal necrosis with separation at the junction of the dermal papilla and matrix cells, and structural changes in the hair shaft resulting in focal destruction with loss of pigment [1, 2]. Scanning electron microscopic studies of hairs revealed focal degenerative changes including longitudinal fissures, loss of cuticle, flattening, and breakage with splintering of the hair shafts. The alopecia is due to breaking off of hair shafts as they emerge from the skin.

The lymphocytic infiltrate in and around hair follicles consists predominantly of $CD8^+$ lymphocytes and smaller numbers of $CD4^+$ cells. These can be eliminated by intralesional steroid injections resulting in regrowth of the hair [1].

Full thickness skin grafts from C3H/HeJ mice with alopecia areata onto C3HSmn.C-*scid/scid* mice partially regrew hair. All hairs that grew back in the graft site were white, not the normal agouti color (Sundberg and Boggess, unpublished data). Preferential regrowth of white hair is typical of human alopecia areata.

Preliminary studies using sera from affected mice in indirect immunofluorescence and Western blot assays have revealed that mice with alopecia areata produce antibodies directed to specific proteins in anagen follicles (Tobin and Bystryn, unpublished data). Densitometric measurements of Western blots (semiquantitative) combined with clinical and histological scoring systems have been developed to grade C3H/HeJ mice. We are currently using this system to select mice to search for linkage in DNA extracted from intercrosses between C3H/HeJ mice with alopecia areata and normal C57BL/6J mice as well as backcrosses of their offspring to C57BL/6J mice.

C3H/HeJ mice are readily available from production colonies at The Jackson Laboratory. However, these mice rarely have alopecia areata at the age of shipment (6-8 weeks of age). Mice have to be aged for 8 to 12 months and followed to determine which animals will develop the alopecia areata.

Acknowledgements

This work was supported by grants from the National Alopecia Areata Foundation (JPS, LEK) and the National Institutes of Health (DK44240, JPS; DK26518, LEK); (JCB/DJT); (DN); XM; and research funds from the Department of Veterans Affairs (LEK).

References

1   Sundberg JP, Cordy WR, King Jr. LE. Alopecia areata in aging C3H/HeJ mice. J Invest Dermatol. 1994; 102: 847-856
2   Sundberg JP. Handbook of mouse mutations with skin and hair abnormalities: animal models and biomedical tools. CRC Press, Boca Raton. 1994
3   Sundberg JP, Valle CM, King Jr. LE. Alopecia areata in aging C3H/HeJ Mice. Handbook of mouse mutations with skin and hair abnormalities: animal models and biomedical tools CRC Press, Boca Raton. 1994; 499
4   Oliver R, Jahoda CAB, Horne KA, Michie HJ, Poulton T, Johnson BE. The DEBR rat model for alopecia areata. J Invest Dermatol. 1991; 96: 97S
5   Sundberg JP, Boggess DL, Montagutelli X, Hogan ME, King Jr. LE. The C3H/HeJ mouse model for alopecia areata. J Invest Dermatol. 1995; 104(5): 17-18
6   Conroy JD. Alopecia areata. In: Andrews EJ, Ward BC, Altman NH (eds.). Spontaneous animal models of human disease. Vol. II. Academic Press, New York. 1979; 30-31
7   Muller GH, Kirk RW, Scott DW. Small animal dermatology. 3rd ed., WB Saunders Co., Philadelphia. 1983; 589-592

Double blind placebo controlled study of Dapsone in the treatment of alopecia areata

S. Macdonald Hull and W.J. Cunliffe

Department of Dermatology, Leeds General Infirmary, Leeds, United Kingdom

Introduction

The anti-inflammatory and immunomodulatory effect of Dapsone on regrowth of scalp hair in patients with alopecia areata was studied as a double blind placebo controlled trial over 6 months. The efficacy and incidence of side effects were comparatively evaluated as an estimate of the therapeutic index

Materials and methods

Patients

30 patients with severe alopecia areata (13 patients) or alopecia totalis/universalis (17 patients) entered the study. There were 5 male and 25 female patients. Their age ranged from 16 to 69 years (average: 43.5 years) with an average duration of alopecia of 8.05 years (range: 0.75 - 20 years).

26 patients had received alternative treatment without success: either topical or intra-lesional steroids, Dithranol, topical minoxidil, UVB or topical immunotherapy (diphencyprone).

Patients of child bearing age were advised not to become pregnant while taking part in the study.

Blood sampling

Pre-study investigations included full blood count, urea and electrolytes, liver function tests, glucose-6-phosphate dehydrogenase, pregnancy test (if appropriate).

Further investigations with full blood count and reticulocytes, urea and electrolytes and liver function tests were checked after 2 weeks and then every 4 weeks.

Test drugs

Dapsone 50 mg bd was prescribed as the active agent. Ascorbic acid 50 mg bd was the placebo. Both tablets were dispensed within an identical outer capsule. Patient randomisation was performed by the Pharmacy Department of Leeds General Infirmary. The study was for 6 months.

Each patient gave informed consent after Ethical Committee approval was given. Patients were reviewed monthly.

Results

15 patients were allocated to Dapsone therapy and 15 patients were allocated to placebo. As 2 patients on Dapsone and 2 patients on placebo failed to proceed after randomisation, 13 patients remained in the Dapsone group and 13 patients remained in the placebo group (see Table 1).

Table 1.
Demographics of treated patients

	Dapsone group	Placebo group
Sex ratio (M/F)	4/9	1/12
Age (years)		
mean	47.6	39.4
range	22-65	16-69
Duration of alopecia (years)		
mean	8.0	8.3
range	0.75-20	2-23

Dapsone group

Side effects

7 of the 13 patients on Dapsone withdrew from the study due to side effects.

One patient developed a generalized macular, papular, pruritic rash after 3 weeks of Dapsone. Malaise was experienced by all 7 patients who withdrew. All patients on Dapsone showed a drop in haemoglobin varying between 1.1-3.4 g/dl at 4 weeks. The drop in haemoglobin was greater in those patients who subsequently withdrew from the study. The difference was not statistically significant (Table 2). Reticulocyte counts were not always given, those received varied between 1.0-6.2%. Platelets and white blood cells showed no significant change throughout the study period.

Hair regrowth

Of the 6 patients who completed 6 months of Dapsone therapy, 3 patients, one female with alopecia universalis and 2 males with extensive alopecia areata, had a generalized growth of terminal scalp hair over the whole scalp, one regrew in the androgenetic pattern and 3 patients had no regrowth at all. These were all females with alopecia areata, alopecia totalis and alopecia universalis.

Table 2.
Comparison of drop in haemoglobin after 4 weeks of therapy for patients on Dapsone who withdrew (A) or not (B) from the study (g/dl). Data not available for 3 patients

	A, n= 7	B, n= 6
1	2.3	1.1
2	2.2	1.9
3	1.5	1.4
4	3.5	2.1
5	3.2	-
6	3.4	-
7	-	

Placebo group

Side effects

None of the placebo group withdrew from the study. There were no significant alterations of the full blood count for any patient in the placebo group. 4 of the 13 patients on placebo had some sparse patchy regrowth of vellus hair on the scalp.

Hair regrowth

No patient from either group showed regrowth of facial or bodily hair after 6 months of therapy.

Conclusion

Dapsone appears to have a stimulatory effect on the regrowth of scalp hair in patients with alopecia areata, totalis and universalis. However significant side effects were experienced by 54% of patients on Dapsone. In each case the side effects related to a marked haemolysis and associated drop in haemoglobin concentration. Although Dapsone could be considered as an alternative treatment for alopecia areata, the side effects of this drug render it unacceptable. However, Cimetidine has been shown to have a stabilizing effect on the haematological changes caused by Dapsone [1]. A further study of combined therapy, Dapsone + Cimetidine, should be considered.

Reference

1   Coleman. Dapsone: modes of action, toxicity and possible strategies for increasing patient tolerance. British Journal of Dermatology. 1993; 129: 507-513

©1996 Elsevier Science B.V. All rights reserved.
Hair research for the next millenium
D.J.J. Van Neste and V.A. Randall (Eds)

Systemic cyclosporine and low dose prednisone in the treatment of chronic severe alopecia areata: a clinical and immunopathologic evaluation

J. Shapiro, H. Lui, V. Tron and V. Ho

University of British Columbia Hair Clinic, Vancouver, Canada

Background

Systemic cyclosporine has been shown to be beneficial in the treatment of severe alopecia areata, but the response was not durable. The combination of low dose prednisone and cyclosporine has been reported to maintain remission even after the cyclosporine has been stopped [1, 2].

Objective

Our purpose was to determine in the long term whether the addition of low dose prednisone to cyclosporine can
1) reduce the dose requirement of cyclosporine,
2) produce a durable cyclosporine-free remission. Immunopathologic evaluation of T cell populations were to be analyzed during treatment.

Materials and methods

8 patients with severe alopecia areata were given prednisone 5 mg per day in combination with an initial dose of cyclosporine of 5 mg/kg/day. The dose was adjusted to determine the lowest dose required to maintain hair growth. After 6 months of combined therapy, the treatment was discontinued and the patients followed. Scalp biopsies were taken at baseline, when new hair growth was seen, and at the end of 24 weeks.

Results

2/8 patients showed cosmetically acceptable hair regrowth. In one successful patient, the hair fell out when the cyclosporine was below 4 mg/kg/day. The other one discontinued cyclosporine after 12 weeks due to persistent elevation of serum transaminase.

Side effects included generalized edema, hypertension, abnormal liver function tests and hypertrichosis. Two patients had to discontinue medication due to side effects. The ratio of CD4 + / CD8 + cells in the scalp biopsy specimens was decreased in 6/8 patients with treatment. The two responders were part of this group.

2/8 patients showed an increase of the ratio.

Conclusion

Combination low dose cyclosporine and prednisone therapy is effective in 25% of patients treated. However, contrary to a previous report, remission was not durable after a discontinuation of cyclosporine despite maintenance treatment with low dose prednisone. Cellular infiltrates showed no significant trends during treatment. In view of the potential adverse effects of chronic cyclosporine therapy, this treatment is not generally recommended.

References

1   Gupta A, Ellis C, Cooper K *et al*. Oral cyclosporine for the treatment of alopecia areata. A clinical and immunohistochemical analysis. J Am Acad Dermatol. 1990; 22: 242-250
2   Teshima H, Urabe A, Irie M *et al*. Alopecia universalis treated with oral cyclosporine A and prednisolone: immunologic studies. International J Derm. 1992; 31(7): 513-516

©1996 Elsevier Science B.V. All rights reserved.
Hair research for the next millenium
D.J.J. Van Neste andV.A. Randall (Eds)

A clinical and psychological study on alopecia in children

C.K. Lee, G.Y. Ahn, Y.W. Cho, M.N. Kim and B.I. Ro

Department of Dermatology, College of Medicine, Chung Ang University,
65-207, 3ka Hangang-ro, Yongsan-ku, Seoul 140-757, Korea

Introduction

Alopecia in children shows variable and unpredictable clinical features, poor prognosis, high recurrence rate, and vulnerability to psychiatric trauma. There have been no clinical studies of alopecia in children in Korea. The authors performed a clinical and psychological study on alopecia in children in order to evaluate its clinical characteristics and psychologic dynamics.

Materials and methods

Eighty-two patients with alopecia under the 15 years old who have visited at the Department of Dermatology, Yongsan Hospital, College of Medicine, Chung Ang University from January 1991 to March 1995 were reviewed.

All patients were evaluated for: incidence, clinical classification, age of first visit and school carrier status, duration of the alopecia and recurrence rate, family history, associated diseases, environmental stress factors, and psychologic problems.

Results

Incidence

The incidence of alopecia in children was 1.03% of the total number of new dermatologic non-resident patients.

Clinical classification

Of the eighty two patients, 51 were males and 31 were females. Among them, alopecia areata was most prevalent (52 cases, 63.4%), followed by alopecia totalis (15 cases, 18.3%), trichotillomania (9 cases, 11.0%), and alopecia universalis (6 cases, 7.3%).

Age of first visit and school carrier status

The mean age of first visit was 9.0 years old. According to school carrier status, 22 patients did not reach school age (26.8%), 41 patients were primary school students (50.0%), and 19 patients were middle school students (23.2%).

Duration of the alopecia and recurrence rate

The mean duration was 19.34 months. Previous episodes of alopecia were observed in 20 cases (24.4%). The recurrence rate was highest in alopecia areata (17 patients), followed by alopecia totalis (1 patient), trichotillomania (1 patient), and alopecia universalis (1 patient).

Family history

Family history of alopecia areata was observed in 11.5% (6/52) of alopecia areata cases, 6.7% (1/15) of alopecia totalis, and 33.3% (2/6) of alopecia universalis cases.

Associated diseases

Associated diseases were observed in 40 patients (48.8%); atopic dermatitis was most common (26.0%), followed by seborrheic dermatitis (6.1%), verruca (3.7%) and congenital heart disease (3.7%), etc (Table 1).

Table 1.
Associated diseases with alopecia in children

Associated diseases	Number of patients
Atopic dermatitis	21
Seborrheic dermatitis	5
Verruca	3
Congenital heart disease	3
Thyroiditis	2
Acanthosis nigricans	1
Nephrotic syndrome	1
Tic	1
Myasthenia gravis	1
Sarcoma	1
Asthma	1
Total	40

Position of childhood alopecia in the family

The most common position of childhood alopecia in the family was the eldest sibling (53.7%), and the others were: the youngest sibling (31.5%), middle sibling (7.3%), and only child (4.9%) in the order of frequency.

Environmental stress factors of children with alopecia

45 patients (54.9%) had an environmental stress factor; in the order of frequency: stress due to family relationship (44.0%), stress due to school task (8.5%), stress due to extracurricular education (1.2%), and friendship discord (1.2%) (Table 2).

Table 2.
Environmental stress factors of children with alopecia

Environmental stress factor	Number of patients	
Parents both working	13	
Family discord	8	36 (44.0%)
Broken family	4	
Conflict with siblings	11	
Stress due to school task	7	
Stress due to extracurricular education	1	
Friendship discord	1	
Total	45	

Psychologic problems

On the neuropsychiatric consult, problematic cases were observed in 54.9% (45/82) patients. Neurotic children were the most common problem (15/45), followed by trichotillomania (9/45), anxiety disorder (7/45), and depression (6/45) (Table 3).

Table 3.
Psychologic problems of children with alopecia

Problems	Number of patients
Neurotic child	15
Trichotillomania	9
Depression	6
Anxiety disorder	7
Habit disorder	3
Personality disorder	2
Maternal deprivation	2
Enuresis	1
Total	45

Conclusion

These results suggested that alopecia in children were predominently developed in primary school students. Atopic dermatitis is the most common associated disease. The relationship between parents and children is an important factor in the development of the disease or may contribute as an aggravating factor.

References

1   Teillac D. Alopecia areata in children. Ann Pediatr Paris. 1988; 35: 327-330
2   Clore ER, Corey A. Hair loss in children and adolescents. J Pediatr Health Care. 1991; 5: 245-250
3   Mehregan AH. Trichotillomania. A clinicopathologic study. Arch Dermatol. 1970; 102: 129-133
4   Esterly NB. Alopecia areata symposium. Pediatric Dermatol. 1983; 4: 136-158
5   Oranje AP, Peereboom WJ, de RD. Alopecia areata in children. Tijdschr Kindergeneesk. 1987; 55: 177-181
6   Mendoza BE. Psychosomatics of alopecia areata: apropos of 43 cases. An Esp Pediatr. 1987; 26: 263-266

Androgens and antiandrogens

Workshop report on:

New views on androgens and scalp hair follicle function

S. Takayasu

Department of Dermatology, Oita Medical University, Hasamamachi, Oita, 879-55, Japan

Introduction

Our understanding of the process of androgenetic alopecia started with the studies of Hamilton. He clearly demonstrated common baldness is caused by androgens in genetically predisposed hair follicles. In androgen target cells, circulating testosterone enters the cell, often undergo reduction by 5α-reductase to dihydrotestosterone (DHT), and binds to the androgen receptor. The activated DHT-receptor complex binds to androgen responsive element and interacts with other transcription factors. Although both testosterone and DHT can bind to the same receptor, the DHT-receptor complex acts upon target genes more actively than the testosterone-receptor complex. Recently, two distinct proteins, termed type I and type II 5α-reductases have been identified in the rat, man and very recently cynomologus monkey. Generally speaking, type I is thought to play a catabolic role and is found in the liver and skin, mostly in the sebaceous gland. type II exerts androgenic effects and is abundant in the prostate, human foreskin and beard dermal papilla cells. The dermal papilla cell, a specialized mesenchymal cell, can induce hair follicles in the epithelium obtained from hairless skin. Also from the endocrinological view point, Cunha *et al.* demonstrated that mesenchyme is the actual target of androgen and a mediator of androgenic effects upon epithelium, using recombinants of these two components obtained from prostates of either wild or androgen insensitive mice.

Summary

Dr. Hodgins talked about localization of androgen receptor in human hair follicles, using different kinds of antibodies. The antibody against the N-terminal domain of human androgen receptor specifically stained the nuclei of dermal papilla cells of occipital hair follicles, whereas the epithelial portion of hair follicles was unstained. In contrast, when the antibody against the fusion protein including the DNA-binding domain was used, a much higher concentration of the antibody was required to stain dermal papilla cells and the staining pattern was largely non-specific. The second interesting point is whether androgen receptor is constitutively expressed in the dermal papilla cells. In the occipital and temporal regions, only dermal papilla cells of small hair follicles are stained, while in larger follicles staining is negative. These findings suggest that dermal papilla cells express androgen receptor after they respond to androgens.

Secondly, Dr. Messenger presented his data on the aromatase activity in cultured dermal papilla cells and skin fibroblasts. This enzyme converts testosterone to estradiol. He proposed a hypothesis that oestrogen might cause common baldness. This hypothesis is based on the inhibitory effect of proestrogen on the hair growth in mice. Aromatase activity was detected in cultured skin fibroblasts, but not in any cultured dermal papilla cells. The presence of oestrogen receptor in the skin has not been proved yet. Thus, this interesting hypothesis on the role of oestrogen awaits further research.

Next, Dr. Uno presented a few slides, showing the inhibitory effect of finasteride, a type II 5α-reductase inhibitor, and RU58841, an androgen receptor blocker, on common baldness of stumptailed monkeys. In contrast, type I inhibitor had no effect on the progression of the baldness. Interestingly, both male and female stumptails develop common baldness, although it is more marked in the male. The differences of serum androgen levels between males and females are similar to those between men and women. Therefore, we should study whether androgen metabolism in the bald skin differs between the male and female monkey. Particularly, we should like to know which type of 5α-reductase is present in the hair follicle and dermal papilla cell of this monkey.

Then Dr. Bergfeld talked about androgen excess syndrome with acne, androgenetic alopecia and hirsutism. The key serum androgen we should measure first is dehydroepiandrosterone which is secreted in large amounts by the adrenal gland. However, since only 15% of the patients show abnormal levels of this androgen, other patients may have an abnormal sensitivity of the skin to androgens. In addition, these patients often suffer from obesity, diabetes mellitus, heart attack and uterine cancer, if they are left untreated. She recommended combined therapy with antiandrogen, oestrogen, dexamethasone and minoxidil.

The last contributor, Dr. Adachi indicated gaps between biological and biochemical findings of androgen dependency, quoting hamster sebaceous glands as an example. His group picked up the gene FAR-17, which disappears after castration. Therefore, this gene is androgen-dependent. However, subsequent studies revealed FAR-17 is not directly activated by androgens. Therefore, Dr. Adachi said we have to look for the genes directly activated by androgens, since such genes must play a key role in the action of androgens.

HAIRAN syndrome

F.M. Camacho and M.A. Muñoz

Department of Medical-Surgical Dermatology, Hospital Universitario Virgen Macarena, Facultad de Medicina, Avda. Dr. Fedriani 3, 41071 Sevilla, Spain

Introduction

«HAIRAN syndrome» is a syndrome of familiar virilization. Patients present as hyperandrogenic women (HA) with insulin resistance (IR) and acanthosis nigricans (AN). It is present in 5-50% of women with hyperandrogenism [1-6].

Hyperinsulinemia stimulates the production of ovarian androgens by means of the interaction of insulin-type growth factor-I (IGF-I) with insulin receptors [7-10]. In the ovary, IGF-I has been shown to stimulate the production of androgens in the ovarian stroma. Although acanthosis nigricans is relatively typical for insulin resistance, it is not a «sensitive marker», as less than 30% of women with insulin resistance also present acanthosis nigricans [11]. Nevertheless, hyperandrogenemia is LH-dependent but not insulin-dependent, although insulin may have an amplifying effect. HAIRAN syndrome belongs to the polycystic ovaries syndrome type II [12, 13]. For this reason we have revised 18 cases of polycystic ovaries in fat women with insulin-resistance. We have also studied 50 patients with SAHA to assess the presence of HAIRAN because we know that natural evolution of seborrhoea, acne, hirsutism, alopecia (SAHA) is polycystic ovarian disease [14].

Materials and methods

We have studied a series composed of 50 patients with constitutional hyperandrogenism (SAHA syndrome) and 20 patients with polycystic ovaries syndrome to assess how frequent the HAIRAN syndrome is in these two groups and when it appears during the evolution of SAHA to polycystic ovaries syndrome.

We have also reviewed the biochemical parameters in the «ovarian SAHA», a hyperandrogenism syndrome induced by the excessive production of ovarian androgens, and also in the «suprarenal SAHA» and «hyperprolactinemic SAHA», to assess if the altered biochemical parameters found by us in the polycystic ovarian type II were already altered in the constitutional SAHA, and if they could be used as evolution markers. All familial SAHA, i.e. those with normal hormonal levels, were excluded from the study.

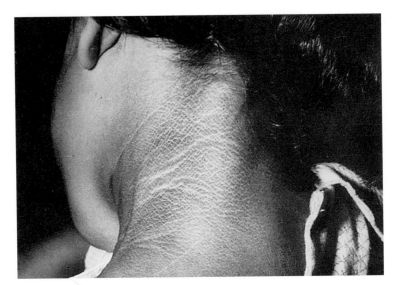

Figure 1. Acanthosis nigricans in a woman with polycystic ovaries syndrome

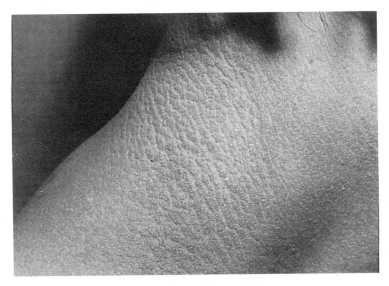

Figure 2. Ovarian SAHA with acanthosis nigricans

Results

We did not find HAIRAN syndrome in any of the 50 cases of SAHA: 18 cases of «ovarian SAHA», 15 cases of «suprarenal SAHA» and 17 of «hyperprolactinemic SAHA». Nevertheless we found 3 cases of acanthosis nigricans amongst the 18 cases of «ovarian SAHA» (Figs. 1 and 2). The biochemical patterns are summarized in Table 1. On the other hand we could verify that 70% of the polycystic ovarian patients presented the whole syndrome, i.e. hyperandrogenism, insulin resistance and acanthosis nigricans; in other words, this was present in those with a longer period of evolution.

Table 1.
Biochemical changes in the 4 patterns of SAHA studied

	SHBG	Δ-4-Androstene-dione	DHEA-S	Prolactin
HAIRAN	N	N or ⬠	N	N
Ovarian SAHA	N	▲	N	N
Suprarenal	N	N	▲	N
Hyperprolactinemia	N	N	N	▲

	Androstane-diol glucuronide	17-hydroxy-progesterone	Free testosterone	Obesity
HAIRAN	N	N or ⬠	N or ⬠	▲
Ovarian SAHA	N or ⬠	N or ⬠	N or ⬠	N or ⬠
Suprarenal	N	*	▲	N
Hyperprolactinemia	N	*	N	N

SHBG: Sex Hormone Binding Globulin
DHEA-S: DehydroEpiAndrosterone-Sulfate
⬠ : *moderately increased*
▲ : *greatly increased*
N: *normal*
*: *not done*

Discussion

We did not find the full HAIRAN syndrome in patients with SAHA. Acanthosis nigricans was only found in those patients with ovarian SAHA and obesity. So acanthosis nigricans is relationed to obesity in SAHA, but it is not a marker of polycystic ovarian disease because we found HAIRAN syndrome in 70% of the fat women with polycystic ovarian disease and insulin-resistance.

References

1 Barbieri RL. Hyperandrogenic disorders. Clin Obstet Gynecol. 1990; 33: 640-654
2 Barbieri RL. Hyperandrogenism: new insights into diagnosis and therapy. Curr Opin Obstet Gynecol. 1991; 3: 316-325
3 Camacho F. Hirsutismo. Diagnostico y tratamiento. Monogr.Dermatol. 1992; 5: 352-373
4 Sperling LC, Heimer WL. Androgen biology as a basis for the diagnosis and treatment of androgenetic disorders in women. I. J Am Acad Dermatol. 1993; 28: 669-683
5 Martin V, Thivelt CH, Bajard L, Thomas L, Faure M. Acanthosis nigricans and insulin resistance in obese patient: a frequent but understimated dermato-endocrinopathy. Eur J Dermatol. 1991; 1: 19-23
6 Gines E, Sotillo I, Herrera E, Camacho F. Acantosis nigricans e insulin resistencia en adolescente. Actas Dermosifiliogr. 1993; 84: 22-24
7 Sharp PS, Kiddy DS, Reed MJ, Anyaoku V, Johnston DG, Franks S. Correlation of plasma insulin and insulin-like growth factor-I with indices of androgen transport and metabolism in women with polycystic ovary syndrome. Clin Endocrinol. 1991; 35: 253-257
8 Mirsa P, Nickoloff BJ, Morhenn VB, Hintz RL, Rosenfeld RG. Characterization of insulin like growth factor-I, somatomedine C receptors on human keratinocyte monolayers. J Invest Dermatol. 1986; 87: 264-267
9 Poretsky L. On the paradox of insulin-induced hyperandrogenism in insulin states. Endocr Rev. 1991; 12: 3-13
10 Pugeat M, Crave JC, Elmidani M, Nicolas MH, Garoscio-Cholet M, Lejeune H, Dechaud H, Tourniaire J. Pathophysiology of sex hormone binding globulin (SHBG): relation to insulin. J Steroid Biochem Mol Biol. 1991; 40: 841-849
11 Cruz PD, Hud JA Jr. Excess insulin binding to insulin-like growth factor receptors: proposed mechanism for acanthosis nigricans. J Invest Dermatol. 1992; 98 (6 suppl): 82S-85S
12 Kahn CR, Flier JS, Bar RS, Ascher JA, Gorden P, Martin MM, Roth J. The syndromes of insulin resistance and acanthosis nigricans. Insulin receptors disorders in man. N Engl J Med. 1976; 294: 739-745
13 Panidis D, Skiadopoulos S, Rousso D, Ioannides D, Panidou E. Association of acanthosis nigricans with insulin resistance in patients with polycystic ovary syndrome. Br J Dermatol. 1995; 132: 936-941
14 Bunker CB, Newton JA, Kilborn J, Patel A, Conway GS, Jacobs HS, Greaves MW, Down PM. Most women with acne have polycystic ovaries. Br J Dermatol. 1989; 121: 675-680

Involvement of androgens *in vivo* and *in vitro* during the dorsal hair growth of castrated rat

A. Ohuchi[1], S. Mitsui[1], M. Hotta[1], M. Hattori[1], R. Tsuboi[2] and H. Ogawa[2]

[1]Biological Science Laboratories, Kao Corporation, 2606, Akabane, Ichikaimachi, Haga, Tochigi, Japan
[2]Department of Dermatology, Juntendo University, 2-1-1, Hongo, Bunkyo-ku, Tokyo, Japan

Introduction

Androgens differentially regulate the growth of human hair, including the beard, axillary hair and frontal scalp hair of genetically predisposed individuals [1]. As for the growth stimulating activity of androgens on the beard, several reports have suggested that androgen receptors are localized in follicular papilla cells, but not in follicular epithelial cells, and that follicular papilla cells secrete soluble mediators to stimulate the proliferation of the epithelial cells in response to androgens [2]. In contrast, androgens regress human frontal scalp hairs, leading to androgenetic alopecia. The growth-inhibiting activity of androgens is poorly understood mainly due to the lack of proper experimental systems. Johnson [3] reported that castration of male rats accelerated the initiation of the third anagen phase in dorsal coat hair, while implantation of testosterone slowed it down, thereby suggesting the androgen-dependent hair growth inhibition in rats. In this study, we developed a castrated rat system by combining it with a culture of isolated hair follicles, and then examined whether androgens affect rat hair growth *in vivo* and *in vitro* so as to analyze the cellular and molecular mechanisms of the androgen-dependent hair regression.

Materials and methods

Castration and testosterone treatment

Male Spraque-Dawley rats were castrated at 6 weeks of age, and were raised with or without testosterone treatment. Testosterone was continuously administered by intraperitoneally implanted osmotic pump, ALZET®. In this system, the rate of testosterone release was approximately 100 μg/day. We histologically observed the morphology of dorsal skin at 8, 9 and 11 weeks of age, and measured the length and the diameter of dorsal hair shafts at 12 weeks of age, when the hair follicles were arrested at the telogen phase. Statistical significance of the difference of two groups was assessed using the Student's t-test.

In vitro study

Hair follicles were prepared from 9-week-old male rats that had been castrated at 6 weeks of age to eliminate the effects of endogenous androgens. For the *in vitro* hair elongation study, hair follicles were isolated and maintained using the method described by Philpott *et al*. [4]. Briefly, hair follicles from dorsal skin dermis were isolated by gentle microdissection, and maintained in serum-free Williams E medium at 31°C, 5 % CO_2-90 % O_2 in 96-well plates, and their length then measured. For DNA synthesis measurement, a large number of hair follicles were prepared from dorsal skin dermis by collagenase treatment (500 units/ml) for 20 min, embedded in collagen gel using 48-well plates and cultured in serum-free Williams E medium. DNA synthesis was measured by ^{3}H-thymidine (1 μCi/ml) incorporation into the cultured hair follicles from day 4 to 6. Total hair DNA content was determined using the fluorometric diaminobenzoic acid method [5].

Immunohistochemistry

Frozen sections of dorsal skin from 9-week-old rats were indirectly stained with a polyclonal anti-androgen receptor antibody as described by Prins *et al*. [6]. Cultured papilla cells prepared from dorsal hair follicles were similarly stained with monoclonal anti-androgen receptor antibody as described by Chang *et al*. [7].

Oligodeoxynucleotides

Phosphorothioate oligonucleotides for a sense (5' GGATGGAGGTGCAGTT AGGGC-3') and its antisense sequence of rat androgen receptor mRNA [8] were used after purification by reverse-phase liquid chromatography. The sense sequence was designed to contain the initiation codon of the rat androgen receptor mRNA. On day 1, the antisense or sense oligonucleotide was added, at a final concentration of 3 μM, to the gel-embedded cultures of the hair follicles prepared from the castrated rats as described above. After 24 hr, 10 ng/ml of testosterone was added to the cultures. As a measure of the hair growth, ^{3}H-leucine (1μCi/ml) incorporation in culture hair follicles from day 4 to 6 was measured.

Results and discussion

We initially examined histologically the *in vivo* effect of castration, with or without testosterone supplement, on the growth of dorsal hair of rat. In the castrated rat, the hair follicle formation had already begun at 8 weeks of age, approximately 1 week earlier than in normal rat, reproducing Johnson's observation [3]. At 9 weeks of age, the hair follicles of the castrated rat were enlarged as compared with those of the normal control. In contrast, the hair follicles of castrated rat supplemented with testosterone had their size reduced to almost that of normal rat. This observation was confirmed by quantitative measurements of the length and the diameter of the hair shafts at 12 weeks of age. Both the length and the diameter in the castrated rat were significantly greater than those of the normal rat, while those of castrated rat supplemented with testosterone were of a similar size to those of normal rat (Table 1). These results indicate that androgens modulate the rat dorsal hair growth in an inhibitory manner.

Table 1.
Effect of castration with or without testosterone supplement, on the size of dorsal hair shafts

Treatment	Length (cm)	Diameter (μm)
Normal rat (n=4)	1.42± 0.10	121.1± 2.6
Castrated rat (n=4)	1.63± 0.06*	167.8± 4.4*
Castrated rat supplemented with testosterone (n=4)	1.44± 0.07**	138.5± 21.6**

* $p<0.05$ *compared with that of normal rat*
** $p<0.05$ *compared with that of castrated rat*

In order to investigate more precisely the role of androgens, we assessed the effect of androgens on the growth of isolated hair follicles. Ten ng/ml of testosterone inhibited the hair follicle elongation by 55 % after 7 days in culture. The DNA synthesis in cultured hair follicles was significantly reduced by the addition of dehydrotestosterone as well as testosterone. Oestradiol-17β and progesterone, however, had little effect on the DNA synthesis. These results suggest that rat dorsal hair follicle is the primary target organ for androgens and that the inhibitory effect might be androgen-specific.

We then examined whether the effect of androgens in hair follicles was mediated by androgen receptors. Immunohistochemical observation of rat dorsal skin revealed androgen receptors in the follicular papilla, but not in the follicular epithelium, which is consistent with the observation in human beard hair follicles [2]. When cultured follicular papilla cells were subjected to immunocytochemical staining with monoclonal anti-androgen receptor antibody, androgen receptors were detected in the nuclei of the papilla cells. The intranuclear localization of the receptor in cultured papilla cells is compatible with that in other typical androgen target cells [6, 7]. These results strongly suggest that papilla cells are the androgen target in the rat dorsal hair follicle.

We further studied the involvement of the androgen receptor in androgen-dependent hair growth inhibition by a functional assay using antisense oligonucleotide complementary to androgen receptor mRNA. Follicular papilla cells were cultured for 24 hours in the presence of 3 μM sense or antisense oligonucleotide. The cells were then reacted with monoclonal anti-androgen antibody and visualized by immunofluorescence. The cells pre-treated with the sense oligonucleotide did not change the fluorescence intensity, while the cells pre-treated with the antisense oligonucleotide dramatically reduced the staining of the nuclei, showing the ability of the antisense oligonucleotide to suppress the expression of androgen receptors in cultured follicular papilla cells. Subsequently, the effect of the antisense oligonucleotide on the testosterone-induced hair growth regression was examined. The pre-incubation with antisense oligonucleotide neutralized the inhibiting effect of testosterone on cultured hair follicles (Table 2). The sense oligonucleotide had no effect on the testosterone-induced protein synthesis inhibition. The pre-incubation with sense or antisense oligonucleotide had no effect on the protein synthesis of cultured hair follicles without testosterone, denying the non-specific toxic effect of the oligonucleotides to the cells at the concentration used. These results suggest that androgen receptors mediate the androgen-dependent growth inhibition of rat dorsal hair.

In summary, these results suggest that circulating androgens regress rat dorsal hair growth through their binding to androgen receptors located in the papilla cells. Considering the importance of epithelial-mesenchymal interaction in hair growth and development [9, 10], we expect that androgens might exert their effect by modulating the interactions between the papilla and the epithelium.

Table 2.
Effect of the antisense oligonucleotide on testosterone-induced protein synthesis inhibition in castrated rat hair follicle

Treatment	Pre-treatment		
	None	Sense oligo	Antisense oligo
No-treatment	83023±7409	79798±4110	81376±5500
Testosterone	67526± 710	62415±1842	77978±4936*

p<0.05 compared with that of pre-treatment with sense oligonucleotide

References

1   Ebling FJG. Clin Endocrinol Metab. 1986; 15: 319-339.
2   Itami S, Kurata S, Sonoda T, Takayasu S. Br J Dermatol. 1995; 132: 527-532
3   Johnson E. J Endocrin. 1958; 16: 351-359
4   Philpott MP, Green MR, Kealey T. Br J Dermatol. 1992; 127: 600-607.
5   Fiszer-Szafarj B, et al. Analyt Biochem. 1981; 110: 165-170.
6   Prins GS, Birch L, Green GL. Endocrinology. 1991; 129: 3187-3119.
7   Chang C, Chodak G, et al. J Steroid Biochem. 1989; 34: 311-313.
8   Chang C, Kokontis J, Liao S. Pro Natl Acad Sci. USA. 1988; 85: 7211-7215
9   Oliver RF. J Embryol Exp Morphol. 1967; 18: 43-51
10 Warren R, Wong TK. Arch Dermatol Res. 1994; 286: 1-5

Hair research for the next millenium
D.J.J. Van Neste and V.A. Randall (Eds)

Androgen induction of follicular epithelial cell growth is mediated via insulin-like growth factor-I from dermal papilla cells

S. Itami, S. Kurata and S. Takayasu

Department of Dermatology, Oita Medical University, Hasamamachi, Oita, 879-55, Japan

Introduction

Androgens are known to regulate the growth of some sorts of hair, including the beard, axillary hair and frontal scalp hair of genetically predisposed individuals [1]. Although the process of regulation of hair growth by these hormones is still unclear beard and axillary dermal papilla cells were recently shown to possess the characteristics of androgen target cells [2-6]. Beard dermal papilla cells possess a higher 5α-reductase activity and a larger amount of androgen receptors than reticular dermal fibroblasts or dermal papilla cells from the occipital scalp [2-5]. Besides, the enzyme found in beard dermal papilla cells appears to be type II 5α-reductase [4], and axillary dermal papilla cells show a low 5α-reductase activity, corresponding to type I 5α-reductase [5]. In contrast, follicular epithelial cells do not have the characteristics of androgen target cells [3, 6, 7]. Although androgen itself does not have a proliferative effect on either type of cells when cultured alone, androgen significantly stimulated the proliferation of follicular epithelial cells which were cocultured with beard or axillary dermal papilla cells [5, 6]. No such effect was observed when dermal papilla cells from occipital scalp hair follicles were used in the cultures. These findings suggest that beard and axillary dermal papilla cells produce androgen-dependent diffusible growth factors which stimulate follicular epithelial cells.

Will the aim of investigating the molecular basis of the action of androgens on beard growth, we studied the influence of androgen on the expression of mRNA of several growth factors which have been reported to affect the growth of hairs in beard dermal papilla cells by reverse transcriptase-polymerase chain reaction (RT-PCR).

Materials and methods

The methods used for isolating and culturing dermal papilla cells and outer root sheath cells are described elsewhere [4-6]. All experiments were performed on cells in the third to fourth passage of subculture. Beard dermal papilla cells were cultured to subconfluence in Dulbecco's modified Eagle's medium (DMEM) supplemented with 10% FCS, then in DMEM with 2% FCS containing 10^{-9}M R1881 and/or cyproterone acetate for 48h. Outer root sheath cells were cultured in KGM. The cells were harvested after 48h and total RNA was isolated by the acid guanidinium thiocyanate-phenol-chloroform method. One hundred nanograms of total RNA of each sample was reverse transcribed and the resultant cDNA was amplified using a thermal cycler in a final volume of 25 µl. The oligonucleotide primers for PCR were based on published mRNA sequences and were summarized in Table 1. PCR amplification was performed for 32 cycles for human insulin-like growth factor-I (IGF-I), basic fibroblast growth factor (bFGF), hepatocyte growth factor (HGF) and keratinocyte growth factor (KGF), 30 cycles for human IGF-I receptor (IGF-I-R) and 18 cycles for glyceraldehyde-3-phosphate dehydrogenase (G3PDH). The products were analyzed on 2% agarose gel electrophoresis.

For the coculture experiments beard dermal papilla cells were cultured in DMEM supplemented with 10% charcoal-treated FCS and then were plated at a density of 0.8×10^4 cells/cm^2 in the lower compartment of Transwell culture dishes. After 24h, beard outer root sheath cells (1×10^4/cm^2) were added to the upper compartment of the dishes. The two types of cells were then cocultured for 5 days in MCDB 153 medium without growth factors in the presence of 10^{-9}M methyltrienolone (R1881) and/or 10^{-7}M cyproterone acetate. In some experiments, various concentrations of neutralizing antibody for human IGF-I was added to such cultures. After culture for 5 days, the total number of cells in each dish was counted by an automatic cell counter.

Table 1.
Polynucleotides used in this study

		Primers	Position	Size (bp)
KGF	Sense	5'-GCAAACAGCGTCACAGCAAC	190 - 209	831
	Anti-sense	5'-GCCATAGGAAGAAAGTGGGC	1001 - 1020	
bFGF	Sense	5'-CTTTGGCTGCTACTTGGAGG	1983 - 2002	975
	Anti-sense	5'-TGTAGAGACGGGGTTTCACC	2958 - 2957	
HGF	Sense	5'-GAATGCATCCAAGGTCAAGC	1011 - 1020	868
	Anti-sense	5'-AATCATCCAGGACAGCAGG	1859 - 1878	
IGF-I	Sense	5'-GGTGGATGCTCTTCAGTTCG	340 - 359	882
	Anti-sense	5'-CCACAGATGGAATCTTGTGG	1202 - 1221	
IGF-I-R	Sense	5'-AATAACATTGCTTCAGAGCTG	1147 - 1167	933
	Anti-sense	5'-GATGGTGCCGTCGGCATACTT	2059 - 2079	
G3PDH	Sense	5'-CCCATCACCATCTTCCAG	250 - 267	577
	Anti-sense	5'-CCTGCTTCACCACCTTCT	809 - 826	

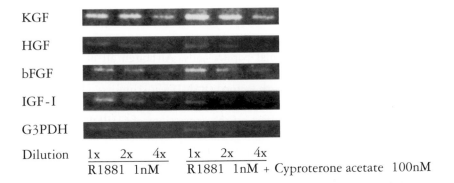

Figure 1. Effect of androgen on the expression of several growth factor mRNAs in beard dermal papilla cells. Cells were treated by R1881 and/or cyproterone acetate. RNAs were serially diluted and reverse transcribed.

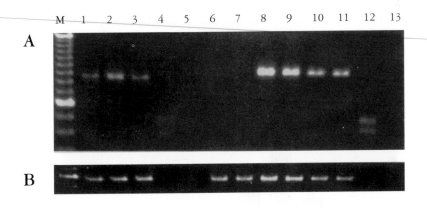

*Figure 2. Expression of IGF-I and IGF-I receptor in dermal papilla cells and outer root sheath cells (**A**). IGF-I expression was detected in beard dermal papilla cells (lanes 1, 2, 3), but not in outer root sheath cells (lanes 6, 7). IGF-I receptor expression was detected in both dermal papilla cells (lanes 8, 9) and outer root sheath cells (lanes 10, 11). Cells were cultured in the presence of R1881 (lanes 2, 7, 9, 11) or R1881 and cyproterone acetate (lane 3). Controls (lanes 1, 6, 8, 10) were prepared as described in Materials and methods. To confirm the identity of the products, aliquots were digested with restriction endonuclease (lanes 4, 12). Lanes 5 and 13 are controls for genomic DNA contamination. M, size markers. The expressions of G3PDH mRNA of each sample were shown in (**B**). (From Itami et al. {8}. Reprinted by permission from Academic Press, Inc.)*

Results and discussion

We examined the effect of androgen on the expression of IGF-I, KGF, bFGF and HGF mRNAs in beard dermal papilla cells. Although all of the growth factor mRNAs were specifically expressed in the beard dermal papilla cells, only the expression of insulin-like growth factor-I (IGF-I) was stimulated by androgen (Fig. 1). Androgen clearly upregulated the IGF-I mRNA expression by beard dermal papilla cells, but had no affect on the expressions of G3PDH in the cells (Fig. 2). This enhancement was antagonized by cyproterone acetate. IGF-I mRNA was not expressed in the outer root sheath cells. Outer root sheath cells and beard dermal papilla cells also specifically expressed IGF-I receptor mRNA; the expression was not affected by the addition of androgen in either type of cell.

When outer root sheath cells were cultured together with beard dermal papilla cells, the proliferation of outer root sheath cells was significantly stimulated by the addition of androgen (Fig. 3). Since cyproterone acetate antagonizes this stimulatory effect of androgen, the effect is apparently mediated by the androgen receptor pathway. In contrast, the proliferation of dermal papilla cells was not affected by the addition of androgen even in a coculture condition. Neutralizing antibody against human IGF-I inhibited the proliferation of outer root sheath cells and antagonized the androgen-elicited stimulative effect on the outer root sheath cells in a dose dependent manner, but did not inhibit the proliferation of beard dermal papilla cells (Fig. 4). Therefore, the stimulatory

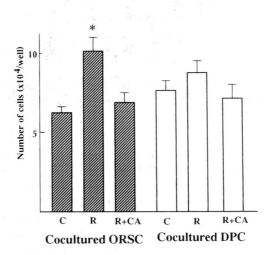

*Figure 3. Effect of R1881 and cyproterone acetate on the proliferation of beard dermal papilla cells and outer root sheath cells. Cells were cocultured in the presence of R1881 (R) or with both R1881 and cyproterone acetate (R+CA). Control cells (C) were cultured with vehicle alone. DPC, dermal papilla cells; ORSC, outer root sheath cells. *$p<0.05$ vs. the respective control.*

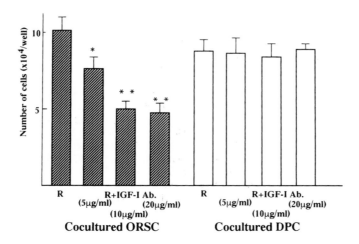

Figure 4. The influence of neutralizing antibody against human IGF-I on the proliferation of androgen-stimulated outer root sheath cells cocultured with beard dermal papilla cells. *p<0.05, **p<0.01 vs. culture without IGF-I antibody. (From Itami et al. {8}. Reprinted by permission from Academic Press, Inc.)

effect of androgen on the growth of outer root sheath cells in our coculture system is probably mediated by IGF-I derived from dermal papilla cells in a paracrine fashion.

Insulin-like growth factor-I (IGF-I) is a paracrine/autocrine growth factor in many organs and its expression is normally limited to mesenchymal cells. IGF-I has been found to stimulate human hair growth *in vitro* at physiological concentrations and to prevent the premature entry of cultured hair follicles into catagen [9]. Null mutant mice for the IGF-I receptor gene show a marked decrease in the absolute number of hair follicles [10]. These observations indicate that the IGF-I receptor pathway is essential for the growth and differentiation of hair follicles. Besides, IGF-I mRNA expression is localized to cells of mesenchymal origin in the skin of human fetus [11]. This finding correlates well with our present data which localized IGF-I mRNA expression in dermal papilla cells, but not in outer root sheath cells. Lack of androgen receptor [3, 6] and the expression of IGF-I mRNA in outer root sheath cells further suggests that androgen exerts its effect on the outer root sheath cells through dermal papilla cells. This is in contrast to the prostate, where both epithelium and stroma possess androgen receptors [12].

In conclusion, our present data show that beard dermal papilla cells are androgen target cells and that IGF-I is a candidate for one of androgen-induced growth factors for follicular epithelial cells produced by dermal papilla cells in a paracrine fashion.

References

1 Hamilton JB. Am J Anat. 1942; 71: 451-480
2 Randall VA, Thornton M, Messenger AG. J Endocrinol. 1992; 133: 141-147
3 Choudhry R, Hodgins MB, Van der Kwast TH, Brinkman AO, et al. J Endocrinol. 1992; 133: 467-475
4 Itami S, Kurata S, Sonoda T, Takayasu S. J Invest Dermatol. 1991; 96: 57-60
5 Itami S, Kurata S, Sonoda T, Takayasu S. Ann NY Acad Sci. 1991; 642: 385-395
6 Itami S, Kurata S, Sonoda T, Takayasu S. Br J Dermatol. 1995; 132: 527-532
7 Sonoda T, Itami S, Kurata S, Takayasu S. J Dermatol Sci. 1993; 6: 214-218
8 Itami S, Kurata S, Takayasu S. Biochem Biophys Res Commun. 1995; 212: 988-994
9 Philpott M, Sanders D, Kealey T. J Invest Dermatol. 1994; 102: 857-861
10 Liu J, Baker J, Perkins AS, Robertson EJ, et al. Cell. 1993; 75: 59-72
11 Han VKM, D'Ercole AJ, Lund PK. Science. 1987; 236: 193-197
12 Prins GS, Birch L, Greene GY. Endocrinol. 1991; 129: 3187-3199

Testosterone inhibits the capacity of cultured balding scalp dermal papilla cells to produce keratinocyte mitogenic factors

N.A. Hibberts and V.A. Randall

Department of Biomedical Sciences, University of Bradford, Bradford, West Yorkshire, BD7 1DP, United Kingdom

Androgenetic alopecia

Androgenetic alopecia or male pattern baldness affects a large number of people, and although this condition is prevalent worldwide, the incidence and severity is dependent upon the individual's racial origin; Caucasian males have a higher incidence of male pattern baldness than Oriental males or American Indians [1]. This condition is characterized by a gradual regression of the frontal hair line, and in severe cases, the central crown regions of the scalp are also affected.

Although the involvement of androgens in male pattern baldness had been frequently speculated upon, it was only when the American anatomist, Hamilton, observed that men who had been castrated before puberty did not go bald, and the balding process was halted in individuals who were castrated in later life, that the correlation between androgens and balding was made [2]. Subsequently, Ludwig [3] used the term androgenetic alopecia, combining «androgen» and «genetic», and stated that «androgen cannot produce common baldness without an inherited genetic disposition, and an inherited genetic disposition cannot produce baldness without androgen.»

Androgens and the hair follicle

The human hair follicle is affected by several hormones, including glucocorticoids [4], thyroid hormones [5] and those involved in pregnancy [6]. However, androgens are the most obvious regulators of human hair growth. At puberty, the growth of the beard is stimulated in males, and in both sexes, a characteristic pattern of axilla and pubic hair growth is observed. Paradoxically, the same levels of circulating androgens may cause the regression of hair follicles in androgen-sensitive scalp hair follicles, whilst appearing to have no effect on non-balding ones (reviewed in [2]). This suggests a differential response to androgens by the hair follicle depending upon the anatomical site (Fig. 1).

The role of the dermal papilla

The hair follicle is a three dimensional tube of epithelial cells which protrudes through the epidermis and dermis containing in its bulb, the mesenchyme-

304

derived dermal papilla. Hair growth is not continuous but cyclic, with a growing anagen phase, a resting telogen phase, and a short transitory catagen phase. It is believed that the dermal papilla plays an important role in the regulation of the hair cycle and in control of human hair growth e.g. hair diameter. Androgens probably act on the hair follicle via the mesenchyme-derived dermal papilla causing the production of soluble mitogenic factors, which then influence the surrounding epithelial cells [7]. Hibberts *et al.* [8] have shown that testosterone is responsible for stimulating beard dermal papilla cells to produce additional mitogenic factors which stimulate skin keratinocytes. In addition, Itami *et al.* [9] have shown that beard dermal papilla cells are capable of increasing the uptake of ^{3}H-thymidine of outer root sheath cells in a co-culture system.

The culture of dermal papilla cells derived from beard, non-balding scalp, axilla and pubic hair follicles is well established [10]. It has been shown that cultured dermal papilla cells *in vitro* retain characteristics that are dependent on their *in vivo* properties. Various authors have demonstrated that beard dermal papilla cells contain higher levels of androgen receptors, the ability to produce additional mitogenic factors and a greater 5α-reductase capacity than non-balding scalp ones [11-13]. Reynolds *et al.* [14] have reported that cultured dermal papilla cells retain the ability to induce hair follicle formation *in vitro*, supporting the validity of studying these cells in culture.

The culture of dermal papilla cells from balding scalp hair follicles has only recently been reported [15]. Balding scalp hair follicles are considerably smaller

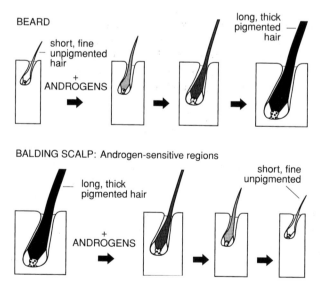

Figure 1. Androgens stimulate changes in hair follicle, gradually increasing the size of those in many areas such as the face, whilst simultaneously inhibiting follicles in androgen-sensitive scalp regions in genetically susceptible individuals

than those from non-balding scalp, hence creating considerable technical difficulties in the culture of these cells. Cultured balding scalp dermal papilla cells have been shown to exhibit typical aggregative behaviour, but grow significantly slower than non-balding scalp dermal papilla cells and show a greater dependency on factors present in human serum. In addition, cultured balding scalp dermal papilla cells have been shown to contain higher levels of specific androgen receptors than those present in non-balding scalp ones [16].

Experimental design

This study was designed to investigate the production of mitogenic factors produced by balding and non-balding scalp dermal papilla cells, using the incorporation of ^{3}H-thymidine by the skin epithelial cell line NCTC 2544. Further investigations were carried out to determine whether testosterone was capable of further stimulating these cells to produce additional factors.

Cell culture

The culture of dermal papilla cells was carried out as described in [15]. Briefly, full depth skin biopsies were obtained from balding and non-balding scalp. Using microdissection techniques, the dermal papilla was removed from each hair follicle and 3-5 such dermal papilla were placed in a sterile 35 mm tissue culture dish containing medium E199 + 20% pooled female human serum. Dishes were examined after 14 days and cells were passaged into 25 cm^2 flasks when sufficient cells were present. Corresponding lines of balding scalp dermal fibroblasts were also established. Dermal papilla cells, dermal fibroblasts and the continuous skin epithelial cell line, NCTC 2544 were routinely subcultured in medium E199 containing 10% fetal calf serum (FCS).

Collection of conditioned medium

Balding and non-balding scalp dermal papilla cells and balding scalp dermal fibroblasts were cultured to confluency in medium E199 containing 10% FCS. Cells were then washed in PBS (x4) and incubated in serum-free medium E199 ± 10 nM testosterone for 24 hours. The conditioned medium was then sterile filtered and stored at -20°C until required.

Analysis of conditioned medium

The incorporation of ^{3}H-thymidine by skin keratinocytes, NCTC 2544 was used to analyze the mitogenic effects of the conditioned medium. The keratinocytes were seeded at 2.5×10^3 cells/well in 96 well plates and incubated for 72h in normal growth medium, cells were washed with PBS (x2) and incubated for 6h in serum free medium E199 before incubation for 18h in test medium containing 500nM cyproterone acetate.

Fresh test medium containing 0.5 µCi/ml ^{3}H-thymidine was added and incubated for 2h. Cells were then washed in PBS (x2), digested in 2M NaOH for 18h at 4°C and the extracts counted in duplicate.

Results

Conditioned medium produced by balding and non-balding scalp dermal papilla cells and balding scalp dermal fibroblasts, in the presence, or absence, of testosterone increased the uptake of ^{3}H-thymidine by the keratinocytes above control levels (p < 0.001; Mann-Whitney U test). However, only medium conditioned by balding scalp dermal papilla cells in the presence of testosterone reduced the uptake by 35% compared to medium conditioned in the presence of the ethanol vehicle alone (p < 0.05).

Discussion

Dermal papilla cells and dermal fibroblasts are capable of secreting soluble mitogenic factors in culture which influence the skin epithelial cell line, NCTC 2544. However, it is only conditioned medium produced by balding scalp dermal papilla cells, in response to physiological levels of testosterone, that has a reduced capacity to stimulate the growth of the keratinocytes. This effect may be due to the dermal papilla cells producing an inhibitory compound, or conversely, reducing synthesis of stimulatory factors. This exciting result is what might be expected from observing the effects of androgens on balding scalp hair follicles *in vivo*. Further analysis of the soluble mitogenic factors in dermal papilla conditioned medium should enable a greater understanding of the roles of androgens in human hair growth.

References

1   Hamilton JB. Ann NY Acad Sci. 1951; 53: 708-728
2   Hamilton JB. Am J Anat. 1942; 71: 451-480
3   Ludwig E. Hautarzt. 1962; 13: 337-339
4   Stenn KS, Paus R, Dutton T, Sarba B. Skin Pharmacol. 1993; 6: 125-134
5   Jackson D, Church RE, Ebling FJ. Br J Dermatol. 1972; 87: 361-367
6   Lynfield YL. J Invest Dermatol. 1960; 35: 323-327
7   Randall VA. Clin Endocrinol. 1994; 40: 439-457
8   Hibberts NA, Quick JR, Messenger AG, Randall VA. Br J Dermatol. 1994; 131(suppl): 427
9   Itami S, Kurata S, Sonoda T, Takayasu S. Br J Dermatol. 1995; 132: 527-532
10 Messenger AG. Br J Dermatol. 1984; 110: 685-689
11 Randall VA, Thornton MJ, Messenger AG. J Endocrinol. 1992; 133: 141-147
12 Randall VA, Thornton MJ, Hamada K, Redfern CPF, Nutbrown M, Ebling FJ, Messenger AG. Ann NY Acad Sci. 1991; 642: 355-375.
13 Itami S, Kurata S, Sonoda T, Takayasu S. J Invest Dermatol. 1991; 96: 57-60
14 Reynolds AJ, Jahoda CAB. Ann NY Acad Sci. 1991; 642: 226-242
15 Randall VA, Hibberts NA, Hamada K. Br J Dermatol. 1996; 134: 437-444
16 Hibberts NA, Randall VA. J Endocrinol. 1993; 137 (suppl); P55

Dermal papilla cells in macaque alopecia trigger a testosterone-dependent inhibition of follicular cell proliferation

N. Obana and H. Uno

Regional Primate Research Center, University of Wisconsin, Madison, Wisconsin 53715, U.S.A.

Introduction

In 1969, Oliver, as a pioneer on experimental works of the dermal papilla, hypothesized that interaction of the dermal papilla cells with follicular epithelial differentiation is probably of the same nature as embryonic induction, continues throughout life and maintains the functional integrity of the adult follicles [1]. Later, his colleagues demonstrated an inductive capacity of cultured dermal papilla cells implanted as pellets into the base of follicles from which the lower halves had been removed [2]. Based on these studies, further work on the mechanism of androgens on the sexual hairs in studies on dermal papilla derived from the beard hair follicle has suggested an important role for the stimulatory actions of androgens [3, 4]. Androgens have paradoxically different effects on human hair follicles depending on their site. They stimulate hair growth in many sites, such as the beard and pubis, but can cause regression on the scalp in genetically disposed individuals [5]. Their inhibitory actions using the cultured dermal papilla cells derived from the bald scalp have not been examined.

The frontal alopecia which develops in postpubertal stumptailed macaques is known as a pertinent model of human androgenetic alopecia [6-8]. We examined the effect of testosterone on interactions between outer root sheath (ORS) cells and dermal papilla (DP) cells derived from the bald frontal scalp skins of stumptailed macaques.

Materials and methods

Both bald frontal (male and female, 7-12 year) and occipital scalp skins (male and female, 6-13 year) were obtained from stumptailed macaques using a 4 mm punch. The DPs were isolated under the microscope (x180) and cultured with Dulbecco's modified Eagle's medium (DMEM) supplemented with Testosterone-free fetal bovine serum (FBS). Cells were subcultured after trypsin treatment 4 weeks after the beginning of primary cell cultures. For the culture of ORS cells, the hair follicles were dissected from the occipital skin and treated with 0.2% collagenase in DMEM for 30 min at 37 °C in order to remove the connective tissues. After rinsing with phosphate buffered saline without calcium or magnesium, the hair follicles were transferred into the dishes and cultured with DMEM supplemented with 10% FBS, epidermal growth factor (10 ng/ml), insulin (5 µg/ml) and hydrocortisone (0.5 µg/ml). On the fourth day, media were changed to keratinocyte growth medium (KGM) containing epidermal growth factor (10 ng/ml), insulin (5 µg/ml), hydrocortisone (0.5 µg/ml), and bovine pituitary extracts. Second- and third-passage cells were used. For coculture of DP cells and ORS cells, DP cells were inoculated at a density of 1×10^4 cells/well into type I collagen coated multiplates and cultured with DMEM supplemented with 10% charcoal-treated FBS. After 24h incubation, the media were discarded and ORS cells (1.5×10^4 cells/well) were added with KGM without bovine pituitary extracts. Some ORS cells were cultured in cell culture inserts coated with type I collagen and those inserts were placed in the wells in which DP cells had been cultured on the bottom, as described above.

Results

The mean longitudinal length of the isolated DP derived from the bald frontal scalp skin (FDP) was 75.0 ± 5.2 µm and that of the occipital scalp skin (ODP) was 153.1 ± 4.8 µm. The mean population doubling time of FDP cells (69.0 ± 5.9 h) was significantly ($p < 0.01$) longer than that of ODP cells (39.5 ± 4.1 h). Testosterone ($10^{-10} \sim 10^{-7}$M) showed no effects on proliferation of either type of cultured DP cells and testosterone (10^{-10}M) had no effect on proliferation of cultured ORS cells. When FDP and ORS cells were cocultured in the same well, their total cell number significantly increased compared to the sum of the number of FDP and ORS cells cultured alone (Fig. 1). Testosterone (10^{-10}M) completely inhibited the cell proliferation enhanced by coculture. RU58841, a potent non-steroidal androgen receptor blocker, antagonized this testosterone-elicited inhibition. The total number of cocultured ODP and ORS cells was not affected by testosterone.

Furthermore, FDP and ORS cells were cocultured using a cell insert, which separated the two cell types by a collagen coated membrane (Fig. 2). The coculture led to increased numbers of ORS cells and testosterone inhibited this stimulation of proliferation. The number of cultured FDP cells was not affected by coculture or testosterone.

Discussion

To our knowledge, this is the first data demonstrating the inhibitory effect of testosterone on proliferation of ORS cells, which were cocultured with DP cells derived from the bald frontal scalp of the macaque. This study showed the inhibitory effect of testosterone only when FDP cells and ORS cells were

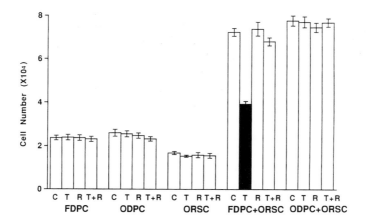

Figure 1. *Effect of testosterone on proliferation of DP cells and ORS cells cocultured in the wells.*
ORS cells with or without testosterone ($T;10^{-10}$ M) and/or RU 58841 ($R;10^{-10}$ M) were added one day after cultivation of DP cells and cells were counted seven days after the start of cultivation. Each value represents the mean ±SE (n=6). C, control; FDPC, bald frontal DP cells; ODPC, occipital DP cells; ORSC, ORS cells.

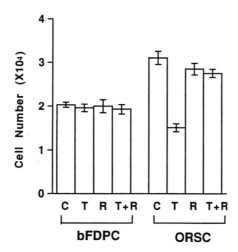

Figure 2. *Inhibitory effect of testosterone on proliferation of ORS cells cocultured with balding frontal DP cells. Cell inserts with ORS cells (ORSC) were placed in the wells in which bald frontal DP cells (FDPC) had been cultured on the bottom. Testosterone ($T;10^{-10}$ M) and/or RU 58841 ($R;10^{-10}$ M) were added one day after cultivation of FDPC. ORSC and FDPC were separately counted 7 days after cultivation of FDPC. Each value represents the mean ± SE (n=6).*

cocultured, although testosterone by itself showed no effects on proliferation of either type of cells cultured alone. These results are comparable with the results, using beard follicles, whereby testosterone showed no effects on [³H] thymidine uptake by the dermal papilla cells cultured alone [3]. Also, DNA synthesis was enhanced by testosterone when the DP cells and ORS cells were cocultured [4], suggesting that the DP cells are primary target cells of androgens. We suggest that testosterone inhibits proliferation of epithelial cells via the FDP cells and this effect is mediated by an androgen receptor. The FDP cells cultured without testosterone can still secrete the soluble substances, which can stimulate proliferation of ORS cells. The involvement of soluble substances provided by DP cells derived from other androgen-sensitive or -insensitive hair follicles has also been demonstrated in *in vitro* studies [4, 9-11]. Although these soluble mitogenic substances are still unknown, there are two possibilities of an inhibitory mechanism of testosterone. Testosterone can combine with its receptors after diffusing the plasma membrane and also may be metabolized intracellularly by the enzyme 5α-reductase to 5α-dihydrotestosterone, which can also bind and activate the androgen receptor. One possibility is that these testosterone-receptor complexes might directly change the gene expressions of FDP cells in order to prevent the production and secretion of soluble mitogenic substances. Another one is that unknown inhibitory substances produced by testosterone-receptor complexes in FDP cells might inhibit the action of mitogenic substances on epithelial cells of hair follicles, although mitogenic substances can still be normally produced from FDP cells like DP cells derived from other types of hair follicles.

Stumptailed macaques are known as a pertinent model of androgenetic alopecia [6-8]. *In vivo* studies using this model showed that finasteride, type II 5α-reductase inhibitor [7] and RU 58841 [8], an androgen receptor blocker, stimulated hair growth. This study reconfirmed that stumptailed macaques are a pertinent model of androgenetic alopecia, showing direct effects of testosterone on epithelial cells cocultured with FDP cells.

References

1 Oliver F. In: Montagna W, Dobson RL, eds. Advances in Biology of Skin, Vol. 9. Pergamon Press, Oxford. 1969; 19-33
2 Jahoda CAB, Horne KA, Oliver RF. Nature. 1984; 311: 560-562
3 Randall VA, Thornton MJ, Hamada K, Messenger AG. J Invest Dermatol. 1992; 98: 86S-91S
4 Itami S, Kurata S, Sonoda T, Takayasu S. Ann NY Acad Sci. 1991; 642: 385-395
5 Ebling FJG, Hale PA, Randall VA. In: Goldsmith L. ed. Biochemistry and Physiology of the Skin, 2nd ed. Oxford University Press, New York. 1991
6 Uno H. In: Speroff L. ed. Seminars in Reproductive Endocrinology: Andrology in Women. Vol. 4. Thieme-Stratton Press, New York. 1986; 131-141
7 Rittmaster RS, Uno H, Povar ML, Mellin TN, *et al.* J Endocrinol Metab. 1987; 65: 188-194
8 Rhodes L, Harper J, Uno H, Gatio G, *et al.* J Endocrinol Metab. 1994; 78: 991-996
9 Reynolds AJ, Jahoda CAB. J Cell Sci. 1991; 99: 373-385
10 Hirai Y, Takebe K, Takashima M, Kobayashi S, *et al.* Cell. 1992; 69: 471-481
11 Limat A, Hunaiker T, Waelti ER, Inaebnit SP, *et al.* Arch Dermatol Res. 1993; 285: 205-210

Testosterone or IGF-1 stimulates hair growth in whole organ culture only in androgen-dependent red deer hair follicles

M.J. Thornton[1], D.G. Thomas[2], T.J. Jenner[1], B.R. Brinklow[2], A.S.I. Loudon[2] and V.A. Randall[1]

[1]Department of Biomedical Sciences, University of Bradford, Bradford, West Yorkshire, BD7 1DP, U.K.
[2]Institute of Zoology, Regent's Park, London, NW1 4RY, U.K.

Function of the hair follicle

Many hair follicles produce different types of hair in response to environmental changes or to the age or sex of the mammal. The hairs formed may significantly change in thickness, length and color. This allows many mammals to adjust to seasonal changes in the climate by altering the thermal insulating properties of their coat, or altering the color of their coat to retain camouflage when the seasons change, as seen in some arctic mammals [1]. This transforming ability of the hair follicle also allows hair changes which allow obvious distinctions between young animals and adults and between the adult sexes [2].

Androgens and the hair follicle

Hormones control the type of hair produced by many mammalian follicles [1-3], but the precise mechanisms are unclear. Androgens are obvious regulators of human hair growth, transforming small vellus follicles into larger terminal follicles [4]. To cause these modifications, androgens must alter, either directly or indirectly, the activity of many components of the hair follicle. The mesenchyme-derived dermal papilla at the base of the follicle plays a major regulatory role in hair growth [5], and there is increasing evidence to suggest that androgens exert their effects via the dermal papilla [4]. Androgen receptors have been measured in both human [6] and red deer dermal papilla cells [7], demonstrating that cells derived from androgen-dependent follicles *in vivo* have a higher androgen receptor content *in vitro*.

The red deer model

The red deer (*Cervus elaphus*) is a good animal model in which to study hair growth because it has a seasonal coat growth cycle with two distinct and separate pelage types each year. Furthermore, in the male, there are localized breeding season related coat changes in the form of a dramatic neck mane, which along with the antlers, clearly distinguishes the male from the female during the breeding season [8]. Since the growth of the mane is androgen-dependent, the red deer also offers an excellent model in which to study the hormonal regulation of hair growth.

In contrast to human hair follicles, the red deer stag hair follicle is subjected to dramatic seasonal fluctuations in androgen levels, the result of which determines the type of hair produced. The neck follicles exhibit an intrinsic ability to react to androgens, which are high during the breeding season, in contrast to other body follicles. The small neck hairs are replaced by long, thick mane hairs when the summer coat is replaced by the winter coat (breeding season), presumably in response to the high levels of circulating androgens. Significantly, these long, thick mane hairs are replaced by short neck hairs that are similar to the rest of the coat when the winter coat is replaced by the summer coat (non-breeding season). Whether this is due to the significantly lower serum androgen levels at this point in the hair growth cycle, or whether other factors are involved is unclear. With these very dramatic variations in serum androgen levels, that correspond to whether a small neck or large mane follicle is produced, it would seem that androgens must control the formation of different types of hairs by the same follicles in successive seasons, i.e. the hormonal response can be switched on and off.

In contrast to human hair growth, the hair cycle in red deer is in synchrony and occurs at a similar time each year. Mane or spring neck/flank follicles offer the possibility of comparing androgen-potentiated and relatively independent tissues. The red deer provides an excellent model, since they offer readily accessible androgen-dependent follicles with much shorter hair growth cycles and with the knowledge of what stage in the cycle the follicles are likely to be. Furthermore, there are clear measurable differences in plasma levels of testosterone and other growth factors such as IGF-1 which may be important in hair growth [9].

The role of IGF-1

There is increasing evidence that IGF-1 may play an important role in hair growth. At physiological levels, IGF-1 has been shown to stimulate the growth of human hairs in whole organ culture [10]. Other workers have demonstrated that the IGF-1 receptor is important in controlling the hair growth cycle [11], and more recently it has been reported that cultured dermal papilla cells secrete IGF-1 (Hibberts, Kato, Messenger and Randall, personal communication; Itami *et al.* elsewhere in this publication).

In the red deer, another prominently visible secondary sexual characteristic, seen only in the male, is the antlers. Like the mane, the antlers are renewed each year with their growth and maturation intrinsically linked to fluctuations in plasma testosterone. Although testosterone is important in antler maturation and cleavage, it would appear that IGF-1 plays a role in the stimulation of antler growth. Plasma levels of IGF-1 are elevated in the spring, which corresponds to the stimulation of new antler growth in red deer stag; recently IGF-1 receptors have been located in the antler tip, with higher numbers in the epidermis [12].

Experimental design

This study was designed to determine whether the growth of androgen-dependent mane hair follicles is stimulated by testosterone via androgen receptors in whole organ culture; control follicles from the flank region taken at the same time from the same animals were also investigated. Further comparisons were made by investigating the growth of hairs (neck and flank) taken from the same animals later in the year when they were growing their summer coat. At this time of year serum androgen levels are low and the mane is not produced.

Parallel punch biopsies (6 mm) were taken from the mane and flank of 5 adult stags during the breeding-season and then from the same 5 animals during the non-breeding season. Anagen hair follicles were carefully microdissected out, placed in individual 16 mm dishes and washed with sterile phosphate buffered saline before incubating in William's Medium E with 5 mM glucose at 37°C in 5% CO_2 in air, after Philpott et al. [10]. Six follicles from each area of each animal were incubated in serum-free medium containing 10 nM testosterone, or 10 nM testosterone +1 μM of the antiandrogen cyproterone acetate (CPA), or alcohol vehicle alone (0.002%). Growth was measured by micrometry every 24h.

Mane, flank and neck hair growth was linear over 72h under control conditions. Corresponding mane and flank (breeding season) and corresponding neck and flank (non-breeding season) grew at a similar rate. However, non-breeding season hairs grew slightly faster than breeding season hairs. Mane hairs grew faster in the presence of testosterone (0.769 mm ± 0.06 SEM), than under control conditions (0.637 mm ± 0.07 SEM). Testosterone had no effect on

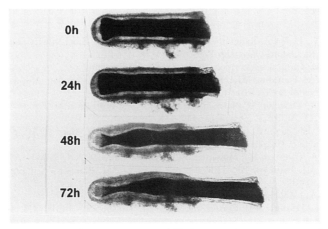

Figure 1. An isolated breeding-season mane follicle (x100) grown in control culture conditions, and photographed every 24h. Reproduced with permission from the Editors of the Third International Congress on the Biology of Deer.

corresponding flank follicles, or non-breeding season neck and flank. The antiandrogen cyproterone acetate prevented the testosterone stimulation of mane hairs. IGF-1 also increased the growth of mane hairs to a similar level as that produced by adding testosterone (0.774 mm ± 0.07 SEM). IGF-1 also had no effect on corresponding flank follicles, or non-breeding season neck and flank.

Discussion

The ability of testosterone to stimulate growth of androgen-dependent mane hairs, but not control flank hairs means that red deer hair follicles' response *in vitro* appears to parallel that *in vivo*; inhibition by the antiandrogen indicates a direct receptor-mediated action. These exciting results demonstrate that this is a unique *in vitro* model system that mirrors hormonal responses *in vivo*. The similar response to IGF-1 suggests this growth factor may have a role in secondary sexual hair growth. Since hair growth involves interactions between various different cell types including the mesenchyme and epithelium, this whole organ red deer model system which correlates with biological activity is an excellent system for studies of hormonal regulation of hair growth.

Acknowledgements

This work was supported by a project grant to Drs BR Brinklow, VA Randall & ASI Loudon from the Agricultural and Food Research Council (A.G. 63/529).

References

1   Ebling FJG, Hale PA, Randall VA. In: Goldsmith LA, ed. Biochemistry and Physiol of the Skin. 2nd ed. Oxford University Press, New York. 1991
2   Randall VA. Clinical Endocrinol. 1994; 40: 439-457
3   Randall VA, Thornton MJ, Messenger AG, Hibberts NA, Loudon ASI, Brinklow BR. J Invest Dermatol. 1993; 101: 114S-120S
4   Randall VA, Thornton MJ, Hamada K, Redfern CPF, Nutbrown M, Ebling FJG, Messenger AG. Ann NY Acad Sci. 1991; 642: 355-375
5   Oliver RF, Jahoda CAB. In: Rogers GE, Reis PR, Ward KA, Marshall RC, eds. The biology of wool and hair, Chapman & Hall, London. 1989; 51-67
6   Randall VA, Thornton MJ, Messenger AG. J Endocrinol. 1992; 133: 141-147
7   Thornton MJ, Brinklow BR, Hibberts NA, Loudon ASI, Randall VA. J Endocrinol. 1993; 137: (suppl) 182
8   Lincoln GA. J Zoology. 1971; 163: 105-123
9   Suttie JM, Fennessy PF, Corson ID, Laas FJ, Crosbie SF, Butler JH, Gluckman PD, J Endocrinol. 1989; 121: 351-360
10   Philpott MP, Green MR, Kealey T. J Cell Science. 1990; 97: 463-471
11   Little JC, Redwood KR, Stones AJ, Granger SP. J Invest Dermatol. 1994; 102 (4): 533
12   Elliott JL, Oldham JM, Ambler GR, Bass JJ, Spencer GS, Hodgkinson SC, Breier BH, Gluckman PD, Suttie JM, J Endocrinol. 1992; 130: 2513-2520

315

Transplantation of vellus hair in male pattern baldness to nude mice

S. Kondo and Y. Hozumi

Department of Dermatology, Yamagata University School of Medicine, Iida, Yamagata-City, Yamagata 990-23, Japan

Introduction

It is known that scalp baldness in androgen dependent alopecia is due to transformation of terminal hair into vellus hair with a very short duration of the growth phase of the hair cycle. Hence, to cure the baldness, the vellus hair should be reverted into the terminal hair. As there is no animal model equivalent to the human vellus hair transformation, we tried to transplant samples of balding scalp containing some vellus hair onto nude mice.

Materials and methods

Explants were obtained from 19 different individuals with male pattern baldness (age ranging from 29 to 75). Samples were collected from the balding frontal or parietal regions. Two to six 2 mm diameter scalp punch biopsies were taken from each subject.

One to three specimens from each donor were transplanted on the head or on the neck of one nude mouse (nu/nu). The specimens were either buried in the mouse skin and after a week the surface was air exposed, or, from the beginning, they were sutured edge to edge with a piece of nylon thread to the mouse skin with the scalp surface exposed as shown in Figure 1.

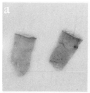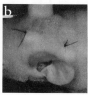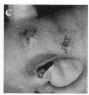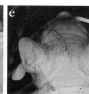

Figure 1. Transplantation of vellus hair bearing explants to nude mice
*2mm punch biopsies with vellus hair (**a**) were burried in the skin (**b**) or sutured on the nude mouse skin (**c**). Hair growth from the graft shown in C after 85 days (**d**) and 140 days (**e**)*

Results

Most of the transplanted specimens showed no necrosis. Especially, when they were buried in the mouse skin at first and then exposed after a week, the whole explants were kept in good condition. The original hair on the explants dropped off soon after transplantation.

So far 31 mice were transplanted, each one bearing one to three explants. 21 had two scalp grafts. In 10 mice, hair growth was noticed (Fig. 1).

The lag phase between grafting and the start of hair growth ranged from 19 to 70 days (Fig. 2). The length of the growing phase ranged from 16 to 86 days (Fig. 2). The length of the hair at the end of the growth phase in the mice was compared with that of the correspondent hair on the scalp (Fig. 3). A paired t test showed no significant difference between hair lengths. The growth rate of the transplanted hair ranged from 0.07 to 0.18 mm/day (Fig. 4).

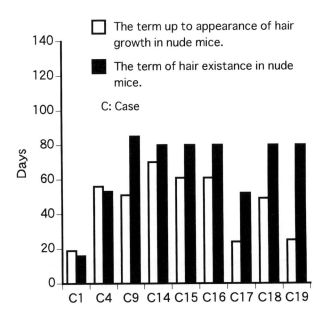

Figure 2. Duration of the lag phase between grafting and the start of new hair growth

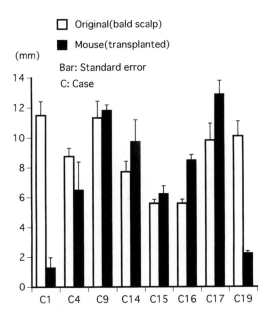

Figure 3. *Comparison of hair length measured in situ and on transplants*

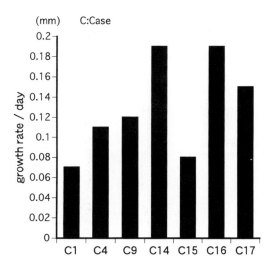

Figure 4. *Growth rate of transplanted vellus hair*

Discussion

To achieve cosmetically acceptable results in the treatment of male pattern baldness, the thin and short vellus hair should be stimulated so as to increase more than 10 times the usual length. So far no agent for treatment of male pattern baldness has met this satisfaction standard. For the purpose of the research, one of the most desirable ways is to establish an in vitro or an animal model of the baldness. We have already reported on an in vitro model for growing human terminal hair of the scalp, beard, axilla and pubis [1, 2]. However we realized that the actively growing terminal hair might be different from vellus hair in many ways. As for an animal model, nude mouse transplantation of human terminal hair is now widely known, but transplantation of vellus hair of male pattern baldness has only rarely been reported [3]. In this report, we could observe the first hair cycle on nude mice, but did not observe a subsequent second hair cycle from the same follicles. The rate and extent of the transplanted hair growth were correlated with but growth rates were slower than those noted in vivo confirming previous reports [3]. Overall, our data suggest that the vellus hair were not substantially modified after transplantation onto nude mice. Accordingly, this animal model may be convenient for various experiments on baldness. As an example, we refer to preliminary observations showing, after application of cyclosporin, some prolongation of the growing phase [4].

References

1   Kondo S, Hozumi Y, Aso K. Arch Dermatol Res. 1990; 284: 4442-4445
2   Kondo S, Hozumi Y, Sato N, Aso K. J Dermatol. 1992; 19: 348-352
3   Van Neste D, de Brouwer B, Dumortier M. Annals NYAcad Sci. 1991; 642: 480-482
4   Hozumi Y, Imaizumi T, Kondo S. J Dermatol Sci. 1994; 7: s33-s38

Testosterone conditioned nude mice: an improved model for experimental monitoring of human hair production by androgen dependent balding scalp grafts

D. Van Neste[1], B. de Brouwer[1], C. Tételin[1] and A. Bonfils[2]

[1]Skin Study Center, Skinterface, Tournai, Belgium
[2]Roussel Uclaf, Romainville, France

Introduction

The interest of clinicians in a condition as common as androgen dependent alopecia became triggered after the discovery of compounds showing some efficacy in «maintaining hair» by reverting a variable proportion of vellus follicles into terminal hair follicles [1]. The enthusiasm was soon implemented by a large number of studies using *in vitro* culture of pilosebaceous units (or parts of it). However, we like to stress that hair follicles only survive a few days in these conditions and that, most of the time, *in vitro* studies focus on one hair growth variable i.e. linear hair growth. Hence, there is much room left for outlining the clinical relevance of existing laboratory tests and/or for developing a model of normal and diseased human scalp including its biological environment. This might be extremely helpful for testing efficacy of compounds on the human target at the earliest stages of drug development i.e. well before phase I studies. The approach using the human scalp graft onto nude mouse mimics *in situ* conditions and appears to us as a serious candidate for this purpose.

In a recent review [2], we dealt with, amongst others, items such as the rate of success of transplantation of human scalp onto nude mice, scalp embryology and hair follicle morphogenesis, amino-acid analysis and protein composition of hairs produced by normal scalp- and by genetically deficient scalp transplants. As far as androgen dependent alopecia is concerned, the experiments reported herein were initiated after regional control of the defect had been elegantly demonstrated by Nordström's experiments. He used autologous transplantation: when affected scalp sites were transplanted to other body sites there was progression of the balding process at the same pace in the donor area and in the transplant [3].

On balding scalp samples that were transplanted onto nude mice, we demonstrated that hair growth continued and could be evaluated over a 6 months period. The distribution of diameters of the hairs collected from the grafted specimens was similar to that of hairs collected *in situ* i.e. on the scalp of subjects affected with androgen dependent alopecia. However the linear hair growth rate was decreased in grafts, terminal and vellus hairs being equally affected [4]. This indicates that the systemic environment exerts some influence. Using histological techniques incipient re-cycling was clearly demonstrated [5] and this eventually resulted in new hairs visible at the scalp surface (unpublished data). As it was not yet known whether human scalp hair production in general and hair cycling in particular were influenced by androgens, we conducted the experiments described in the next section.

Materials and methods

What are testosterone conditioned nude mice (TCNM)?

There were at least 3 reasons to use female rather than male mice for our grafting experiments. Grafting of human scalp specimens was much easier to handle on female than on the more aggressive male nude mice; male mice show wide variation of serum testosterone concentrations; finally, because female mice have much lower endogenous levels of testosterone as compared with males, they appeared more suitable for experiments requesting controlled levels of testosterone. Thus TCNM were female nude mice having a regular topical application of androgens. Preliminary dose-finding studies were conducted in order to find ideal concentration of testosterone to be administered topically in a clinical and pharmacological relevant test (Table 1; Humbert J and Bonfils A, personal communication). Accordingly, a 3 % testosterone propionate solution in ethanol was selected, 10 µl (i.e. 300 µg of testosterone propionate) of which should be applied every week day. This concentration was well tolerated and did not result in significant changes of survival rate of the animals. Testosterone conditioning was started within 6 to 8 weeks after grafting.

Table 1.
Dose finding of topical testosterone

Topical dose of TP (µg/mouse)	Time and results of serum testosterone levels (ng/ml)		
	24 h	48 h	72 h
30	0.13	0.19	0.00
100	0.77	0.04	0.00
300	3.79	0.82	0.24

Three topical doses of testosterone propionate (TP) were used. Serum levels of testosterone were monitored for 72 hours after a single application (3 female Swiss mice per group, average weight 30 g). 300 µg per mouse was found to be the most appropriate to create a systemic hormonal environment (3.79 ng/ml) as close as possible to the physiological testosterone level in human males (5 ng/ml) {6} after a single application. Accumulation of TP was also avoided with the 5 days a week regimen.

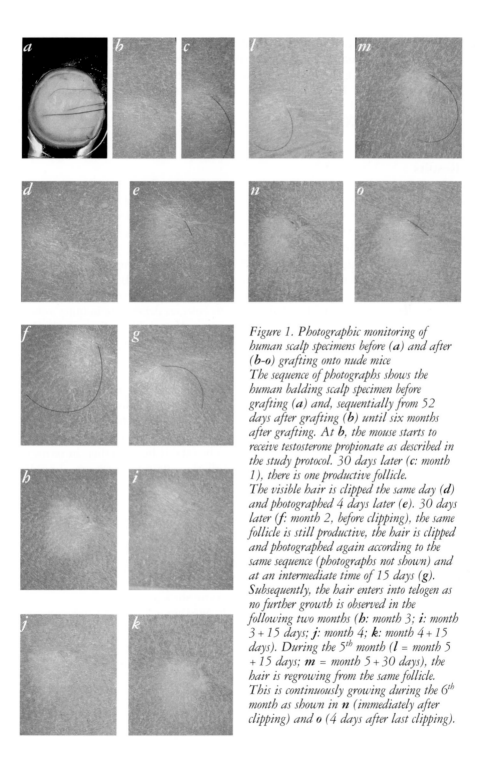

Figure 1. *Photographic monitoring of human scalp specimens before (**a**) and after (**b-o**) grafting onto nude mice*
The sequence of photographs shows the human balding scalp specimen before grafting (**a**) and, sequentially from 52 days after grafting (**b**) until six months after grafting. At **b**, the mouse starts to receive testosterone propionate as described in the study protocol. 30 days later (**c**: month 1), there is one productive follicle.
The visible hair is clipped the same day (**d**) and photographed 4 days later (**e**). 30 days later (**f**: month 2, before clipping), the same follicle is still productive, the hair is clipped and photographed again according to the same sequence (photographs not shown) and at an intermediate time of 15 days (**g**). Subsequently, the hair enters into telogen as no further growth is observed in the following two months (**h**: month 3; **i**: month 3 + 15 days; **j**: month 4; **k**: month 4 + 15 days). During the 5ᵗʰ month (**l** = month 5 + 15 days; **m** = month 5 + 30 days), the hair is regrowing from the same follicle. This is continuously growing during the 6ᵗʰ month as shown in **n** (immediately after clipping) and **o** (4 days after last clipping).

Inhibition of hair production in TCNM?

Productive specimens were defined as follows: one visible hair at least at one point in time during the 6 months observation period. Ten productive grafts in untreated mice and 10 similar grafts in the testosterone conditioned mice were evaluated. The grafts were monitored monthly by photographic (Fig. 1 and **colour plates XV-XVI**) and micrometric methods.

Results

In this study, we observed a reduction of the number of second hair cycles recorded during the six months period: 7,14% of the follicles on TCNM (2/28 follicles) as compared with 12,12% of those on control mice (4/33 follicles).

Hence, the inhibition of balding human scalp hair recycling mimics the changes observed *in situ* suggesting that TCNM might be considered as a reasonably acceptable candidate model for androgen dependent alopecia. Besides, the findings from *in vitro* studies show that testosterone influences cellular events at the molecular level [7]. However, because hair follicle *in vitro* cultures degenerate in quite a short time, it is hard to extrapolate whether testosterone effects will result in increased or decreased hair production or changes in the duration of the hair growth cycle.

Future of the model

There is preliminary evidence from various sources that grafting of human scalp onto nude mice is a reasonable experimental approach for the study of hair follicle physiology and pathology. Cycling of human hair from balding scalp grafted on TCNM appears to be a potential measuring tool for evaluation of testosterone receptor blockers. It remains to be established whether, in terms of industrial development, it really answers all the questions that are clinically relevant for drug screening programmes.

References

1   Dawber R, Van Neste D. Martin Dunitz, London, 1995; pp 1-262
2   Van Neste D. Dermatologic Research Techniques. H.I. Maibach (Ed.). CRC Press, Boca Raton. 1996; pp 37-49
3   Nordström REA. Acta Derm Venereol (Stockh). 1979; 59: 266-268
4   Van Neste D, de Brouwer B, Dumortier M. In Molecular and structural biology of hair. K.S. Stenn, A.G. Messenger, H.P. Baden (Eds.). Annals New York Academy of Sciences. 1991; 642: 480-482
5   Van Neste D, Warnier G, Thulliez M, Van Hoof F. In Trends in human hair growth and alopecia research. D. Van Neste, J.M. Lachapelle, J.L. Antoine (Eds.). Kluwer Academic Publ (Dordrecht). 1989; pp 117-131
6   Neumann F, Töpert M. In Hair and hair diseases. Eds. C.E. Orfanos, R. Happle. Springer Verlag, Berlin. 1990; pp 791-826
7   Thornton MJ, Messenger AG, Elliott K, Randall VA. J Invest Dermatol. 1991; 97: 345-348

Hair research for the next millenium
D.J.J. Van Neste and V.A. Randall (Eds)

An easy method to detect candidate genes associated with androgenetic alopecia

C. Gerst and B.A. Bernard

L'Oréal, Hair Biology Research Group, 92583 Clichy Cedex, France

Introduction

Male Pattern Baldness (MPB) is a multifactorial and probably a multigenic disease because of the variability of the clinically observed phenotypes.

MPB could be caused at least in part by a disorder of androgen biosynthesis or metabolism and by an over-expression or -activity of the androgen receptor (AR) that regulates the expression of androgen-responsive genes.

In order to investigate the genetics of MPB, we compared a control population of non-alopecic males with an affected population of alopecic males on two candidate genes. We focused our interest on: (i) the steroid 17α-hydroxylase gene ($CYP\ 17$) for which A2 allele has been shown to be associated with Polycystic Ovaries (PCO) syndrome and MPB [1] and (ii) the AR gene for which the length of the Glutamine (Gln) polymorphism repeat located in the transactivation domain seems to influence the $in\ vitro\ AR$ activity. The longer the strech (> 40 repeats), the lower the AR activity [2, 3]. The description and the localization of the polymorphisms of CYP17 and AR genes are given in Figure 1. We used a non-invasive method in which DNA was directly extracted from plucked hairs and the genomic DNA region of interest was amplified by PCR with specific primers.

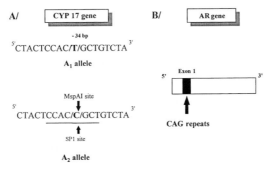

Figure 1. CYP17 and AR polymorphisms
A) The -34 bp mutation site where a T (A1 allele) is replaced by a C (A2 allele) creates a MspAI site and a SP1 site in the 5' region of the CYP 17 gene.
B) The polymorphic CAG (Gln) stretch is located in the exon 1 of the AR gene.

324

Materials and methods

Genomic DNA was extracted from plucked hairs. 80 volunteers were men aged between 35 and 60. They were classified in two main categories.

NON-ALOPECIC PHENOTYPE

ALOPECIC PHENOTYPE

PCR amplifications

The *CYP17* PCR amplification was performed directly on 1 plucked hair mixed with PCR reagents (Amersham). Primers (F: 5'-CATTC GCACTCTGGAGTC-3', R: 5'-AGGCTCTTGGGTACTTG-3') have been described previously as well as the PCR conditions [1]. 1/3 of the PCR amplification product was submitted to digestion with MspAI and electrophoresis on a 5% polyacrylamide gel. DNA fragments were visualized by ethidium bromide staining. A1 allele gave a 459 bp fragment while A2 allele, due to the presence of a MspA1 restriction site, gave 2 fragments of 235 bp and 124 bp.

For the AR PCR, the genomic DNA was extracted from plucked hairs after water boiling for 10 min and phenol/chloroform/isoamylic alcohol (25/24/1) extraction. Primers: F1: 5'-GAATCTGTTCCAGAGCGTCCGC-3'; R1: 5'-CT GCCTTACACAAC TCCTTGGCG -3', 1 cycle at 95°C, 1 min; 35 cycles at 94°C, 1 min; 57°C, 1 min; 72°C, 1 min. 1 µl of the first PCR was used for re-amplification with primers F2: 5'-CACCTCCCGGCGCCAGTTTGCT GCTGCTGC -3'; R2: 5'-TGCTGCTGCTGC CTGGGGCTAGTCTCTTG-3'. 1 cycle at 95°C, 1min; 30 cycles at 94°C, 1 min; 61°C, 1 min; 72°C, 1 min. DNA fragments were electrophoresed on a 6% polyacrylamide gel and the exact length of the PCR-amplified fragments were determined with Bio-Profil software (Vilbert-Lourmat). The scale was given by molecular weight marker V of Boehringer. The allele size ranged from 79 bp (7 CAG repeats) to 141 bp (28 CAG repeats).

Results

a) CYP17 Restriction fragment length polymorphism

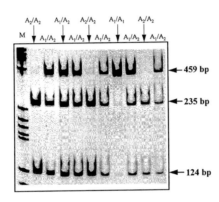

Figure 2. CYP17 amplified products were analyzed on a 5% polyacrylamide gel. 3 patterns are observed. One 459 bp fragment corresponds to the A1/A1 homozygous genotype. 2 fragments of 235 bp and 124 bp correspond to the homozygous A2/A2 genotype. The presence of 3 fragments of 459 bp, 235 bp and 124 bp corresponds to the A1/A2 heterozygous genotype. Genotype and allele frequencies of CYP17 stand as displayed in Table 1.

Table 1.

Subject group	Genotype frequency				Allele frequency		
	A1/A1	A1/A2	A2/A2	Total	A1	A2	Total
Non alopecic (n=47)	0.32	0.64	0.04	1	0.64	0.36	1
Alopecic (n = 34)	0.15	0.65	0.2	1	0.47	0.53	1

$$\chi^2 = 7.07, p < 0.05$$

b) AR length polymorphism

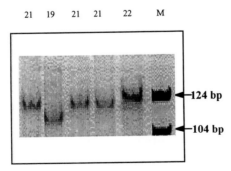

Figure 3. 19, 21 and 22 represent the number of CAG repeats in the AR amplified products analyzed on a 6% polyacrylamide gel. This figure shows that it is easy to detect a difference of one CAG repeat in the amplified fragment of AR exon 1. When the distribution of the number of CAG repeats was studied in alopecic and non-alopecic groups, no significant difference can be displayed (see Fig. 4).

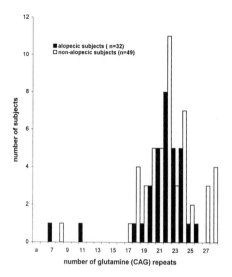

Figure 4. Polyglutamine stretch in the AR genes of alopecic and non-alopecic subjects

Discussion

Study of the CYP17 polymorphism within the two populations shows that the A2 allele is significantly more frequent in the alopecic group than in the non-alopecic group. Our results confirm those from previous studies which showed the association of A2 allele to PCO syndrome and MPB. This enzyme catalyses the rate limiting step in androgen biosynthesis in both the gonads and adrenal gland. A single base change in the 5' promoter region creates an additionnal SP1-type promoter site which may cause increased expression of 17 α-hydroxylase and consequently an increased synthesis of androgens. In the case of the *AR* gene, we show that the polymorphic CAG triplet repeat region encoding a polyglutamine stretch in the N-terminal region (exon 1) of the *AR* gene is similar within the two populations. The polyglutamine tract may be important in transcriptionnal regulation but can be excluded as a possible cause of alopecia. In conclusion we show that the use of a non-invasive method to obtain a source of genomic DNA is easy and convenient to assess the association of MPB with a given DNA polymorphism.

Acknowledgements

We are grateful to Miss C. Olivry for the preparation of the figures.

References

1 Carey A, *et al.* Human Molecular Genetics. 1994; 3: 1873-1876
2 Jenster G, *et al.* Biochemistry. 1994; 33: 14064-14072
3 Macke J, *et al.* Am. J Hum Genet. 1993; 53: 844-852

RNA-levels of 5α-reductase and androgen receptor in human skin, hair follicles and follicle-derived cells

W. Eicheler, A. Huth, R. Happle and R. Hoffmann

Department of Dermatology, Philipp University, Deutschhausstraße 9, 35033 Marburg, Germany

Introduction

Many androgen-dependent processes in the skin are driven by the 5α-reduced metabolite of testosterone, dihydrotestosterone (DHT). 5α-reductase isoenzymes type I and II supply target cells with DHT by activation of testosterone (T). Local differences in androgen sensitivity, e.g. balding versus non-balding scalp, seem to be intrinsic features of the single hair follicle, because the special androgen sensitivity is maintained after transplantation to other body sites [1].

The physiological role of a local modification of the hormonal signal and its role in androgen related disorders such as male pattern baldness or female hirsutism is not clear yet. Several lines of evidence led to the concept of a higher local 5α-reductase activity in these conditions [2]. Enzyme activities of 5α-reductase in complete skin samples [3] and hair follicles [4] were shown to be elevated in balding scalp areas compared to non-balding areas, but no data had been available yet on the level of RNA expression. We applied a semiquantitative RT-PCR technique with high sensitivity and specificity to get more insight into the expression of the key proteins in androgen action in cultivated single hair follicles and follicle-derived cell lines.

Materials and methods

Single anagen hair follicles were dissected from scalp biopsies [5]. They were cultivated for up to ten days in William's medium E containing 0 to 1 µM testosterone. The follicle length was measured using a video imaging system. Primary cell lines of outer root sheath keratinocytes were established from isolated hair follicles and subcultivated in a low-calcium medium. Papilla cell lines were obtained from microdissected dermal papillae and were subcultivated in Chang's medium [6]. 5α-reductase enzyme activity was determined by incubating hair follicles or cells with ^{3}H-testosterone. Metabolites were extracted, separated by thin layer chromatography, and quantified using a linear scanner. The metabolites were identified by comparison with ^{3}H-reference steroids.

RNA was extracted with phenol-chloroforme [7] and quantified

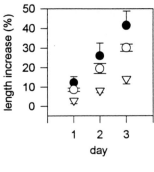

control
0,1µM t
1,0µM t

Figure 1a. Growth of cultivated hair follicles is inhibited by testosterone in a dose- dependent manner. Donor: male, age 24

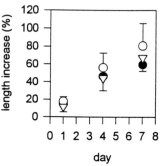

Figure 1b. Hair follicles of another donor show no significant growth inhibition by testosterone. Donor: male, age 25

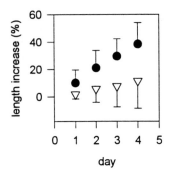

Figure 1c. Growth inhibition by testosterone is also observed in female hair follicles from of some, but not all donors. Donor: female, age 51,occipital scalp, alopecia androgenetica

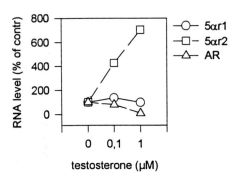

Figure 2. RNA levels in the hair follicles shown in Figure 1a collected at day 3 quantified by RT- PCR and normalized to the β-actin levels. The level of 5 α—reductase type II-RNA is higher in testosterone-treated follicles,whereas AR- and 5 α—reductase type I-RNAs are not changed. Donor: male, age 24

spectroscopically. Equal amounts of RNA were reversely transcribed and subjected to the polymerase chain reaction (PCR) with oligonucleotide primers specific for 5α-reductase type I, 5α-reductase type II, androgen-receptor (AR), and β-actin. Specificity of the primers was confirmed by restriction mapping. The PCR-products were quantified with reverse phase HPLC [8]. All data were normalized to the corresponding β-actin mRNA expression.

Results

With respect to the *in vitro* growth, two types of hair follicles were identified; androgen-sensitive follicles showed a dose-dependent inhibition of length growth by testosterone (Figs. 1a and 1c), whereas in androgen-insensitive follicles no effect of testosterone was observed (Fig. 1b). Both types of follicles were found in male and in female donors aged between 15 and 51 years. Also, in hair follicles of the occipital scalp, androgen sensitive as well as androgen insensitive follicles were found. In androgen sensitive follicles, RNA levels of 5α-reductase type I and AR were not significantly affected by testosterone, but 5α-reductase type II-RNA levels were increased in these follicles (Fig. 2). In isolated hair follicles, ^{3}H-testosterone was mainly metabolized to 4-androstene-3,17-dione and subsequently to the 5α-reduced metabolites 5α-androstane-3,17-dione, 5α-androstane-17β-ol-3-one (DHT), and 5α-androstane-3β-ol-17-one (androsterone). Differences were seen between hair follicles originating from the frontal and occipital scalp. Frontal hair follicles showed a higher 5α-reductase activity compared to occipital hair follicles (Table 1).

Table 1
Enzyme activity in plucked hair follicles from the frontal and occipital male scalp

	5α-reductase (pmol/h)	17β-HSOR (pmol/h)
frontal	0,054	0,046
occipital	0,001	0,005

Frontal hair follicles show higher enzyme activities (expressed as pmol/h per follicle) of 5α-reductase and 17β-HSOR as compared with occipital follicles.
Donor: male, age 30, with androgenetic alopecia.

In most samples of complete skin, hair follicles and follicle-derived cell lines, RNA for both 5α-reductase isoenzymes and the androgen receptor were detected. 5α-reductase type I-RNA was abundant in all samples, whereas 5α-reductase type II-RNA levels were very low, or not even detectable.

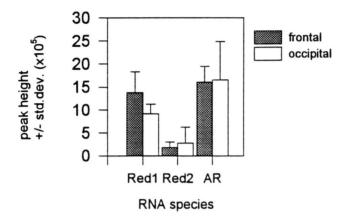

Figure 3 RNA levels in papilla cell lines from male occipital and frontal scalp. Levels of 5α-reductase I-mRNA are higher in frontal cells. Donor: male, age 30

In cultivated follicular keratinocytes, 5α-reductase type I-RNA was constitutively expressed and showed only minor sensitivity to testosterone treatment. AR-RNA was downregulated by T, whereas 5α-reductase type II-RNA was induced in these cells. In papilla-cells, 5α-reductase type I-RNA was again expressed constitutively and the AR-RNA was downregulated by T. Even after stimulation with T, 5α-reductase type II-RNA was very low. In papilla cell lines derived from male frontal and occipital scalp hair follicles, mRNA-levels of 5α-reductase type I were higher in the frontal papilla cells (Fig. 3).

Discussion

The presence of both 5α-reductase isoenzymes and the androgen receptor in human skin, hair follicles, and follicle derived cell lines indicate that they are potential targets for androgen action. They possess the enzymatic apparatus to modulate and enhance the hormonal signal. The influence of androgens on hair growth shows local differences, e.g. between frontal and occipital areas of the male scalp, or between the beard and scalp hair region. Because subjects with an inherited lack of 5α-reductase type II, but normal 5α-reductase type I isoenzyme neither go bald nor grow a beard [9], a key role of the 5α-reductase type II isoenzyme in the local control of hair growth was proposed. On the other hand, serum DHT, originating from tissues with high 5α-reductase type II levels, e.g. the prostate, could exert systemic effects on skin and its appendages. The first hypothesis would presume differences in the 5α-reductase levels in hair follicles of different origin. In complete skin samples and hair follicles, these differences have been described [3, 4], but could not be shown with immunochemical methods [10, 11]. Hair growth and balding are very slow processes, which spread over a period of months or years. Possible differences in androgen metabolizing enzymes with physiological effects on hair growth could therefore be very small and difficult to detect. The described method of semiquantitative PCR-analysis may provide a new tool with high sensitivity and specificity and could be very useful in detecting even small differences in the expression levels of androgen-mediating enymes.

Cultivated hair follicles seem to provide an appropriate model for the study of androgen action. The different testosterone-sensitivity of follicle growth *in vitro* could reflect the *in vivo* sensitivity to androgens and a possible predisposition to androgenetic alopecia. Interestingly, hair follicles with a different expression pattern of the key enzymes of androgen action and a different *in vitro* sensitivity of follicle growth were found in the occipital scalp. One may speculate that these differences reflect a potential androgen sensitivity *in vivo* e.g. a predisposition for later androgenetic disorders.

The relative mRNA levels of 5α-reductase type I and II showed a differential sensitivity to testosterone treatment. 5α-reductase type I was the predominant isoenzyme in all samples examined and was hardly changed by testosterone treatment. The 5α-reductase type I levels were higher in frontal hair papilla cell lines compared to occipital lines, whereas 5α-reductase type II mRNA levels showed no marked differences and were low in both cell types. On the other hand, the induction of 5α-reductase type II-mRNA by testosterone in hair follicles could indicate a physiological function in androgen sensitive hair follicles. If so, inhibition of this isoenzyme would be a reasonable approach to treat alopecia androgenetica.

References

1   Orentreich N. Ann N Y Acad Sci. 1959; 83: 463-479
2   Ebling FJG. In: Champion RH, Burton JL, Ebling FJG, eds. Textbook of Dermatology. Oxford: Blackwell. 1992; 125-155
3   Dallob AL, Sadick NS, Unger W, Lipert S, Geissler LA, Gregoire SL, Nguyen HH, Moore EC, Tanaka WK. J Clin Endocrinol Metab. 1994; 79: 703-706
4   Schweickert HU, Wilson JD. J Clin Endocrinol Metab. 1974; 38: 811-819
5   Philpott MP, Green MR, Kealey T. Br J Dermatol. 1992; 127: 600-607
6   Warren R, Chestnut MH, Wong TK, Otte TE, Lammers KM, Meili ML. J Invest Dermatol. 1992; 98: 693-699
7   Chomczynski P, Sacchi N. Anal Biochem 1987; 162: 156-159
8   Henninger HP, Hoffmann R, Grewe M, Schulze-Specking A, Decker K. Biol Chem Hoppe-Seyler. 1993; 374: 625-634
9   Imperato-McGinley J, Guerrero L, Gautier T, Peterson RE. Science. 1974; 186: 1213-1215
10 Thigpen AE, Silver RI, Guileyardo JM, Casey ML, McDonnell JD, Russell DW. J Clin Invest. 1993; 92: 903-910
11 Eicheler W, Dreher M, Hoffmann R, Happle R, Aumüller G. Br J Dermatol. 1995; 133: 371-376

Expression of androgen receptor, type I and type II 5α-reductase in human dermal papilla cells

J. Nakanishi[1], S. Itami[2], K. Adachi[1], Y. Nakayama[1] and S. Takayasu[2]

[1]Shiseido Research Center, 2-12-1 Fukuura, Kanazawa-ku, Yokohama, 236 Japan
[2]Department of Dermatology, Oita Medical University, Hasama-machi, Oita, 879-55 Japan

Introduction

Androgens affect the growth of human hair and the response of hair to the hormone is variable depending on the site of the follicle. Although the mechanism of androgen mediated hair growth has been largely unclear, beard and axillary dermal papilla cells (DPCs) were shown to possess the characteristics of androgen target cells [1-5]. Beard dermal papilla cells possess a higher 5α-reductase activity than DPCs from occipital scalp hair, and the enzyme found in beard DPCs appears to be type I and type II 5α-reductase [2, 6]. In contrast, axillary DPCs show a low activity of type I 5α-reductase, akin to the enzyme of DPCs from occipital scalp hair [7]. Besides, androgen receptors were detected in DPCs of beard, axillary and frontal scalp hair, but not in DPCs of occipital scalp hair by the immunohistochemical studies [4, 5]. Androgen receptors were also detected in the nuclei of cultured beard and axillary DPCs, but DPCs from occipital scalp hair showed little staining [5].

In the present study, we examined the mRNA levels of 5α-reductase and androgen receptor in cultured dermal papilla cells from several body sites, in order to investigate the cellular basis of the androgen action in hair follicles.

Materials and methods

Isolation and culture of dermal papilla cells

The methods used for isolating and culturing dermal papilla cells have been described elsewhere [2, 8]. Skin specimens were obtained at plastic surgery, and dermal papilla cells were isolated from the skin samples of 23 men aged 16-47 years. These samples included beard, axillary, frontal scalp and occipital scalp skin from 5, 5, 7 and 6 individuals, respectively.

Isolation of total RNA

Total RNA was isolated from each culture of dermal papilla cells at confluency after the 3rd-6th subculture by the AGPC method [9].

Reverse transcription-polymerase chain reaction (RT-PCR)

cDNA was synthesized from 1 µg of total RNA. The reverse transcription mixture contained 2.5 µM random hexamer, 5 mM $MgCl_2$, 50 mM KCl, 10 mM Tris-HCl, pH8.3, 1 mM each deoxynucleotide triphosphate, 1U/µl RNase inhibitor, and M-MLV reverse transcriptase. The mixture was incubated at 25°C for 10 min, followed by 42°C for 45 min, 99°C for 5min, then 4°C for 5 min. The resultant cDNA was amplified using 2mM $MgCl_2$, 50mM KCl, 10mM Tris-HCl, pH8.3, 0.025U/µl Taq DNA polymerase, and 0.5 µM each of the forward and reverse primers. The PCR primers were based on published mRNA sequences and were as follows: type I 5α-reductase, 5'-TTACCCGTTT CTGATGCGAG-3' and 5'-GTTCTCCACTTACACACAGC-3'; type II 5α-reductase, 5'-GGCCTCTTCTGCGTACATTA-3' and 5'CTAAGAAGCAA CTGTCGCCA-3'; androgen receptor, 5'GGTAAGGGAAGTAGGTGGAA-3' and 5'-CCTTCTAGCCCTTTGGTGTA-3'; and for glyceraldehyde-3-phosphate dehydrogenase (G3PDH), 5'-CCCATCAC CATCTTCCAG-3' and 5'-CCTGCTTCACCACCTTCT-3'. 28 cycles for type I 5α-reductase, 38 cycles for type II 5α-reductase, 33 cycles for androgen receptor, and 18 cycles for G3PDH were performed, with each cycle comprising 1 min at 94°C, 1 min at 60°C, and 1 min at 72°C. The PCR products were analyzed on 2% agarose gels stained with ethidium bromide. Each product was digested with restriction endonuclease to confirm its identity.

Results

The mRNA levels of 5α-reductase and androgen receptor in cultured dermal papilla cells (DPCs) from beard (Be), axillary hair (Ax), frontal scalp hair (FS) and occipital scalp hair (OS) were examined by RT-PCR (Fig. 1, Table 1). Both type I 5α-reductase and androgen receptor were expressed in all samples of DPCs from each site, with the order being Ax>Be>OS=FS. On the other hand, the expression of type II 5α-reductase varied depending on the samples or the site of

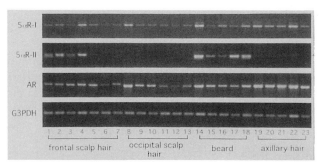

Figure 1. Expression of 5α-reductase and androgen receptor in cultured dermal papilla cells from various body sites

biopsy. In DPCs from beard (5/5 samples), frontal scalp hair (5/7) and axillary hair (4/5), the expression was observed with the order being Be>FS>>Ax. In contrast, the expression was not observed in DPCs from occipital scalp hair. The differences in the mRNA levels of type II 5α-reductase in the same site might be caused not only by the individual variation, but also by the variation of passage number. In fact, we observed that the mRNA level of type II 5α-reductase decreased with passage, although the levels of type I 5α-reductase and androgen receptor did not change (data not shown).

We also examined the effect of androgens on the expression of 5α-reductase and androgen receptor in beard dermal papilla cells. The cells were treated with 10^{-9} M methyltrienolone (R1881) or with both 10^{-9} M R1881 and 10^{-6} M cyproterone acetate for 48 h before the isolation of total RNA. The mRNA levels of 5α-reductase and androgen receptor were not affected by these treatments (Fig. 2). The same results were obtained using the DPCs from axillary, frontal scalp hair and occipital scalp hair (data not shown).

Table 1.
mRNA levels of 5α-reductase and androgen receptor in cultured dermal papilla cells from various body sites

	5α-reductase I	5α-reductase II	androgen receptor
Frontal scalp hair	58 ± 40	73 ± 28	62 ± 31
Occipital scalp hair	63 ± 43	N.D.	79 ± 55
Beard	100 ± 57	100 ± 65	100 ± 16
Axillary hair	152 ± 34	9 ± 5	168 ± 44

The results of densitometric analysis (5α-reductase or androgen receptor vs. G3PDH) are shown. The values of beard DPCs were taken as 100%. means ± S.D. N.D.: not detected

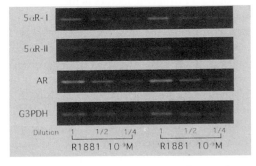

Figure 2. Effect of cyproterone acetate on the expression of 5α-reductase and androgen receptor

Discussion

The present study has provided the profile of 5α-reductase and androgen receptor gene expression in cultured dermal papilla cells from beard, axillary hair, frontal scalp hair and occipital scalp hair. In beard dermal papilla cells, high levels of these gene expression, especially the highest level of type II 5α-reductase, were observed. These results were consistent with the previous findings that beard DPCs possess a several-fold higher 5α-reductase activity and an acidic pH optimum which are characteristics of type II 5α-reductase present in androgen target cells [6, 10], and a larger amount of androgen receptors than reticular dermal fibroblasts or DPCs from the occipital scalp [3-5]. These results suggest that androgen exerts its effects on beard follicles through the receptor system in DPCs, as occurs in the embryonic urogenital sinus [11]. We did not detect the effect of androgen on the expression of androgen receptor, type I and type II 5α-reductase. Androgen receptor mRNA has been reported to be down-regulated by androgens in LNCaP cells, while the expression do not respond to the treatment in genital skin fibroblasts [12]. This difference in the response may be due to the difference of the cell type or to the difference of the culture conditions. In axillary DPCs, the highest levels of type I 5α-reductase and androgen receptor gene expression among DPCs from the four sites and a low level of type II 5α-reductase were observed. In spite of such a high mRNA level of type I 5α-reductase, axillary DPCs show low enzyme activity, akin to that of DPCs from occipital scalp hair [7]. The results of androgen receptor mRNA expression were consistent with the immunohistochemical study. These data may explain why the patients with type II 5α-reductase deficiency show scanty beard growth but normal axillary hair growth at puberty [10, 13]; i.e. the beard growth requires the presence of both androgen receptors and type II 5α-reductase in DPCs, whereas testosterone itself may stimulate the growth of axillary hairs by binding to the androgen receptors of DPCs, as occurs in skeletal muscle and the embryonic Wolffian duct [10, 13, 14]. Besides, it has been shown that beard and axillary DPCs produce diffusible factors which stimulate follicular epithelial cells. The production of such mitogenic factors is increased by androgens [5], and IGF-1 has been found to be one of these androgen-dependent growth factors [15]. In DPCs from frontal scalp hair, the mRNA levels of type I 5α-reductase and androgen receptor were similar to those of DPCs from occipital scalp hair. On the other hand, a high level of type II 5α-reductase was observed in DPCs from frontal scalp hair, which is in contrast to the undetectable level in DPCs from occipital scalp hair. These data suggest that the balding on the frontal scalp of genetically predisposed individuals after puberty requires DHT-receptor binding pathway like beard growth [5]. Further studies using samples with or without the genetic background of androgenetic alopecia are required.

In conclusion, our present study shows that the sensitivity of hairs to androgen is partially controlled by the site specific expression of 5α-reductase and androgen receptor in dermal papilla cells.

References

1 Itami S, Kurata S, Takayasu S. J Invest Dermatol. 1990; 94: 150-152
2 Itami S, Kurata S, Sonoda T, Takayasu S. J Invest Dermatol. 1991; 96: 57-60
3 Randall VA, Thornton MJ, Messenger AG. J Endocrinol. 1992; 133: 141-147
4 Choudry R, Hogins MB, Van der Kwast TH, Brickman AO, et al. J Endocrinol. 1992; 133: 467-475
5 Itami S, Kurata S, Sonoda T, Takayasu S. Br J Dermatol. 1995; 132: 527-532
6 Andersson S, Berman DM, Jenkins EP, Russell DW. Nature. 1991; 354: 159-161
7 Itami S, Kurata S, Sonoda T, Takayasu S. Ann NY Acad Sci. 1991; 642: 385-395
8 Messenger AG. Br J Dermatol. 1984; 110: 685-689
9 Chomczynski M, Sacchi N. Anal Biochem. 1987; 162: 156-159
10 Wilson JD. Biol Reprod. 1992; 46: 168-173
11 Cunha GR, Taguchi O, Shannon JM, et al. In: Serio M, Motta M, Zainsi M, Martini L, eds. Sexual differentiation. Basic and Clinical Aspects. New York: Raven Press. 1994; 33
12 Wolf DA, Herzinger T, Hermeking H, Blaschke D, Hörz W. Mol Endocrinol. 1993; 7: 924-936.
13 Imperato-McGinley J, Guerrero L, Gautier T, Peterson RE. Science. 1974; 186: 1213-1215
14 Perez-Palacios G, Chávez B, Méndez JP, et al. J steroid Biochem. 1987; 27: 1101-1108
15 Itami S, Kurata S, Takayasu S. Biochem Biophys Res Commun. 1995; 212: 988-994

Expression of steroid 5α-reductase I and II in scalp skin in normal controls and in androgenetic alopecia

D.W. Russell, E.L. Wiley and D.A. Whiting

Dallas, Texas, USA

Introduction

Conflicting evidence exists regarding the relative roles of the isozymes of 5α-reductase [1] in human scalp. Although 5α-reductase type I isozyme predominates over 5α-reductase type II isozyme in human scalp skin [2], the absence of 5α-reductase type II isozyme is known to prevent androgenetic alopecia [3]. So far, a significant concentration of 5α-reductase I activity and an insignificant concentration of 5α-reductase type II activity has been found in sebaceous glands of the human scalp [4]. Normal sebum excretion rates in men with inherited 5α-reductase type II deficiency suggest that 5α-reductase type I modulates androgenic activity in sebaceous glands [5]. Recent work confirmed the presence of 5α-reductase type I in sebaceous glands, but also indicated its presence in epidermis, sweat glands and hair follicles in human skin; 5α-reductase type II was also found in human scalp, but in sites that did not correlate well with recognized sites of androgen receptors [6].

This study was designed to show, by immunohistochemical assay, the specific cell types in human scalp skin in normal controls and in androgenetic alopecia which expressed types I and II 5α-reductase.

Materials and methods

Paired 4 mm punch biopsies of scalp vertex skin were obtained from 22 normal controls (13 males, 9 females), 30 males with androgenetic alopecia and 30 females with androgenetic alopecia. Polyclonal antisera were obtained by synthesizing segments of 25 amino acids of each isozyme of the 5α-reductase molecule (amino acids 232-256 of the type I isozyme, and amino acids 227-251 of the type II isozyme), and injecting them into rabbits to raise antipeptide sera. The antisera were purified by affinity chromatography on the starting antigen [7, 8]. The type I antisera proved to be selective for type I 5α-reductase, but the type II antisera recognizes both isozymes, although with a slight preference for the type II protein. It was shown that the 5α-reductase type II staining of sebaceous glands was due to a cross reaction with 5α-reductase type I and did not indicate the presence of 5α-reductase type II. Formalin-fixed tissue sections were stained.

The staining intensity in sebaceous glands, hair shafts and roots was rated from 0 to 4, and stained cells in hair follicles and stained dermal spindle cells were counted, per slide.

Results

5α-reductase type I was expressed strongly only in sebaceous glands in both normal controls and androgenetic alopecia. 5α-reductase type II was also expressed in hair follicles and in interfollicular dermal spindle cells. In normal controls the average slide stained for 5α-reductase type II showed a staining intensity of 0.45 in hair shafts and 0.1 in hair roots, with 6.7 stained cells in hair follicles and 1.4 stained dermal spindle cells; in androgenetic alopecia the average slide stained for 5α-reductase type II showed a staining intensity of 0.4 in hair shafts and 1.9 in hair roots, with 9.2 stained cells in hair follicles and 13.1 stained dermal spindle cells.

Conclusions

It is suggested that 5α-reductase type I regulates sebaceous activity and 5α-reductase type II affects hair growth. 5α-reductase type II staining shows almost a 3-fold increase in androgenetic alopecia as compared to normal controls.

References

1   Thigpen AE, Silver RI, Guileyardo JM, Casey ML, et al. J Clin Invest. 1993; 92: 903-910
2   Andersson S, Russell DW. Proc Natl Acad Sci USA. 1990; 87: 3640-3644
3   Andersson S, Bermann DM, Jenkins EP, Russell DW. Nature. 1991; 354: 159-161
4   Thiboutot D, Harris G, Iles V, Cimis G, et al. J Invest Dermatol. 1995; 105: 209-214
5   Imperato-McGinley J, Gautier T, Cai LQ, Yee B. J Clin Endocrinol Metab. 1993; 76: 524-528
6   Eicheler W, Dreher M, Hoffmann R, Happle R, et al. Brit J Dermatol. 1995; 133: 371-376
7   Silver RI, Wiley EL, Thigpen AE, Guileyardo JM, et al. J Urol. 1994; 152: 438-442
8   Silver RI, Wiley EL, Davis DL, Thigpen AE, et al. J Urol. 1994; 152: 433-437

A comparison of the hair growth characteristics of Thai and Caucasian men with male pattern baldness

A. Sivayathorn[1], T. Perkins[2], P. Pisuttinusart[1], T. Hughes[2], J. Hughes[2], P. Sunthornpalin[1] and W. Gibson[2]

[1]Department of Dermatology, Siriraj Hospital, Mahidol University, Bangkok, Thailand
[2]Unilever Research, Colworth House, Sharnbrook, Bedford UK

Introduction

As far as we are aware no comparative racial studies have been carried out on the hair growth characteristics of balding men using the phototrichogram. The objective of the study was to provide data on similarities or differences between Thai and European Caucasian hair growth characteristics by comparing the data obtained from a hair growth study carried out at the Siriraj Hospital, Bangkok with data obtained from a group of similar aged Caucasians at similar stages of baldness in Northern Europe.

Materials and methods

Sixteen healthy Thai men aged between 19 and 55 years and varying in baldness (classified from II to V on the Hamilton Index as modified by Katz *et al.* [1]) were recruited for the study at the Siriraj Hospital, Bangkok.

Two 1 cm^2 sites were chosen for evaluation in an apparently thinning region within the fronto-vertex region of the scalp and one site in the occipital region which is not usually prone to hair loss. The thinning region was defined as the hairy margin of the bald spot. Hair growth was assessed using a modification of the phototrichogram [2, 3] using scalp immersion photography [4] and the following hair growth parameters were measured:

1. Mean diameter (width in μm)
2. Total density (hairs/cm^2)
3. Non-vellus density (hairs > 40 μm in width/cm^2)
4. % anagen (growing) hairs
5. Linear growth rate (μm/day)

Data from the two fronto-vertex sites were combined and compared with data from the corresponding occipital region using Students' paired t-test.

Data from this study were compared with data obtained from similar regions of the scalp of Caucasians taking part in a study at Unilever Research Colworth

342

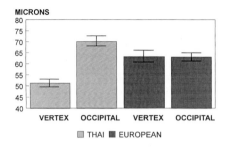

Figure 1. *Mean diameter*

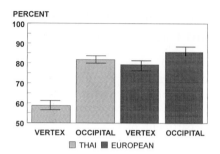

Figure 2. *% anagen*

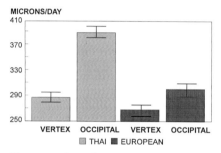

Figure 3. *Growth rate*

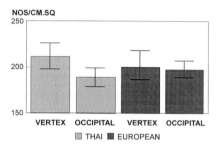

Figure 4. *Total density*

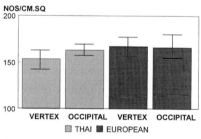

Figure 5. *Non-vellus density*

House, Sharnbrook, England. Subjects were matched in age and stage of baldness and compared using Students' unpaired t-test. Results were considered significant if the p-value was equal or less than 0.05.

Results

Both groups were similar in age and stage of baldness, they did not differ significantly (Table 1).

Significant differences were found between the fronto-vertex and occipital regions in the Thai data for diameter, % anagen and growth rate (Figs. 1, 2 and

3, Table 2). There were no significant differences in total hair density between the fronto-vertex and the occipital regions of the Thai scalps (Fig. 4, Table 2) although the fronto-vertex sites tended to contain the highest number of hairs. No significant differences in total density between the two regions were found in the European data either (Fig. 4, Table 2). If the vellus hairs are excluded the non-vellus density was lower in the fronto-vertex sites of the Thai subjects although not significantly so (Fig. 5, Table 2).

Table 1.
Distribution of age and stage of baldness of Thai and European subjects

Age range (years)	Thai	Europeans
18-30	5	4
31-45	10	11
46+	1	1

Hamilton range	Thai	Europeans
II - < III	2	5
III - < IV	8	6
IV - < V	2	1
V - < VII	4	4

Table 2.
Mean and standard error for Thai and European subjects according to variable and site location

Variable	Thai		European	
	fronto-vertex	occipital	fronto-vertex	occipital
Mean diameter (µm)	51.3 ± 1.8	70.4 ± 2.3 [3]	63.4 ± 2.7	63.1 ± 1.8
% anagen	58.8 ± 3.0	81.8 ± 1.9 [3]	78.8 ± 2.4	86.1 ± 2.3 [2]
Linear growth rate (µm/d)	288 ± 8.0	392 ± 9.0 [3]	267 ± 9.0	300 ± 10.0 [3]
Total density (n/cm²)	212 ± 14.0	189 ± 10.0 [1]	203 ± 16.0	198 ± 9.0
Non-vellus density (n/cm²)	153 ± 10.0	163 ± 6.0	168 ± 10.0	167 ± 13.0

significant differences between fronto-vertex and occipital sites
[3] *p≤0.001*
[2] *p≤0.01*
[1] *p≤0.05*

In the European men significant differences were seen between fronto-vertex and occipital regions for % anagen and growth rate (Figs. 2 and 3, Table 2) but, using a larger sample size, we have previously found significant differences between these regions for diameter and non-vellus density in Caucasian subjects.

When comparing Thai with Caucasian data from the occipital region diameter was significantly thicker and growth rate faster in the Thai subjects. In the fronto-vertex regions % anagen and diameter were significantly lower for Thai data.

Overall there were marked differences in the Thai subjects between fronto-vertex and occipital regions of the scalp. These differences tended to be greater in Thai subjects than in the comparable Caucasian subjects.

Discussion

In occipital regions of the scalp Thai hair was thicker and grew more rapidly in comparison with the Europeans. The increased growth rate is a novel finding and could be either genetic or climatic [5] in origin.

In the fronto-vertex regions the hairs were finer and a lower proportion of them were growing in the Thai men as compared with the Caucasians. However this region was sampled in the hairy margin of the balding spot and the outcome is more likely to be influenced by the precise choice of site.

References

1 Katz HI, Hien NT, Prawer SE, Goldman SJ. J Am Acad Dermatol. 1987; Suppl. 10, 16: 711-718
2 Saitoh M, Usaka M, Sakamoto M. J Invest Dermatol. 1970; 54: 65-81
3 Bouhanna P. Hair and Aesthetic Medicine. Rome: Salus Internazionale. 1984; 277-280
4 Van Neste D, Dumortier M, de Brouwer B, De Coster W. J Eur Acad Dermatol Venereol. 1992; 1: 187-191
5 Randall VA, Ebling FJG, Constable GM. Br J Dermatol. 1985; 113: 769

Effects of a topical type I 5α-reductase inhibitor, LY-191704, on scalp hair growth and sebum in balding stumptail macaques

A.E. Buhl[1], C.J. Mills[1], K.L. Shull[1], M.J. Zaya[1], C.H.L. Shackleton[2], M.N. Brunden[3], K.E. Kappenman[1], T.T. Kawabe[1], D.J. Waldon[1] and A.R. Diani[1]

[1]Biochemistry or [3]Biostatistics, The Upjohn Company, Kalamazoo, MI, USA
[2]Mass Spectrometry Facility, Children's Hospital, Oakland, CA, USA

Introduction

Dihydrotestosterone (DHT) is central to the causal mechanisms of acne and androgenic alopecia. DHT, a 5α-reduced androgen with a high affinity for the androgen receptor, is formed from nonreduced androgens through the action of steroid 5α-reductase. Different genes for this enzyme encode for a type I and type II isozyme [1]. Both isozymes are distributed throughout the body; type II in the urogenital system with some skin activity while type I predominates in the scalp and sebaceous gland [2, 3]. Castration halts the progression of balding in men while replacement androgens reinitiate the progression of hair loss [4]. The congenital absence of a functional type II enzyme is reported to be associated with decreased acne and a lack of androgenic alopecia [5].

Oral treatment with the type II 5α-reductase inhibitor finasteride induces hair growth while reducing systemic levels of DHT. In balding stumptail macaques oral finasteride caused hair regrowth and decreased serum DHT by more than 50% in males [6,7]. Clinical trials in men also demonstrated regrowth of hair on the balding scalp and reductions in serum DHT [8].

We tested the effects of a topical type I specific 5α-reductase inhibitor on hair growth and sebaceous gland activity in balding stumptail monkeys. type I inhibitors have not previously been tested for dermatological uses *in vivo*. We used the potent and selective type I inhibitor LY-191704 (LY) for this study. LY is a 5000 fold more potent inhibitor of the type I than the type II isozyme [9]. Topical therapy with a type I selective agent may avoid drug induced reductions in systemic DHT levels and reproductive side effects.

Materials and methods

The adult stumptail macaques were studied under a protocol approved by the Upjohn Animal Use Committee. Groups of 5-6 monkeys were treated by applying approximately 250 µl of drug or vehicle to each of two 1 square inch areas of scalp 5 days / week for 16 weeks using a paint brush. Treatments included 100% propylene glycol vehicle, LY, 5% minoxidil (MNX), or MNX + LY. Hair growth was measured on the dosed frontal balding area by weighing the amount of hair grown during the experiment [6]. Biopsies and hair sebum measurements were done on the more posterior site. The monkeys were sedated with ketamine during all the sampling procedures.

Drug effects on scalp sebaceous glands were determined at the end of the 16 weeks experiment. Sebum on 0.5 g samples of hair was extracted with ethyl ether then dried and weighed. Effects on sebocytes were monitored by measuring the volume density of the smooth endoplasmic reticulum vesicles using morphometric analysis. Scalp biopsies were processed, then thin sections of sebaceous gland were photographed at 70,000 x using an electron microscope. Stereologic analysis was done on 10 randomly selected sebocytes from one sebaceous gland of each male monkey.

Radioimmunoassays of serum and scalp skin androgens were done by Nichols Institute, San Juan Capistrano, CA. Blood samples were taken at week 0 (immediately before the first drug dose) and week 16 (24 hr after the last drug dose). Three-six mm biopsies were taken from treated scalp of vehicle and 50 mM LY-191704 treated monkeys at week 16.

The ratios of $5\alpha/5\beta$ urinary steroids from the urine of 50 mM LY and vehicle treated monkeys were examined by gas chromatography mass spectrometric analysis. Ratios of androsterone/etiocholanolone, 11 β-hydroxyandrosterone / 11 β-hydroxyetiocholanolone, 5α-tetrahydrocorticosterone / tetrahydrocorticosterone, and 5α-tetrahydrocortisol / tetrahydrocortisol were measured. The 24-hr urine samples were collected between weeks 10 and 16 of the study.

Excretion of LY in urine was measured in samples from vehicle and 50 mM LY treated monkeys. Drug was extracted on Bakerbond spe C-18 and cyano columns then assayed by HPLC using an Intertsil ODS-2 column with an isocratic 45:30:25 water:acetonitrile:methanol mobile phase. LY was detected by UV at 210 nm. The sensitivity limit of this methodology was 1 ng/ml.

5α-reductase activity of LY was tested *in vitro* using cynomolgus scalp skin. One cm^2 pieces of cynomolgus scalp skin were cultured with sufficient William's E medium to maintain a dry epidermal surface. Ten μl of drug or vehicle was applied to the skin surface without contaminating the media and 30 min later the skin was rinsed in saline, blotted dry, cut into 0.5 cm^2 pieces. After cultured in DMEM with ^{3}H-testosterone for 18 hr at 37°C the skin was homogenized, extracted, and ^{3}H-androgens were assayed using HPLC. 5α-reductase activity was determined by the conversion of ^{3}H-testosterone to ^{3}H-5α-reduced products.

Data are presented as mean ± SEM. Analysis of variance followed by nonparametric t-tests was used for non-paired data while paired data were analyzed with paired t-tests. Significance was set at $p < 0.05$.

Results

There were no apparent deleterious effects of LY on the appearance of treated scalp in any monkeys. No change in the animals general health nor reductions in body weight were observed in any group.

Hair growth was not affected by any LY dose but MNX induced hair regrowth with or without LY treatment. Females grew 3-4 fold more hair than males.

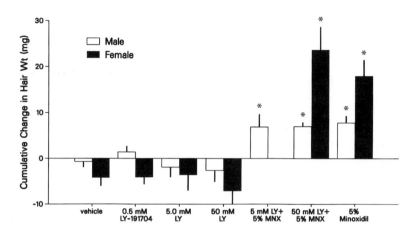

*Hair growth effects of LY-191704 and minoxidil. *Significant effect vs. vehicle.*

Scalp sebaceous gland function was not altered by either LY or MNX. Although the amount of sebum on scalp hair was easily measurable, hair sebum was not influenced by drug treatment. Similarly, comparisons of sebocyte vesicle volume showed no differences between the vehicle and 50 mM LY groups.

Serum DHT, androstenedione, and androstanediol glucuronide were not affected by drug treatment. Serum testosterone in males was also not changed but in females there was an unexplained increase in the vehicle and 50 mM LY groups. Androstanediol, measured only at the end of the study, showed decreases only in the MNX treated male groups.

Scalp concentrations of androstenedione and androstanediol were not affected by LY. DHT was below the sensitivity limit of the assay in all biopsies from both sexes.

Analysis of α/β ratios of urinary steroids showed no systemic 5α-reductase effects of LY when the vehicle and 50 mM LY groups were compared.

Measurement of LY in 24 hr urine samples demonstrated systemic absorption of approximately 1% of the applied daily dose. In the 50 mM LY group drug levels were 53 ± 9 and $27 \pm 5 \mu g/24$ hr for the males and females while in the 50 mM LY + MNX group levels were 79 ± 25 and 40 ± 8. MNX treatment had no effect on drug absorption.

In vitro data showed that topical application of 50 mM LY inhibited 5α-reductase activity in cultured cynomolgus skin. The amount of 5α-reduced androgens was reduced in cultured scalp from both males and females.

Discussion

Although topical treatment with LY had no apparent effects on hair growth or sebaceous glands, our data show that LY was percutaneously absorbed and is a potent 5α-reductase inhibitor in cultured scalp. Approximately 1% of the topical applied drug was present in urine. We know of no other data on drug metabolism or pharmacokinetics for LY.

The lack of hair and sebum effects may be due to several factors. First, the drug concentrations of LY delivered to the pilosebaceous unit and/or the drug residence time in the skin may have been insufficient. Although LY was obviously effective in cultured skin, both clearance and metabolism may be much different *in vivo*. Previous studies show that MNX has a slow transit time through skin and that 5 day/week dosing is sufficient for MNX effects in stumptails. This may not be true for LY. Second, local production of DHT in the pilosebaceous unit may not be critical for androgen effects in the presence of normal systemic concentrations. Thus, even with LY inhibiting all local DHT production circulating levels of DHT would be sufficient to inhibit hair growth and stimulate sebaceous glands. Third, sufficient type II 5α-reductase may be present in the skin to maintain skin concentrations of DHT at normal levels thus supporting baldness and sebaceous gland function. Clearly, further work will be needed to assess the usefulness of type I inhibitors for dermatologic purposes. Topical application to limit systemic exposure is an appealing concept that will require careful testing.

Acknowledgements

We thank Robert C. Gadwood and Bharat V. Kamdar for preparation of the drug; Kim A. Heath and Kenneth C. Kloosterman for their expertise with the monkeys; and Paula W. Lupina for her superb secretarial assistance.

References

1   Russell DW, Wilson JD. Annu Rev Biochem. 1994; 63: 25-61
2   Thigpen AE, Silver RI, Guileyardo, *et al.* J Clin Invest. 1993; 92: 903-910
3   Thiboutot D, Harris G, Iles V, *et al.* J Invest Dermatol. 1995; 105: 209-214
4   Hamilton JB. Am J Anat. 1942; 71: 451-480
5   Imperato-McGinley J, Guerroro L, Gautier T, *et al.* Science. 1974; 186: 1213-1215
6   Diani AR, Mulholland MJ, Shull Kl, *et al.* J Clin Endocrin Metab. 1992; 74: 345-350
7   Rhodes L, Harper J, Uno H, et al. J Clin Endocrin Metab. 1994; 79: 991-996
8   Kaufman KD, DeVillez R, Roberts J, *et al.* J Invest Dermatol. 1994; 102: 615
9   Hirsch KS, Jones CD, Audia JE, *et al.* Proc Natl Acad Sci. 1993; 90: 5277-5281

Stimulation of follicular regrowth by androgen receptor blocker (RU58841) in macaque androgenetic alopecia

H. Uno[1], N. Obana[1], A. Cappas[1], A. Bonfils[2], T. Battmann[2] and D. Philibert[2]

[1]Wisconsin Regional Primate Research Center, Univ. of Wisconsin, 1223 Capitol Court, Madison, WI 53715, USA
[2]Department of Endocrinology, Roussel Uclaf, 111 Route de Noisy, 93230, Romainville, France

Introduction

Our previous studies have revealed that the two hypertrichotic drugs, minoxidil and diazoxide, have successfully shown regrowth of terminal hairs in the bald scalps of stumptailed macaques [1-4]. We also revealed that the antiandrogens, 5α-reductase inhibitor (4MA) and finasteride, demonstrated both prevention of alopecia in periadolescent macaques and regrowth of hair in the bald scalps of adult macaques [5-8].

After topical application of either minoxidil (5%) or diazoxide (5% solution) on the bald scalps of adult macaques, regrowth of terminal hairs appeared after 3 to 4 months of treatment and the hairs grew continuously as long as treatment continued. Microscopically, small vellus follicles in the bald scalp enlarged to terminal size and DNA synthesis in the follicular germinal cells in early and late anagen follicles was enhanced.

Antiandrogens, both topical 5α-reductase inhibitor (4MA) and oral finasteride (Proscar, Merck), have also stimulated hair growth in the bald scalps of adult stumptailed macaques. Either a suppression of intrafollicular conversion of testosterone (T) to dihydrotestosterone (DHT) by topical 4MA or a significant reduction of serum DHT level by oral finasteride appeared to reduce production of follicular suppressive factors in the dermal papilla cells of these androgen-sensitive follicles [9]. The gene(s) for the follicular suppressive factor, yet to be determined, are activated by increased levels of T/DHT.

Although the presence of type II reductase in both human and macaque bald follicles has not been demonstrated, an inhibitor of type I showed no effect on regrowth of hair in the macaque bald scalp [10].

In 1994 Battmann et al. introduced a nonsteroidal blocker of androgen receptors, RU58841, which, upon topical application, induced a potent dose-dependent regression of the hamster flank organ [11]. Hypothetically, the use of an androgen receptor blocker appears to be more efficient for complete blocking of androgenetic action in hair follicles than the inhibition of intrafollicular DHT production by 5α-reductase inhibitors, because a substantial amount of circulatory DHT can directly reach the receptors. To examine this hypothesis, we studied the effect of topical RU58841 on hair regrowth and follicular changes in the bald scalps of adult stumptailed macaques.

Results

In observing monthly photographs of the frontal scalp, all four animals in the 5% RU58841 group exhibited a remarkable regrowth of hair (Fig. 1) as early as 2 months after start of treatment. The most significant regrowth was seen in a female juvenile monkey in the early stage of alopecia. The hair in the frontal bald area grew progressively thicker and longer until 7 to 9 months.

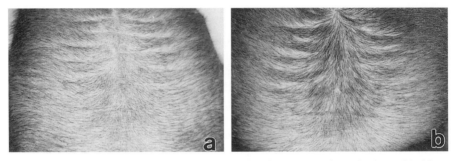

Figure 1. An 8.2-year-old male, showing marked hair regrowth in the frontal bald scalp after 4 months (b) compared to pretreatment scalp (a)

Thereafter, these regrown hairs maintained their length and density without further noticeable growth until 17 months. At 17 months, a second wave of hair growth was noticed in all monkeys; the hairs grew longer and denser than those of the preceding months. The postwithdrawal regression of these grown hairs appeared 3 months after treatment was stopped.

In the 0.5% RU58841 group, three monkeys exhibited a minimal degree of hair regrowth around 2 to 3 months after the start of treatment. Thereafter, these modestly grown hairs maintained their length and density throughout the course of treatment. The postwithdrawal regression of hairs was not noticeable after 5 months.

Three monkeys in the vehicle group showed no signs of hair growth throughout the entire course of treatment. One animal in this group showed a regressive change of hairiness in the frontal scalp during the course.

The folliculogram analysis revealed that all 4 cases treated with 5% RU58841 showed a marked progressive pattern of folliculograms at 4 and 5 months. However, the folliculograms at 11 months indicated no continuous progressive patterns; the population of anagen follicles was slightly reduced and that of telogen follicles was rather increased, but the overall size of the follicles showed no change (Fig. 2). These changes in follicular patterns suggested that a majority of the preexisting anagen follicles turned into the telogen phase of a new succeeding cycle. In two monkeys treated with 5% solution the treatment was stopped at the 13th month and after 5 months the folliculogram patterns showed typical postwithdrawal regression, increased telogen follicles and reduction of follicular size.

The serum levels of T, DHT, and luteinizing hormone were within the normal ranges in all monkeys treated with 5% and 0.5% RU58841 and vehicle, although the levels of these hormones showed some degree of fluctuation during the treatment and postwithdrawal periods. There were no steady increases or decreases in the serum levels of androgens and luteinizing hormone.

The hematological and blood chemistry tests showed no abnormal values in all monkeys treated with RU58841 and vehicle.

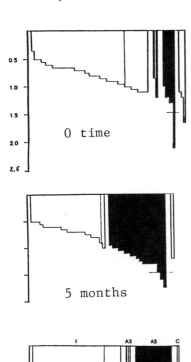

Figure 2. Consecutive folliculograms showing increased population and size of anagen follicles (black bar) at 5 months compared to those of time 0. At 11 months telogen follicles increased, but overall size of follicles remained the same as that of 5 months

Discussion

A potent blocker of androgen receptors, RU58841, induced a significant regrowth of hair in the bald frontal scalps of adult stumptailed macaques. The effect was clearly dose dependent. The degree of hair growth with 5% RU58841 was very dramatic and it occurred as early as 2 months after the start of treatment, but only a modest effect was shown with 0.5% RU58841.

In this preliminary observation, we noticed that 5% RU58841 induced the most significant degree and the earliest response of hair regrowth compared to those induced by the hypertrichotic agent, minoxidil, or by 5α-reductase inhibitors, although direct comparison of the effects between androgen receptor blocker and reductase inhibitors is difficult because of the route of application, topical (RU58841) versus oral (finasteride), dose, total period of time, and method for evaluations. The rate of follicular regrowth by quantitative folliculogram analysis at 6 months showed that RU58841-treated cases had a much higher rate of cyclic progression from telogen to anagen follicles, and greater enlargement of follicular size compared to those of finasteride-treated cases [8].

Interestingly, RU58841 induced the most remarkable effect on hair regrowth in an adolescent female monkey in the early stage of alopecia. The serum levels of androgens in adult females are approximately 10-fold lower in testosterone and 2-fold lower in DHT than those of male monkeys, yet alopecia develops at the same age and to a similar degree in both sexes. The sensitivity of androgenic follicular regression in female monkeys may be higher than in male monkeys.

The other interesting result observed in blocking androgen receptors was that the initial response of hair regrowth was much faster than with the hypertrichotic agent, minoxidil. However, despite such an early and marked effect, progressive hair growth stopped around 7 months, even though treatment continued. This was shown in both gross photographs and folliculogram patterns. However, a second wave of hair regrowth appeared around 17 months. These findings suggest that blocking of androgen receptors induced a rather rapid removal of follicular regressive factors which were produced in the follicular cells by DHT-androgen receptor-gene modulation. Indeed, our recent studies using a co-cultured cell system revealed that when the outer root sheath cells were co-cultured with the dermal papilla cells obtained from the frontal scalps of macaques, the number of outer root sheath cells was decreased after adding testosterone in the medium. This suppressive effect of testosterone was abolished by adding RU58841 in the medium [9], whereas the dermal papilla cells obtained from the nonbald occipital scalp showed no such effect.

Unlike the hypertrichotic agent, minoxidil, the androgen receptor blocker may not have a direct stimulatory effect on follicular cells [2]. Our long term treatment of macaques with minoxidil showed a continuous effect of hair growth demonstrated by both gross observation and folliculogram analysis [2]. However, the effect of the receptor blocker, RU58841, was manifested in a periodic, wavy fashion. This implies that RU58841 by itself has no direct proliferative effect on the follicular cells, unlike minoxidil. During the early anagen phase in a hair cycle, the follicles can grow larger than the follicles in the previous cycle if the suppressive factors are removed by blocking androgenic action. However, fully grown follicles in the late anagen phase remain the same size until the cycle turns over to the next early anagen phase. Overall, cyclic turnover of the macaque scalp follicles occurs once per year [6]. Thus, we observed that the second wave of hair growth appeared approximately 12 months after the cessation of the first growth.

The effect of antiandrogens, including both androgen receptor blockers and reductase inhibitors, on hair growth seems to occur in a periodical fashion. Since we have no data for the cyclic growth period of human bald follicles, the antiandrogen-induced rate and periodicity of hair growth in human androgenetic alopecia is difficult to predict, though the effect of growth is undoubtedly positive. The effect of minoxidil is progressive but as long as androgenic regressive actions exist, the degree of follicular growth is limited [2]. Indeed, a combination of minoxidil and reductase inhibitor enhanced the effect of hair growth [12].

References

1   Uno H. In: Maibach HI, Lowe NJ, eds. Models in Dermatology, Vol. 3. Basel: S. Karger AG. 1987; 159-169
2   Uno H, Cappas A, Brigham P. J Amer Acad Dermatol. 1987; 16: 657-668
3   Uno H, Kurata S. J Invest Dermatol. 1993; 101: 143S-147S
4   Uno H, Kemnitz JW, Cappas A, Adachi K, Sakuma MS, Kamoda H. J Dermatol Science. 1990; 1: 183-194.
5   Uno H. In: Speroff L ed. Seminars in Reproductive Endocrinology: Andrology in Women. Vol 4. Thieme-Stratton Press, New York. 1986; 131-141
6   Rittmaster RS, Uno H, Povar ML, Mellin TN, Loriaux DL. J Endocrinol Metab. 1987; 65: 188-193
7   Rhodes L, Harper J, Uno H, Gaito G, Audette-Arruda J, Kurata S, Berman C, Primka R, Pikounis B. J Clin Endocrinol Metab. 1994; 78: 991-996
8   Uno H, Obana N, Cappas A, Rhodes L, Bonfils A. J Invest Dermatol. 1995; 104: 658
9   Obana N, Uno H. J Invest Dermatol. 1995; 104: 577
10 Rhodes L, Primka R, Berman C, Gato G, Audette-Arruda, Pikounis B, Matuzewska B, Harper J. J Invest Dermatol. 1995; 104: 658
11 Battmann T, Bonfils A, Branche J, Humbert J, Goubet F, Teutsch G, Philibert D. J Steroid Biochem Molec Biol. 1994; 48: 55-60
12 Diani AR, Mulholland MJ, Shull KL, Kubicek MF, Johnson GA, Schostarez HJ, Brunden MN, Buhl AE. J Clin Endocrinol Metab. 1992; 74: 345-350

Hair research for the next millenium
D.J.J. Van Neste and V.A. Randall (Eds)

RU58841 a new therapeutic agent affecting androgen receptor molecular interactions in human hair follicles

M.E. Sawaya

University of Florida Health Science Center, Gainesville, FL 32610, USA

RU58841, a new N-substituted arylthiohydantoin, non-steroidal antiandrogen from Roussel Uclaf, Romainville, France [1, 2], has been tested for inhibiting the androgen receptor (AR) in human hair follicles.

AR has been localized in human hair follicles and found to play a major role in androgenetic alopecia, acne, and hirsutism [3, 4]. RU58841 displayed an excellent activity profile when tested with AR purified from human scalp hair follicles, giving a calculated K_i 0.4 nM, inhibiting 70% dihydrotestosterone (DHT)/R1881 binding, showing RU58841 to be 20% more effective in AR binding than cyproterone acetate.

In short term culture studies we developed cell free systems using nuclei prepared from human scalp versus genital skin to assess binding of AR-58841-inhibitor complexes to nuclear chromatin acceptor sites. Following this binding interaction, transcription was assessed by measuring stimulation or inhibition of RNA polymerase II activity in scalp versus genital hair follicles [5].

AR-58841 complexes bind specifically to nuclear chromatin acceptor sites in both scalp and genital tissue. This results in > 60% reduction in RNA polymerase II in genital tissue, in comparison to control levels of androgen, DHT, whereas, incubated scalp tissue showed 15–20% increase in polymerase activity [5].

The study of beard and scalp hair follicles of 6 male donors in longer term culture (up to 14 days) appeared to be an interesting model. The whole follicles were mounted in a collagen matrix. The study revealed significant differences ($p<0.005$) when the follicles were cultured in DHT (10 nM and 100 nM) in the absence or presence of 1 µM RU58841 added, i.e.:

a) in the presence of RU58841 hair follicle growth rates were found to be increased by 23% for scalp follicles but a 16% decrease was noted in beard follicles

b) protein, DNA and RNA polymerase II activity revealed increases in scalp (25%, 12% and 12% respectively) and respectively equivalent relative decreases in beard hair follicles

c) thioredoxin reductase activity, a sulfhydryl-reducing enzyme important for keratin protein synthesis, increased by 16% in scalp follicles after 14 days in culture but decreased by 10% in beard hair follicles.

Focusing on the binding interactions of RU58841 with the AR, human AR segments produced from full length human AR were constructed [6]. AR region/domains were also tested for RU58841's ability to form a stable domain-complex able to bind to the ARE (androgen response elements).

Gel mobility shift assays were performed using P^{32}-labeled C3-ARE probe. AR segment domains (460-704), (521-704), (460-626), (521-626), were incubated with various ligands: CYP = cyproterone acetate, DHT = dihydrotestosterone, RU58841, versus no ligand, as control. The densitometric scanning of the gels (Fig. 1) show specific AR domains binding to various structural ligands, and the ability of each AR-ligand complex to bind to the ARE-probe.

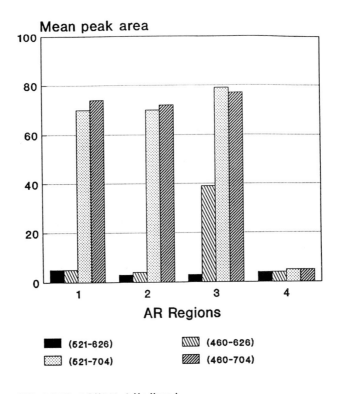

1=CYP, 2=DHT, 3=RU841, 4=No ligand

Figure 1 . AR regions required for AR-ligand complex binding to bind to ARE

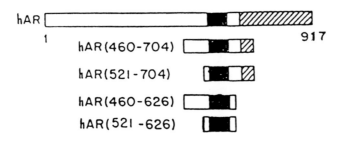

Figure 2. hAR segments produced from full length AR

Figure 1 and 2. AR regions required for AR-ligand complex binding to bind to P^{32}-labeled C3-ARE probe
Human AR segments were produced from full length human AR as previously described
{6}. Mobility shift assays were performed using P^{32}-labeled C3-ARE probe. AR
segments were incubated with various ligands, CYP = cyproterone acetate, DHT =
dihydrotestosterone, RU58841 = RU841, or no ligand = negative control. 5%
Nondenaturing PAGE lanes contained each binding reaction where AR fragments were
preincubated (0.5 μg protein, with 0.5 μM ligand), with later added poly(dI-dC) at
4 °C, then followed by P^{32}-label ARE (0.02 pmol) added for incubation of 15 min
each at 20 °C, then 4 °C. Unbound ARE probe migrated to bottom of gel.
Densitometric scanning was performed indicating mean peak area of the specific AR
regions.

Important is the affinity of RU58841 binding to the (460-626) AR segment.
Deletion of amino acids (460–520) just at the NH_2-terminal of the AR-DNA
binding domain produced (521-626), which RU58841 did not bind to initiate
affinity to the ARE probe.

Therefore, a region encompassing amino acids 460-520 in the NH_2-terminal
domain of AR interacts with RU58841 and with enough affinity to initiate
binding of the DNA domain to the ARE probe. It is known that the large NH_2
terminal domain is essential for full AR activity, since this domain contains
highly acidic regions that potentiates receptor activity [7]. The presence of this
region reduced nonspecific DNA binding and may be crucial in discriminating
between specific and nonspecific activation of transcription, since binding of
RU58841 to this small amino acid segment was specific for the recognition
sequences of ARE.

Conclusion

From kinetic studies we find this compound to be a very unique inhibitor, with binding to the ligand domain, as well as the regulatory domain of AR displaying allosteric binding characteristics, which may be a new and novel approach for antiandrogen treatment of skin disorders, such as androgenetic alopecia, acne and hirsutism.

The model system using human hair follicles from scalp and beard in a 14 days culture system is a novel approach in testing drugs and compounds for their effectiveness in stimulating scalp or inhibiting beard hair growth. Although these studies using human hair follicles *in vitro* were preliminary, other ongoing studies using animal models such as the teddy bear hamster [8], mouse androgenetic alopecia model [8], and macaque monkey [9] and other human models (see elsewhere in this volume) revealed similar findings with regard to RU58841. Testing compounds and drugs using all of these different systems simultaneously (human hair follicles, hamster, mouse and monkey) may be an approach for future drug discovery.

References

1   Battmann T, Bonfils A, Branche C, *et al*. J Steroid Biochem Molec Biol. 1994; 48(1): 55-60
2   Teutsch G, Goubet F, Battman T, *et al*. J Steroid Biochem Molec Biol. 1994; 48(1): 111-119
3   Choudry R, Hodgin MB, Van der Kwast, *et al*. J Endocrin. 1992 ; 133: 467-475
4   Sawaya ME. J Invest Dermat. 1992; 98: 92s-96s
5   Sawaya ME, Roth WI, Hevia O, Flowers FP. J Invest Dermatol. 1995; 104(4): 606
6   Kupfer SR, Marschke KB, Wilson EM, French FS. J Biol Chem. 1993; 268(23): 17519-17527
7   MacLean HE, Choi W, Rekaris G, *et al*. J Clin Endocrin Metab. 1995; 80: 508-516
8   Matias JR, Gaillard M. J Invest Dermatol. 1995; 104(4): 577, 135
9   Uno H, Obana N, Cappas A, *et al*. J Invest Dermatol. 1995; 104(4): 658, 621

Topical 0.05% finasteride significantly reduced serum DHT concentrations, but had no effect in preventing the expression of genetic hair loss in men

D.H. Rushton[1], M.J. Norris[1] and I.D. Ramsay[2]

[1]School of Pharmacy and Biomedical Sciences, University of Portsmouth, Portsmouth, U.K.
[2]Department of Endocrinology, North Middlesex Hospital, London, U.K.

Introduction

The largest cause of hair loss in men is genetic in origin (also known as androgen-dependent alopecia, androgenetic alopecia, androgenic alopecia, common baldness, or male pattern baldness). The extent and rate of hair loss varies between and within individuals, and a significant number of men are affected before the age of 50. While the genetic basis is complex, the inherited predisposition is thought to require male hormone (androgen) mediation. Classically the temporal and vertex areas are involved in patterns described by Hamilton [1], while a diffuse pattern similar to that found in women affects about 5%. Changes may appear as early as 14, but it is during the mid-twenties that most become aware of their loss of hair. This can lead to loss of confidence and an obsession so intense it has resulted in suicide.

In general the medical profession has paid little, or no, attention to hair loss. Recently however, several major pharmaceutical companies have started investigating therapies specifically developed to treat genetic hair loss.

The relationship between genetic hair loss and endogenous androgen secretion is generally accepted [2-4]. Hamilton [2] demonstrated that males castrated before puberty did not become bald, while in castrated adults who are partially bald the process is arrested. However, the administration of testosterone to these groups initiates or continues the balding process providing a suitable genetic background is present. Data from normal men further supports this view where the balding process was reversed following 12 months of oral medroxyprogesterone acetate therapy, while in untreated controls the loss of hair continued (Rushton and Mortimer unpublished data).

It appears that tissue sensitivity to circulating androgens and, in particular, the role of 5α-reductase activity within the hair follicle is of primary importance in the expression of genetic hair loss [5].

From studies in benign prostatic hyperplasia (BPH), a condition known to be mediated by dihydrotestosterone [6], it has been postulated that finasteride might be effective in treating genetic hair loss in men. However, because of the presence of finasteride in seminal fluid during oral therapy, we elected to investigate topically applied finasteride in five men exhibiting genetic hair loss.

Materials and methods

Initial dosing studies were designed to establish the most effective topical concentration of finasteride with respect to serum DHT 5mg Proscar® tablets were crushed to prepare the appropriate concentration suitable for topical dosing studies.

Males with genetic hair loss were selected on a named patient basis, and all gave their informed consent. Following a baseline blood test and medical examination, hair variables were assessed with the Unit Area Trichogram [7] (a method with proven reproducibility [8, 9]) basely and, from the same sites, 12 months later. All blood tests were performed before 11 am following a 12 hr fast, with follow-up blood tests and medical examinations after 1, 4, and 12 months of therapy.

Results

Hormonal changes during dosing studies

The dosing study data are presented in Table 1 and Table 2. The results show that a twice daily application of 0.05% finasteride solution (2 x 2 ml) significantly lowers the serum DHT concentration, with only a marginal increase in DHT suppression being observed when the concentration was increased from 0.05% to 0.075% (data not presented).

Table 1.
Dosing data (mean, n = 2) for topical 0.01% finasteride (2 x 2 ml daily) over a four week duration

	Week 0	Week 1	Week 4	% Change
Testosterone (nmol/L)	25.0	31.0	25.0	0%
DHT (nmol/L)	2.9	1.7	1.7	-31%

Table 2.

Dosing data (mean ± sd, n = 9) for topical 0.05% finasteride (2 x 2 ml daily) over a four week duration

	Week 0	Week 4	% Change	(paired t-test)
Testosterone (nmol/L)	20.2±5.1	19.4±7.8	-4%	NS
DHT (nmol/L)	1.8±0.9	1.1±0.5	-39%	p<0.003

Hormonal and hair changes during topical 0.05% finasteride therapy (Table 3)

During the treatment period significant suppression of the serum DHT was achieved in all individuals, with each remaining below the lower limit of normal (1.3 to 2.5 nmol/L) throughout treatment. In addition, no significant reduction in circulating serum testosterone or oestradiol concentration was found. The mean values obtained for total hair density (hair per cm^2) and non-vellus hair density are also presented. A vellus hair was defined as a hair ≤ 40 μm in diameter, ≤ 30 mm in length.

Table 3.

Mean hair densities and hormonal values from 5 subjects treated with topical 0.05% finasteride for 12 months

Time (months)	0	12	Significance	Normal Range
Total hair per cm^2	256	248	NS	(256 - 359)
Non-vellus hair per cm^2	174	158	NS	(232 - 325)
Testosterone (nmol/L)	15.0	14.0	NS	(10.0 - 35.0)
DHT (nmol/L)	1.42	0.85	p<0.01	(1.3 - 2.5)

(Statistical test: Student's t-test, paired samples)

Discussion

Until recently the medical profession has paid little or no attention to hair loss in men. While genetic hair loss is considered pathologic in women, many physicians still believe it normal in men and something they should learn to live with. However, a significant body of medical and scientific opinion now believes that hair loss adversely affects an individual's quality of life and, as such, demands intervention. Consequently, several pharmaceutical companies have now turned their attention to investigating genetic hair loss in both men and women.

The role of androgens in the pathogenesis of genetic hair loss is well established, but the use of oral non-specific anti-androgen therapy, in men at least, is not without problems. With the development of finasteride it was hoped that a specific treatment for genetic hair loss might at last be available. However, it now transpires that the enzyme 5α-reductase exists as isozymes, with a type-I found in scalp hair follicles and the type-II form being present in prostate. Since finasteride was developed as a 5α-reductase inhibitor for BPH, the efficacy of a type-II inhibitor in genetic hair loss would therefore depend upon the presence of this isozyme (type-II) within scalp hair follicles (to date frequency distributions for the isozymes have yet to be published).

In this study we employed a topical formulation of 0.05% finasteride in view of its presence in seminal fluid of subjects receiving oral therapy. Despite achieving serum DHT levels 40% lower than baseline, no hair regrowth occurred. Additional data from 10 males showed no further loss of hair in two subjects while on treatment; however the remaining eight withdrew after 12 months due to lack of efficacy (unpublished data).

These findings suggest that in individuals in whom hair follicles have little or no type-II 5α-reductase activity, topically applied inhibitors like finasteride are unlikely to be effective. Oral Proscar® (5 mg finasteride) is also unlikely to be effective unless metabolites with different specificity to 5α-reductase isozymes are produced. We therefore eagerly await the arrival of a type-I or mixed 5α-reductase inhibitor.

References

1   Hamilton JB. Patterned loss of hair in man: types and incidence. Annal NY Acad Sci. 1951; 53: 708-728

2   Hamilton JB. Male hormone stimulation is a prerequisite and incitant in common baldness. Am J Anat. 1942; 71: 451-480

3   Winkler K. Anti-androgens in dermatology. Arch Klin Exp Derm. 1968; 233: 296-302

4   Rushton DH, Ramsay ID. The importance of adequate serum ferritin levels during oral cyproterone acetate and ethinyl oestradiol treatment of diffuse androgen-dependent alopecia in women. Clin Endocrinol. 1992; 36: 421-427

5   Sawaya ME, Mendez AJ, Lewis LA, Hsia SL. Two forms of androgen receptor protein in human hair follicles and sebaceous glands: Variation in transitional and bald scalp. J Invest Dermatol. 1988; 90: 606

6   Vermeulen A, Giagulli VA, De Schepper P, Buntinx A. Hormonal effects of 5α-reductase inhibitor (Finasteride) on hormonal levels in normal men and patients with benign prostatic hyperplasia. Eur Urol. 1991; 20 (Suppl): 82-86

7   Rushton DH, James KC, Mortimer CH. The unit area trichogram in the assessment of androgen-dependent alopecia. Br J Dermatol. 1983; 109:429-437

8   Rushton DH, Ramsay ID, James KC, Norris MJ, Gilkes JJH. Biochemical and trichological characterization of diffuse alopecia in women. Br J Dermatol. 1990; 123: 187-197

9   Rushton DH, de Brouwer B, de Coster W, Van Neste DJJ. Comparative evaluation of scalp hair by phototrichogram and unit area trichogram analysis within the same subjects. Acta Derm Venereol (Stockh). 1993; 73: 150-153

Clinical studies on the effects of oral finasteride, a type II 5α-reductase inhibitor, on scalp hair in men with male pattern baldness

K.D. Kaufman*

Merck Research Labs, Rahway, NJ, USA
*on behalf of the Finasteride Male Pattern Baldness Study Group

Introduction

Ever since the clinical observations of James Hamilton over fifty years ago [1], investigators have sought the identification of the specific androgens responsible for the development of male pattern baldness (androgenetic alopecia). In 1974, the description of men with genetic deficiency of type II 5α-reductase shed further light on this issue [2]. These men were found to have low serum dihydrotestosterone, normal or slightly elevated serum testosterone, and no prostate enlargement or male pattern baldness. This led to the search for 5α-reductase inhibitors as potential pharmacologic agents for treatment of disease in man.

Clinical studies

Finasteride, an orally-active type II 5α-reductase inhibitor, was the first such agent developed for clinical use in man. Clinical trials conducted for the treatment of men with benign prostatic hyperplasia established the excellent safety profile of this compound [3]. Studies were subsequently initiated for the treatment of men with male pattern baldness. Concurrently, finasteride administration was shown to result in increased hair growth in the stumptail macaque [4], and to lower scalp skin dihydrotestosterone in balding men [5].

We conducted two separate, placebo-controlled clinical trials to evaluate the safety and efficacy of finasteride in men age 18 to 35 years old with Hamilton classification III vertex and IV male pattern baldness. Finasteride 5 mg/day or placebo was administered orally for 12 months in one study, while finasteride 1 mg, 0.2 mg, or 0.01 mg/day or placebo was administered for 6 months in a second study.

Materials and methods

Objective improvement in hair growth in men with male pattern baldness was determined by analysis of haircounts from macrophotographs taken of a 1 inch diameter circle (5.1 cm^2) of scalp hair centered at the leading edge of the vertex bald spot.

Subjective improvement was determined by analysis of:

1) a self-administered patient hair growth questionnaire (HGQ);

2) investigator clinical assessment (ICA) of hair growth; and

3) assessment of global photographs (GPA) by a panel of expert dermatologists.

Results

Table 1 summarizes the results of these studies. Patients treated with finasteride at 5 mg, 1 mg or 0.2 mg/day showed improvement in hair growth at 6 months (M6) or at 12 months (M12), while treatment with 0.01 mg/day was similar to the placebo. Serum dihydrotestosterone (DHT) was reduced to castrate levels in patients receiving finasteride at 5 mg, 1 mg or 0.2 mg/day, while serum testosterone (T) remained in the normal range. No significant safety issues were identified in patients receiving finasteride at any dose.

Table 1.
Summary of results

Hair Growth Assessment (Change from baseline)	Placebo M6 (N=86)	0.01 mg M6 (N=93)	0.2 mg M6 (N=84)	1 mg M6 (N=95)	Placebo M12 (N=80)	5 mg M12 (N=74)
Haircount (1 inch circle)	-7	-3	61*	77*	-10	95*
HGQ (% improved appearance)	32%	36%	48%*	54%*	29%	71%*
ICA (% increased hair)	53%	49%	70%*	75%*	47%	76%*
GPA (% increased hair)	15%	15%	41%*	58%*	2%	51%*
DHT (median % change)	-3.9%	-10.8%*	-61.7%*	-68.7%*	0.0%	-69.2%*
T (median % change)	8.8%	13.2%	23.9%*	21.5%*	-2.8%	23.0%*

$p<0.05$ vs placebo

Conclusions

In these studies, oral treatment with finasteride at doses from 0.2 to 5 mg/day resulted in clinically significant improvement in hair growth in men with male pattern baldness. These studies are currently ongoing at the 1 mg dose of finasteride to obtain longer term data.

References

1 Hamilton, JB. Male hormone stimulation is prerequisite and an incitant in common baldness. Am J Anatomy. 1942; 71: 451

2 Imperato-McGinley T, Guerrero L, Gautier T, Peterson RE. Steroid 5α- reductase deficiency in man: an inherited form of male pseudohermaphroditism. Science. 1974; 186: 1213-1215

3 Gormley GJ, Stoner E, Bruskewitz RC *et al.* The effect of finasteride in men with benign prostatic hyperplasia. N Engl J Med. 1992; 327: 1185-1191

4 Rhodes L, Harper J, Uno H, *et al.* The effects of finasteride (Proscar®) on hair growth, hair cycle stage, and serum testosterone and dihydrotestosterone in adult male and female stumptail macaques (Macaca Arctoides). J Clin Endocrinol Metab. 1994; 79: 991-996

5 Dallob AL, Sadick N, Unger W, *et al.* The effect of finasteride, a 5α-reductase inhibitor, on scalp skin testosterone and dihydrotestosterone concentrations in patients with male pattern baldness. J Clin Endocrinol Metab. 1994; 79: 703-706

Sebaceous gland

Workshop report on:

The sebaceous gland

T. Kealey

Were a bomb to have landed on Brussels between the 8th and 10th October 1995, the progress of hair research would have been gravely impeded. But the progress of sebaceous research would have been even more grievously arrested, since practically everybody who is anybody in sebaceous gland research worldwide occupied the Hotel Metropole conference hall between 13h00 and 14h00 on Tuesday, October 10th 1995.

Dr Kealey of Cambridge University, the workshop organizer, started the workshop with a brief review of the history of the isolation, organ maintenance and cell culture of the sebaceous gland. He referred only very briefly to the clinical work of Professor Cunliffe (Leeds University), to the work on the cell biology of the rat preputial gland of Dr Rosenfield (Chicago University), to the work on the organ maintenance of the human sebaceous gland of Dr Guy (Cambridge University), and to the work on the molecular biology of androgens within the hamster flank organ of Drs Seki, Adachi *et al.* of Shiseido, since they had already spoken during the plenary sessions, and they attended the workshop. Similarly, Dr Zouboulis' cell culture work on the human sebaceous gland had largely been covered by his poster, though he kindly elaborated on it. Dr Kealey noted with regret that Drs Doran and Shapiro, late of Roche, were no longer culturing human sebocytes, and he also noted with regret that Dr Downing of Iowa University had apparently abandoned sebaceous lipogenesis for epidermal lipogenesis.

Miss Cheryl Smythe and Miss Michaela Tillmanns, both of Cambridge University, briefly reviewed current knowledge on sebaceous lipogenesis, and reference was also made to the work of Dr Middleton (of Nottingham University). Dr Malcolm Hodgins of Glasgow University made some pertinent points.

Perhaps the most animated general discussion focussed on Dr Rosenfield's informing us that a mouse had now been bred that incorporated the large SV40 antigen in its genome (but only activated at 32°C) which might make *in vitro* immortalization very easy in future, and not just for the sebaceous gland. There was general agreement that an immortalized sebocyte cell line that demonstrated no de-differentiation *in vitro* was probably the most urgent need in sebaceous gland research today.

General satisfaction was expressed that sebaceous research seemed to be progressing satisfactorily, if slowly, but that an initial mass of researchers had apparently been achieved. The major political event that emerged was a general consent to Dr Zouboulis' suggestion that he canvass the world of sebaceous research with the suggestion that he could organize a stand-alone international sebaceous forum in Berlin next year (the world's first) and that he would also canvass for answers to the following questions:

1) has the time come for a regular international sebaceous meeting?

2) should it stand alone or be associated with an established meeting?

3) if so, which? (Dr Valerie Randall put in a passionate plea for an association with the EHRS).

Anyone who wishes should contact Dr Zouboulis in Germany on:

Fax no 49-30 8445-4262

Finally, profound thanks were expressed to Dr Dominique Van Neste and to Dr Valerie Randall and the other organizers for the opportunity to hold the sebaceous gland workshop. It was deemed a success, and no bombs fell.

Characterization of FAR-17a, androgen regulated gene expression in sebaceous glands

T. Seki[1], J.A. Rothnagel[2], D. Bundman[2], D.R. Roop[2] and K. Adachi[1]

[1]Shiseido Research Center, 2-12-1, Fukuura, Kanazawa-ku, Yokohama, 236, Japan
[2]Department of Cell Biology, Baylor College of Medicine, One Baylor Plaza, Houston, TX 77030, U.S.A.

Introduction

Sebaceous glands of several mammalian species respond to sex hormones [1]. It is known that androgens stimulate the growth, differentiation and secretion of sebaceous glands of human and other mammals. We have used flank organs of Golden Syrian hamsters as an androgen-regulated model system for human sebaceous glands and hair follicles regulated by androgens. The flank organs are paired-pigmented spots on their backs, which consist of large sebaceous glands, hair follicles and dermal pigment [2, 3]. The flank organs of male hamsters are larger and heavier than those of females. After castration of male hamsters, the size of the flank organ decreases and subsequent androgen administration restores their normal size. Similarly, the flank organs of females can be stimulated by androgens.

To elucidate the mechanism of androgen regulation of gene expression in sebaceous glands and hair follicles, we have recently isolated a cDNA clone from the flank organs-cDNA library by differential hybridization [4]. It was termed FAR-17a, whose expression was found to be highly sensitive to androgens. FAR-17a mRNA of 1.8 kb was reduced after castration and reappeared after stimulation with testosterone. Among several tissues examined, *FAR-17a* gene was expressed at a high level in flank organ and a low level in earlobe and testis [4]. However, various topical steroid applications to the flank organ of castrated male hamsters, showed a full re-activation of mRNA by testosterone and dihydrotestosterone, partial re-activation by androstanedione and androstenedione, and no activation by androstanediol nor dehydroepiandrosterone by dot blot hybridization [5]. As the result of southern blot analysis, it was suggested that *FAR-17a* gene was phylogenetically conserved. This FAR-17a cDNA has 1,637 nucleotides and 693 nucleotides in the coding region. The coding sequence provides a protein of 231 amino acids with a molecular weight of about 27 kDa having basic properties. The data bank did not reveal a strong, significant homology of these cDNA and amino-acid sequences with any published DNA and amino acids sequences [4].

Materials and methods

A primer for reverse transcriptase reaction was FAR-T2: 5'pG665GACACCGCGATGAGAGT682OH3'. Primers for PCR were FAR-T1: 5'pA147CAGAAGCCATGACGAGG164OH3' and FAR-T2 (the same above). Synthetic peptide A was D30DEKLKEFHDGGRSKYL46 GGC (hydrophilic region) and synthetic peptide B was CGGN215HWKWGATVKPLMKKKK231 (C-terminal region). GGC and CGG were used as a hinge. These primers and synthetic peptides were obtained by Protein Chemistry Core Facility, Baylor College of Medicine (Houston, TX).

Hormone treatment of animals

Male and female hamsters (8 weeks after birth, weighing 110 to 130 g) were used in the study. Male hamsters were castrated bilaterally via the scrotal route. 14 days-postcastrated and female hamsters were injected intramuscularly daily with DHT(5α-dihydrotestosterone) 5 mg in sesame oil.

RNA isolation and RT-PCR

Total cellular RNA for RT-PCR was isolated from hamster flank organs by AGPC extraction [6]. Competitive PCR for quantification of mRNA was done according to a procedure previously described [7].

Immunoblot analysis and double-label immunofluorescence identification

Rabbits were used for immunization against the synthetic peptides FAR-17a (A) , FAR-17a(B) coupled to keyhole limpet hemocyanin. Peptide(A) is the hydrophilic region and peptide(B) is the C-terminal region of the deduced FAR-17a protein. These two kinds of rabbit serums were purified by affinity column chromatography with Affi-Gel 102 coupled with each peptide independently. Immunoblot analysis was done as described previously [8, 9]. In the immunofluorescence, the antibodies used were anti FAR-17a (A) antibody, anti FAR-17a(B) antibody, anti mouse keratin K14 C terminal antibody [10] and anti human keratin K14 antibody [11, 12].

Results and discussion

Among several examined, *FAR-17a* gene was expressed at a high level in flank organ and low level in testis and earlobe. However, it was not clear whether *FAR-17a* gene was expressed or not in skin excluding flank organ. In skin of normal male hamsters, the expression of FAR-17a was detected by RT-PCR. By daily subcutaneous injection of androgen to female hamsters, the expression of *FAR-17a* gene could be detected in the female skin. The expression in skin of hamsters was also androgen-regulated. It seemed very important to examine whether this gene had a role only in special tissues like flank organs and earlobes and in a special portion in these tissues. Recent studies have shown that the dermal pigment and the underlying sebaceous gland may respond quite independently to androgenic stimulation [13, 14]. The hair follicles in the flank organ are more sensitive to testosterone than are dermal pigment or sebaceous glands [15]. But the expression was also detected in skin excluding flank organs. Although the expression of FAR-17a mRNA is androgen-regulated, we do not know its biological significance.

We produced two different monospecific antibodies against two kind of peptides of the deduced FAR-17a protein in order to analyze the expression and localization. These polyclonal antibodies were purified by affinity column chromatography. These two anti FAR-17a antibodies detected in a male flank organ a protein, of the same size, about 27 kDa, as that of the deduced FAR-17a protein. The expression of FAR-17a protein was decreased after castration and the protein expression could not be detected in the flank organs of 14 days post-castrated male hamsters . However, the expression of FAR-17a protein increased after injection of androgen time-dependently. It was proved that the expression of FAR-17a protein was also androgen-regulated.

These anti FAR-17a protein antibodies stained sebaceous glands especially and sheath of hair follicle faintly in a male flank organ. Anti mouse keratin K14 antibody stained epithelial cells like epidermis, sebaceous glands and outer root sheath of hair follicles of a male flank organ. We tried to stain hair follicles of human scalp tissues with the anti FAR-17a antibody and anti human keratin K14 antibody by double-label immunofluorescence identification. Anti human keratin K14 antibody stained outer root sheath of hair follicles [12] and anti FAR-17a (B) antibody stained inner root sheath, just inside of outer root sheath which anti human keratin K14 antibody stained.

As FAR-17a mRNA and protein were expressed at high level in sebaceous glands, these may be involved in lipid synthesis. However, this androgen-regulated FAR-17a protein (homologue) was located in the epithelial cells of human hair follicles (inner root sheath cells). On the other hand, sex hormones and antiandrogens influenced *in vitro* growth of dermal papilla cells and outer root sheath keratinocytes of human hair follicles [15, 16]. There is a possibility that FAR-17a protein is involved in the epithelial differentiation of hair follicles.

References

1   Strauss JS, Pochi PE. Recent Prg Horm Res. 1963; 19: 385-444
2   Hamilton JB, Montagna W. Am J Anat. 1950; 86; 191-234
3   Takayasu S, Adachi K. J Invest Dermatol. 1970; 55: 13-19
4   Seki T, Ideta R, Shibuya M, Adachi K. J Invest Dermato.l 1991; 96: 926-931
5   Hisaoka H, Ideta R, Seki T, Adachi K. Arch Dermatol Res. 1991; 283: 269-273

6   Chomczynski P, Sacchi N. Anal Biochem. 1987; 162: 156-159
7   Rappolee DA, Mark D, Banda M J, Werb Z. Science. 1988; 241: 708-712
8   Laemmli UK. Anal Biochem. 1976; 72: 248-254
9   Burnette W N. Anal Biochem. 1981; 112: 195-203
10 Roop DR, Cheng CK, Titterington L, Meyers CA, Stanley JR, Steinert PM, Yuspa SH. J Biol Chem. 1984; 259: 8037-8040
11 Caselitz. J Pathol Anat. 1986; 409: 725
12 Woodcock-Mitchell JR, Eichner R, Nelson WG, Sun TT. J Cell Biol. 1982; 95: 580-588
13 Lucky AW, McGuire J, Nydrof E, Halpert G, Nuck BA. J Invest Dermatol. 1986; 86: 83-86
14 Vermorken AJM, Goos CMAA, Wirtz P. Br J Dermatol. 1982; 106: 99-101
15 Kiesewetter F, Arai A, Hitzenstern JV, Schell H. Arch Dermatol Res. 1991; 283: 476-479
16 Kiesewetter F, Arai A, Schell H. J Invest Dermatol. 1993; 101- 98S-105S

©1996 Elsevier Science B.V. All rights reserved.
Hair research for the next millenium
D.J.J. Van Neste and V.A. Randall (Eds)

Preputial cell culture as a model system to study sebocyte development

R.L. Rosenfield

Departments of Pediatrics and Medicine, Section of Pediatric Endocrinology, University of Chicago Pritzker School of Medicine, Wyler Children's Hospital, 5841 S. Maryland Ave., Chicago, IL 60637, U.S.A.

Introduction

The preputial glands are readily accessible, paired sebaceous glands located in the prepuce of rodents [1]. They consist predominantly of sebaceous cells (sebocytes), with a few other cell types such as duct cells. This sebaceous gland, like those of man, contains sebocytes in an encapsulated acinar arrangement at different maturational stages [1, 2]. Electron microscopy also shows the rodent and human glands to be similar in the morphology of organelles, such as abundant and sometimes atypical mitochondria, many perinuclear lysosomes with crystalline inclusions, peroxisomes and lipid droplets of various sizes [3, 4]. Sebocytes are specialized epithelial cells which proliferate primarily in the undifferentiated and early differentiated stages located in the basal and parabasal layers [4, 5], as in skin. They differentiate into lipid-laden cells which rupture when fully mature, giving rise to the holocrine secretion, sebum.

The development of the preputial gland, like that of human sebaceous glands, has long been known to be dependent on androgen action [1, 2]. The preputial gland grows at puberty to achieve a weight of about 0.125 g in the adult rat. This growth does not occur in the androgen-resistant rat [6, 7]. Testosterone administration is known to stimulate preputial sebocyte proliferation [8] and lipid production [9], and antiandrogen reverses this effect [8]. As also appears to be the case in human sebaceous glands [10], testosterone is converted to the more potent androgen dihydrotestosterone (DHT) by the type I isoform of 5α-reductase rather than the type II isoform that predominates in the classic androgen target tissues of the genital tract (D. Deplewski, S. Liao, and R. L. Rosenfield, unpublished).

More than androgen appears to be involved in regulating the growth and development of the preputial gland, as in human sebaceous glands [1, 2]. For example, retinoids cause atrophy and decreased lipid production [11, 12], antagonizing the effects of testosterone, while catechols stimulate lipogenesis [13].

Preputial cells in primary monolayer culture differentiate as sebocytes

Preputial cells were initially evaluated for the study of sebocyte differentiation by Wheatley *et al.* [13]. Because of limited viability, the effects of hormones and drugs could only be evaluated in incubations of under 3 hr. Lipogenesis was found to be stimulated by epinephrine, cyclic adenosine monophosphate (cAMP), and prostaglandin E_2, and it was inhibited by levodopa as well as antilipemic drugs such as nicotinic acid and clofibrate. However, no effect could be elicited from androgens or retinoic acid, apparently because the time-span of hormone exposure was too short to elicit a cellular response.

In order to assess the interactions of androgens with other hormones in the differentiation of sebocytes, we developed a primary preputial cell culture system. Single cell suspensions are prepared from preputial glands by a modification of the method of Wheatley *et al.* [13]; filleted glands are sequentially treated with Dispase (bacterial neutral protease, Type II) and trypsin [14]. Then these cells are cultured in an epithelial cell culture system on a feeder layer of mitomycin-treated J2 3T3 fibroblasts in medium containing fetal calf serum and epithelial cell growth factors [14]. We routinely use 10% fetal calf serum (FCS) with choleratoxin (10^{-10} M) and cortisol (10^{-6} M); insulin (10^{-6} M) is optional [15]. From fractionation of preputial sebocytes on a Percoll gradient, it appears that undifferentiated sebocytes grow fastest in culture, immature sebocytes retain the capacity to proliferate, and mature sebocytes are not capable of growth [14].

Preputial cells develop epithelial colonies similar to those formed by epidermal cells when observed by phase contrast microscopy. However, preputial cells can be identified as a unique epithelial cell population by the naked eye [15]: compared to epidermal cells they form a smaller number of larger colonies, grow more slowly, and develop domes before confluence.

Further characterization has shown that cultured preputial cells form very few cornified envelopes relative to epidermal cells [15]. In addition, they express a variety of keratins, including a specific cytokeratin of acinar preputial cells, K4, which is found in human sebaceous glands [16] but not in epidermis [17].

Treatment with β-adrenergic agents causes a more prominent cAMP-dependent protein kinase response in preputial cells than in epidermal cells *in vitro*, as *in vivo*, and brings about a distinctive pattern of protein kinase regulatory subunit predominance [3]. This indicates the presence of adenylate cyclase-coupled β-adrenergic receptors and a specific signal transduction pathway.

All-trans-retinoic acid inhibits proliferation of these sebocytes *in vitro* by 31% at 10^{-7} M and arrests it at 10^{-6} M, while having no such effect on epidermal cells [18]. These results indicate that the entire signal transduction pathway involved in retinoid action on sebocytes is expressed in cultured preputial cells.

The androgen receptor (AR) content of preputial cells is similar to that of the prostate gland, with 10-fold greater mRNA abundance than in epidermal cells [19]. When preputial sebocytes were separated according to their state of differentiation by gradient density centrifugation, sebocytes in the 1.080 density fraction contrasted with the more buoyant fractions in expressing significantly less AR, as determined both by immunocytochemistry and RNase protection assay. These results suggest that there is little if any *AR* gene expression in undifferentiated preputial sebocytes (which comprise about 8% of cells in the 1.080 fraction), modest expression of AR in early differentiated sebocytes (which comprise about 40% of the 1.080 fraction), and maximal *AR* gene expression in mid-to late-differentiated sebocytes (which constitute 80% or more of the cells in the more buoyant fractions). In monolayer culture sebaceous epithelial cells express AR mRNA to the same extent as in the 1.080 fraction of freshly dispersed sebocytes, which is about half that of mature sebocytes (p < .02), but about 5-fold greater than that of epidermal cells (p < .01).

Preputial sebocyte differentiation is incomplete in monolayer culture

Preputial sebocytes do not completely differentiate in monolayer culture. By light microscopy, only occasional preputial cells in culture accumulate the fused lipid droplets that are characteristic of mature sebocytes [14]. By electron microscopy it can be seen that preputial cells indeed form abundant tiny lipid droplets, but these droplets fuse in only a very few cells at the center of colonies [14]. These data indicate that preputial sebocytes undergo early differentiation in culture, but seldom reach the stage of mid-differentiation at which intracytoplasmic lipid droplets fuse. The level of *AR* gene expression also indicates that sebocytes do not mature fully in the preputial cell culture system.

Androgen has a paradoxical effect in this system [20]. Androgen inhibits preputial sebocyte proliferation via an AR-dependent mechanism: DHT 10^{-7} M inhibited proliferation of sebocytes (63.8 ± 6.8, SEM, % of control; p < .005), but not of epidermal cells, and the antiandrogen hydroxyflutamide competitively blocked the DHT effect. Furthermore, hydroxyflutamide alone stimulated sebocyte growth, apparently by blocking the action of the nanomolar amount of androgens present in fetal calf serum. We hypothesize that these results indicate that androgen acts to switch early differentiated preputial sebocytes from a proliferative mode to a more differentiated mode, but the latter cannot be expressed because an inhibitory influence upon lipogenesis is imposed by the tissue culture system. Whether DHT exerts its effect on the sebocyte or the feeder layer is unknown.

A certain sequence in the development of hormonal responsiveness during sebocyte differentiation may be deduced from these studies (Table 1):

1) full responsiveness to retinoic acid occurs early in sebocyte differentiation,

2) the β-adrenergic and androgen signal transduction pathways seem to be in place within this stage of differentiation, but

3) full responsiveness of sebocyte lipogenesis to androgen and catechols does not become possible until later in differentiation.

Table 1.
Proposed model of structure-function relationships in sebocyte development

Sebocyte stage	Lipid formation	Hormonal responsiveness
Undifferentiated	None	None
Early differentiated	Perinuclear droplets	Retinoid responsiveness β-adrenergic signal transduction Androgen signal transduction
Mid-differentiated	Fused droplets	Enhancement of lipogenesis
Late differentiated	Drops	Induction of endonuclease?

The challenge of attaining complete sebocyte differentiation in culture

Recent progress in human sebocyte research is pertinent to the developmental biological issues in preputial cell culture. Akamatsu, *et al.* recently reported that human sebocyte proliferation in culture is stimulated by androgen [21]. DHT stimulated the growth of sebocytes from the face and thigh in a dose-dependent manner, with significant stimulation being observed at doses of 10^{-8} M or more. The antiandrogen spironolactone reversed the DHT effect [22]. There are many differences between their study system and ours: human vs rat, secondary vs primary culture, absence vs presence of serum growth factors, and absence vs presence of a stromal feeder layer.

In order to study preputial sebocyte development in the absence of a feeder layer, we have recently turned to the use of conditionally immortal mouse preputial cells. Preputial cells have been grown from a transgenic mouse homozygous for a temperature sensitive strain of the simian virus large tumor antigen which is linked to an interferon-inducable promoter [23]. These cells attach and grow well without a feeder layer in the presence of 10% FCS, choleratoxin, cortisol and γ-interferon. Our preliminary data indicate that they are capable of differentiating further than wild type preputial cells: they develop more fused lipid droplets than epidermal cells similarly prepared according to Nile Red fluorescence. This is a promising system for the further study of sebocyte growth and development.

References

1 Wheatley VR. Jarrett A, ed. Physiology and Pathophysiology of Skin. New York: Academic Press. 1986; Vol 9
2 Thody AT, Shuster S. Physiol Rev. 1989; 69: 383-415

3 Ellis RA. Baccaredda-Boy, Morretti G, Frey JR (eds). Biopathology of pattern alopecia. Karger, Basel. 1968; 146-154
4 Mednieks MI, Laurent SJ, Hand AR, Rosenfield RL. J Invest Dermatol. 1991; 97: 517-523
5 Jenkinson DM, Elder HY, Montgomery I, Moss VA. Tissue & Cell. 1985; 17: 683-698
6 Sherins RJ, Bardin CW. Endocrinol. 1971; 89: 835-841
7 Yarbrough WG, Quarmby VE, Simental JA, Joseph DR, Sar M, Lubahn DB, Olsen KL, French FS, Wilson EM. J Biol Chem. 1990; 265: 8893-8900
8 Ebling FJ. Acta Endocrinol. 1973; 72: 361-365
9 Mesquita-Guimaraes, Coimbra A. Arch Dermatol Res. 1981; 270: 325-331
10 Luu-The V, Sugimoto Y, Puy L, Labrie Y, Solache IM, Singh M, Labrie F. J Invest Dermatol. 1994; 102: 221-226
11 Boris A, Hurley J, Wong CQ, Comai K, Shapiro S. Arch Dermatol Res. 1988; 280: 246-251
12 Gomez EC, Martinez CA. J Am Acad Dermatol. 1982; 6: 746-750
13 Wheatley VR, Brind JL. J Invest Dermatol. 1981; 76: 293-296
14 Rosenfield RL. J Invest Dermatol. 1989; 92: 751-754
15 Laurent SJ, Mednieks MI, Rosenfield RL. In vitro Cell Dev Biol. 1992; 28A: 83-89
16 Latham JAE, Redfern CPF, Thody AJ, de Kretser TA. J Histochem Cytochem. 1989; 37: 729-734
17 Moll R, Franke W W, Schiller DL, Geiger B, Krepler R. Cell. 1982; 31: 11-24
18 Rosenfield RL, Deplewski D. Am J Med. 1995; 98 (suppl 1A): 80S-88S
19 Miyake K, Ciletti N, Liao S, Rosenfield RL. J Invest Dermatol. 1994; 103: 721-725
20 Rosenfield RL, Miyake K, Ciletti N, Liao S. Clin Res. 1993; 41: 257A
21 Akamatsu H, Zouboulis C, Orfanos CE. J Invest Dermatol. 1992; 99: 509-511
22 Akamatsu H, Zouboulis C, Orfanos CE. J Invest Dermatol. 1993; 100: 660-662
23 Jat PS, Noble MD, Ataliotis P, Tanaka Y, Yannoutsos N, Larsen L, Kiousis D. Proc Natl Acad Sci (USA). 1991; 88: 5096-5100

The improved organ maintenance of the human sebaceous gland: modelling *in vitro* the effects of epidermal growth factor and steroid hormones

R. Guy, C. Ridden and T. Kealey

Department of Clinical Biochemistry, University of Cambridge, Addenbrooke's Hospital, Hills Road, Cambridge, CB2 2QR, UK

Introduction

The sebaceous gland *in vivo* demonstrates a number of responses to external stimuli. Androgens cause the gland to develop at puberty [1], oestrogens reduce the rate of sebum excretion in both humans [2] and in animal models [3], 13-*cis* retinoic acid will dramatically reduce sebaceous gland size and sebum excretion [4], while trauma [5] and epidermal growth factor [6] promote an injury response. To help understand the mechanism of these responses, we need to model them *in vitro*, and sebaceous glands maintained as whole organs should provide an optimal system [7]. We have previously reported that human sebaceous glands can be maintained for up to fourteen days as whole organs with full retention of the physiological rate and pattern of new cell formation, but we also reported that the newly formed cells did not differentiate normally, causing a progressive loss of lipogenesis *in vitro* [8]. We now show that this abnormal sebocyte differentiation was attributable to the presence of epidermal growth factor (EGF) and phenol red, the pH indicator used in William's E medium, in our maintenance medium. In their absence human sebaceous glands apparently differentiate normally and respond physiologically to external agents.

Materials and methods

Isolation and maintenance of viable human sebaceous glands

Samples of normal midline chest skin (5mm x 80mm) were obtained from male patients aged between forty and seventy-five undergoing cardiac surgery at Papworth Hospital, Papworth Everard, Huntingdon, UK. Both ethical committee permission and patient consent had been granted for this technique. Glands were isolated by shearing [9] and maintained overnight, floating on polycarbonate filters (pore size 0.45 μm) in 5ml of William's E medium at 37°C supplemented with 2 mM L-glutamine, 100 units/ml penicillin and streptomycin, 2.5 μg/ml Fungizone®, 10 μg/ml insulin, 10 ng/ml EGF, 10 μg/ml transferrin, 10 ng/ml hydrocortisone, 10 ng/ml sodium selenite, 3nMtriiodothyronine, 1% (v/v) trace elements mix, 10 μg/ml bovine pituitary extract, and buffered in a humidified 5% CO_2/95% air atmosphere. In the text this will be referred to as supplemented William's E medium. Where glands are maintained in supplemented, phenol red-free, William's E medium without the addition of EGF this will be referred to in the text as new supplemented William's E medium.

Where appropriate, 1 μm 13-*cis* retinoic acid, 1nM testosterone, 1nM DHT or 600pM water soluble 17-β oestradiol was added. The concentrations of testosterone, DHT and 17-β oestradiol are all in the physiological range [10]; 1 μM 13-*cis* retinoic acid is the clinical therapeutic concentration [11] and the lowest concentration that has previously given maximal inhibition of lipogenesis in the isolated sebaceous gland [8]. Where these additions were absent from control experiments, an equal volume of vehicle was added.

Rates of lipogenesis, DNA synthesis and pattern of lipogenesis

The rate and pattern of [U-14C] acetate incorporation and the rate of [methyl-3H] thymidine incorporation was determined as previously described [8].

Light microscopy

Glands were fixed in phosphate buffered saline containing 4.25% glutaraldehyde for twenty-four hours. The glands were then processed by standard methods, followed by staining with haematoxylin and eosin.

Results

On isolation, glands demonstrated typical *in situ* morphology and the three distinct sebocyte cell types were seen: peripheral undifferentiated cells, partially differentiated cells, and mature differentiated sebocytes containing many lipid droplets (Fig. 1a).

After seven days' maintenance in supplemented William's E medium, there was a large increase in the number of undifferentiated cells. Mature sebocytes were only present centrally, there was hyperkeratinisation of the luminal surface of the gland and the rate of lipogenesis fell (Table 1).

All supplements had been previously added arbitrarily on the assumption that all were necessary for gland maintenance. To establish which of these supplements were essential, and to exclude those that had no effect or were inhibitory, we maintained glands with each of the supplements removed in turn, with all the others still present. Removing EGF caused increased rates of lipogenesis over seven days (Table 1). In addition, the pattern of lipogenesis was very similar to that seen in freshly isolated glands (data not shown). This improvement was achieved without an increase in the rate of cell division (Table 1). The subsequent, individual, removal of the other supplements from the medium, however, all resulted in lower rates of lipogenesis (data not shown).

When glands were maintained for seven days in new supplemented William's E medium (without phenol red and EGF) there was apparently almost perfect retention of *in situ* morphology (Fig. 1b). The three distinct sebocyte cell types were seen. This suggests that normal gland function is maintained over seven days in culture in this medium. In addition, we found that maintaining glands in phenol red-free medium further improved rates of lipogenesis, such that they did not fall over seven days in culture (Table 1). The pattern of lipid synthesis in glands maintained for seven days in this new supplemented William's E medium was similar to that of freshly isolated glands (data not shown). There was, moreover, no change in the rate of cell division. When phenol red was returned to the medium, there was a reduction in the rate of lipogenesis back to control levels (Table 1).

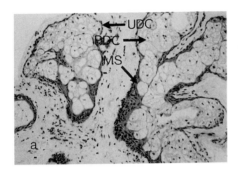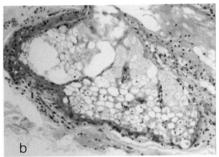

Figure 1.(a) A freshly isolated human sebaceous gland. The three distinct sebocyte cell types can be seen: peripheral undifferentiated cells (UDC) partially differentiated cells (PDC) and mature differentiated sebocytes (MS).
Figure 1(b) A sebaceous gland maintained for seven days in new supplemented William's E medium.

When glands were maintained for seven days in new supplemented William's E medium, further supplemented with 600pM 17-β oestradiol, there was a thickening of the undifferentiated basal cell layer and some luminal keratinisation. In addition, the rate of lipogenesis fell over seven days but there was no change in the rate of cell division (Table 1). This indicates, therefore, that 17-β oestradiol is altering the normal pattern of differentiation of the newly formed sebocytes. When glands were maintained for seven days in new supplemented William's E medium further supplemented with 1nM testosterone there was no apparent change in gland morphology and no change in the rate of lipogenesis (Table 1). Similarly the addition of 1nM DHT had no effect (Table 1) indicating that the lack of an effect with testosterone is not simply due to a lack of active 5α-reductase in the gland. These findings suggest, therefore, that androgens are not necessary for short-term stimulation of lipogenesis. When glands were maintained for seven days in new supplemented William's E medium further supplemented with 1 μM 13-*cis* retinoic acid, there was a thickening of the peripheral undifferentiated cells layer of the gland, a small degree of luminal keratinisation and a significant fall in the rates of lipogenesis and cell division (Table 1).

Table 1.
Rates of lipogenesis and DNA synthesis in isolated sebaceous glands

Condition of maintenance	Rates of lipogenesis pmols/mg wet weight/.hour (mean±SEM)		Rates of cell division fmols/mg wet weight/.hour (mean±SEM)	
	Fresh	*Seven days*	*Fresh*	*Seven Days*
Supplemented William's E	1131.5 ±129.3	201.9 ±38.6¶		
Supplemented William's E without EGF	1275.2 ±117.0	643.2 ±150.7†	168.2 ±15.9	160.4 ±17.2
New Supplemented William's E	1545.2 ±283.9	1512.8 ±175.4	154.9 ±17.9	147.6 ±18.4
+10mg/ml Phenol Red	1361.7 ±131.6	788.7 ±140.4*	152.5 ±19.5	149.9 ±21.2
+600pM Oestrogen		891.5 ±153.1**		155.8 ±33.2
+1nM Testosterone		1527.0 ±163.1		145.1 ±25.8
+1nM DHT		1593.0 ±181.3		151.4 ±39.2
+1μM 13-*cis* Retinoic Acid		783.8 ±133.7**		94.1 ±18.1**

n=5 subjects for all conditions, 5 glands per subject per time point.
¶ *indicates a significant difference (p<0.01)with regard to fresh glands maintained in supplemented William's E medium,*
† *indicates a significant difference (p<0.01) with regard to fresh glands maintained in supplemented William's E medium without EGF and glands maintained for seven days in supplemented William's E,*
* *indicates a significant difference (p<0.01) with regard to glands maintained for seven days in new supplemented William's E medium and fresh glands maintained in new supplemented William's E, further supplemented with 10mg/ml phenol red,*
** *indicates a significant difference (p<0.01) with regard to glands maintained for seven days in new supplemented William's E medium by Student's paired t-test.*

Discussion

In this study we have described significant improvements in the maintenance of the isolated sebaceous gland. We have shown that in this improved model, where we are able to apparently retain normal sebaceous gland function over seven days, we can apparently model the *in vivo* actions of steroids and EGF.

The *in vitro* effects of EGF on the sebaceous gland may be significant as there is extensive evidence for a significant role for EGF in skin development and maintenance. *In vivo*, human skin has high concentrations of the EGF receptor in the basal cells of the epidermis and in the skin appendages [12] and we have shown that EGF stimulates a population of dividing cells in the hair follicle [13]. This, and our own data suggest that EGF may play an important physiological role in sebocyte differentiation.

The *in vitro* effect of 17-β oestradiol complements current *in vivo* data. Oestrogens have been shown to inhibit lipogenesis in the human sebaceous gland [2] and the rat preputial gland [3]. Phenol red has been described as having oestrogen-like effects [14] which may explain its effects on gland morphology and lipogenesis and why they are very similar to those of 17-β oestradiol. When we added testosterone to this improved model we were unable to observe any effect. This was not due to a lack of 5α-reductase activity since DHT was also found to have no effect. These *in vitro* effects apparently mimic those *in vivo* since pharmacological doses of testosterone over a number of weeks in adult males causes only a small rise in the rate of sebum secretion [2]. In addition, the anti-androgen 17-α-propyltestosterone has no effect on sebum excretion rate over twelve weeks in man [15] and it is only after much longer term treatment of up to thirty-seven months that sebum excretion rates are reduced with the antiandrogen cyproterone acetate [16]. Therefore, whilst androgens are clearly essential for sebaceous gland development at puberty [1] and for the long term maintenance of sebum secretion, they do not appear to be necessary for short-term stimulation of lipogenesis.

The *in vitro* effects of 13-*cis* retinoic acid have been described *in vivo* [4, 17] and demonstrate that we are apparently able to model its therapeutic action.

Acknowledgements

We thank the surgeons at Papworth Hospital for supplying us with skin. We thank Mr. C Burton of the Department of Histopathology for his assistance with the photography and Mr. D Thompson for technical assistance. We thank Dr. A Evenson, Dr. W Gibson, Dr. M Green and Mr. C Harding of Unilever and Dr. M Philpott of our own group for stimulating discussions. This work was supported by Unilever Research and, in its earlier phase, by the MRC, Glaxo and Mrs. Ellie Barker.

References

1   Pochi P E, Strauss J S, Downing D T. J Invest Dermatol. 1979; 73: 108-111
2   Strauss J S, Kligman A M, Pochi P E. J Invest Dermatol. 1962; 39: 139-155
3   Ebling F J, Skinner J. J Invest Dermatol. 1983; 81: 448-451
4   Landhaler M, Kummermehr J, Wagner A, Plewig G. Arch Dermatol Res. 1980; 269: 297-309
5   Irvin T T. Wound Healing Principles and Practice. Chapman and Hall. 1981; 25-28
6   Moore G P M, Panaretto B A, Carter N B. J Invest Dermatol. 1985; 84: 172-175
7   Freshney I R. Culture of Animal Cells. Wiley-Liss. 1987; 297-307
8   Ridden J, Ferguson D, Kealey T. J Cell Science. 1990; 95: 125-136
9   Kealey T. Methods Enzymol. 1990; 190: 338-345
10 Cook B, Beastall G H. In: Green B and Leake R E (eds). Steroid hormones, a practical approach. IRL Press. 1987; 1-65
11 Colburn W A, Gibson D M. Clin Pharmacol Ther. 1985; 37: 411-414
12 Green M R, Couchman J R. J Invest Dermatol. 1985; 85: 239-245
13 Philpott M P, Kealey T. J Invest Dermatol. 1994; 102: 186-191
14 Leake R E, Freshney R I, Munir I. In: Green B and Leake R E (eds.) Steroid hormones, a practical approach. IRL Press. 1987; 205-218
15 Franz T J, Lehman P A, Pochi P, Odland G F, Olerud J. J Invest Dermatol. 1989; 93: 475-479
16 Burton J L, Laschet U, Shuster S. Br J Dermatol. 1973; 89: 487-490
17 Jones D H, King K, Miller A J, Cunliffe W J. Br J Dermatol. 1983; 108: 333-345

Human sebocyte cultures are an appropriate model for studying sebaceous gland function at the cellular level

Ch. Zouboulis

Department of Dermatology, University Medical Center Benjamin Franklin, The Free University of Berlin, Berlin, Germany

Introduction

The development of methods for cultivation of human sebocytes *in vitro* [1] (Fig. 1) makes studies at the cellular and molecular level possible, leading to the establishment of new concepts in understanding sebaceous gland function.

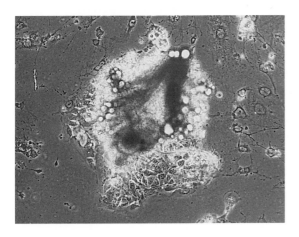

Figure 1. Primary sebocyte culture outgrowing from an isolated sebaceous gland

Sebocyte activity and lipids

Despite the preservation of several markers of sebocyte differentiation *in vitro* [2, 3], cultured sebocytes were shown to produce low amounts of squalene and only exhibit a moderate increase of cell size during differentiation [4, 5] (Table 1). These findings confirm *in vivo* results of a positive correlation of squalene amounts with cell size, especially in acne-involved sebaceous glands [6]. It is likely, that sebaceous glands follow *in vivo* the saturated side chains metabolic pathway (Kandutsch-Russel pathway), so that they do not metabolize squalene to cholesterol. On the other hand, total lipid synthesis and squalene metabolism to cholesterol are antagonistic NADPH-dependent phenomena. Therefore, squalene in sebum could be a reliable marker of sebocyte activity and terminal differentiation *in vivo* and *in vitro*.

In contrast to previous concepts, which supposed free fatty acids as a product of triglyceride metabolism induced by follicular bacteria, it was found that human sebocytes *in vitro* synthesize low amounts of free fatty acids [4]. One of them, linoleic acid, shown to suppress neutrophil oxygen metabolism and phagocytosis, stimulated sebocyte proliferation *in vitro* [7] (Fig. 2). Therefore, linoleic acid may play a role in the induction of acne lesions.

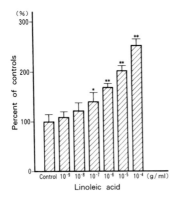

*Figure 2. Linoleic acid stimulates sebocyte proliferation. *p<0.05, **p<0.01*

Sebocytes and androgens

Sebocytes cultured from different body parts (face and upper legs) were found to respond to androgens in a distinct way [8, 9]. Testosterone inhibited the proliferation of sebocytes derived from the legs and decreased intracellular total lipids, while it stimulated the proliferation of facial sebocytes (Fig. 3). In contrast, 5α-dihydrotestosterone stimulated proliferation and lipid synthesis of sebocytes from both face and legs. These findings confirm the recently detected

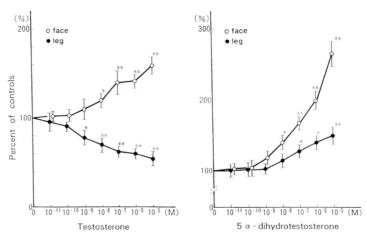

*Figure 3. Effects of androgens on the proliferation of human sebocytes. *p<0.05, **p<0.01*

Table 1.
Characteristics of sebocyte differentiation *in vitro*

Morphology
- Polymorphic epithelial appearance not resembling a cobble-stone pattern (**A**)
- Presence of cells in several stages of sebocytic differentiation with moderate increase of cell size (**B-D**)
- Abundant cytoplasmic lipid droplets in differentiated sebocytes (**E**)
- Lack of desmosomes in intercellular contacts

Activity
- Slower proliferation than epidermal keratinocytes of the same subjects
- Decreasing number of proliferating cells after subcultivation
- Lipid synthesis during cell proliferation (**F**)
- 4-8 times higher lipid content than keratinocytes
- Synthesis of squalene, wax esters, and free fatty acids (**G**)

Antigen phenotype
- Expression of human polymorphous epithelial mucin epitopes, Sebaceous Gland Antigen (SGA) and MAM-6c
- Expression of keratins 4, 13 and 7 (**H, I, J**)
- Enhanced expression of keratin 19 compared to keratinocytes (**J**)
- No expression of keratins 1 and 2
- Low expression levels of involucrin and formation of small numbers of cornified envelopes

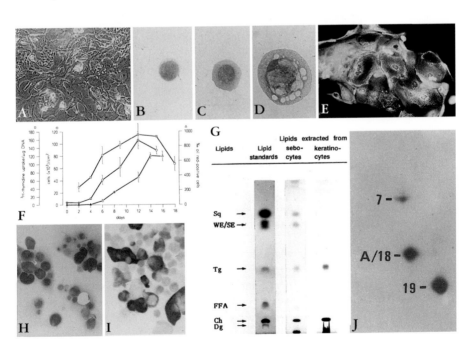

390

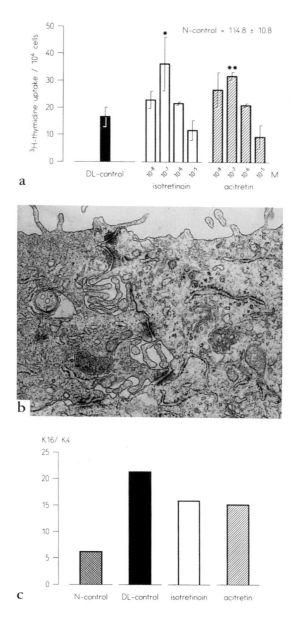

Figure 4. Sebocytes maintained under serum-free (vitamin A-free) conditions.
(a) Prominent decrease of proliferation.
(b) Electron microscopy shows narrow intercellular spaces and abundant desmosomes.
(c) Keratin 16:4 ratio, which negatively correlates with sebocyte differentiation, increased.
Retinoids partially restored the altered sebocyte functions. *p<0.05, **p<0.01

higher 5α-reductase activity in acne-prone skin than in skin from arms, abdomen and legs, especially in the sebaceous glands [10]. They also could explain the predisposition of certain areas of the body to acne lesions.

Sebocytes and retinoids

Vitamin A and retinoids have been shown to produce considerable morphological and biochemical changes to sebaceous glands *in vivo*; *in vitro*, vitamin A was found essential for sebocyte activity and differentiation [11]. Cultivation of sebocytes under serum-free (vitamin A-free) conditions resulted in prominent decrease of proliferation (Fig. 4a), number of intracellular lipid droplets, synthesis of total lipids, especially triglycerides, squalene, and wax esters, and labeling with monoclonal antibodies identifying progressive and late-stage sebocyte differentiation. Intercellular spaces narrowed and cell-to-cell contacts were established by abundant desmosomes (Fig. 4b). The keratin 16: 4 ratio which negatively correlates with sebocyte differentiation, increased (Fig. 4c). Both nonaromatic (isotretinoin) and aromatic (acitretin) retinoids partially reversed the effects of delipidization (vitamin A depletion) on sebocytes in a similar way (Fig. 4a).

In contrast, the same retinoids exhibited distinct, clinical-like effects under normal culture conditions [4, 12]. Nonaromatic retinoids (isotretinoin, tretinoin) decreased sebocyte proliferation in a dose-and time-dependent manner, while acitretin was only active in high concentrations (Fig. 5a). Furthermore, isotretinoin was the most potent inhibitor of lipid synthesis, decreasing triglycerides, wax/sterol esters, free fatty acids, and squalene (Fig. 5b).

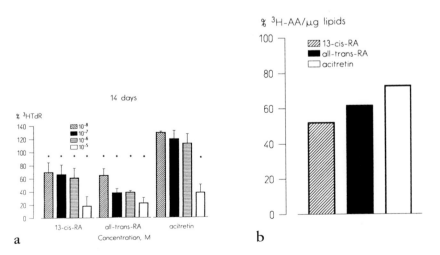

Figure 5. Retinoids and human sebocytes. (a) Inhibition of proliferation by nonaromatic retinoids, (b) quantitation of sebocyte lipids.$*p<0.05$

These results indicate that differentiated retinoid action on the sebaceous gland could rather be an effect of the interaction of synthetic retinoids with vitamin A and/or with other molecules.

References

1   Xia L, Zouboulis Ch, Detmar M, *et al.* J Invest Dermatol. 1989; 93: 315-321
2   Zouboulis ChC, Xia L, Detmar M, *et al.* Skin Pharmacol. 1991; 4: 74-83
3   Zouboulis ChC. In vitro Cell Dev Biol. 1992; 28A: 699
4   Zouboulis ChC, Xia L, Korge B, *et al.* In: Saurat J-H, ed. Retinoids 10 years on. Basel: Karger. 1991; 254-273
5   Zouboulis ChC, Krieter A, Gollnick H, Orfanos CE. Exp Dermatol. 1994; 3: 151-160
6   Stewart ME, Sears JK, Downing DT. J Invest Dermatol. 1991; 96: 594A.
7   Akai Y, Akamatsu H, Ri S, *et al.* Jpn J Dermatol. 1994; 104: 647-649
8   Akamatsu H, Zouboulis ChC, Orfanos CE. J Invest Dermatol. 1992; 99: 509-511
9   Zouboulis ChC, Akamatsu H, Stephanek K, Orfanos CE. Skin Pharmacol. 1994; 7: 33-40
10 Thiboutot D, Harris G, Iles V, *et al.* J Invest Dermatol. 1995; 105: 209-214
11 Zouboulis ChC, Korge BP, Mischke D, Orfanos CE. J Invest Dermatol. 1993; 101: 628-633
12 Zouboulis ChC, Korge B, Akamatsu H, *et al.* J Invest Dermatol. 1991; 96: 792-797

©1996 Elsevier Science B.V. All rights reserved.
Hair research for the next millenium
D.J.J. Van Neste and V.A. Randall (Eds)

Is the sebaceous gland important for inner root sheath breakdown?

M.P. Philpott, D.A. Sanders and T. Kealey

Department of Clinical Biochemistry, University of Cambridge, Addenbrookes Hospital, Cambridge CB2 2QR, United Kingdom

Introduction

The inner root sheath (IRS) is believed to play a supporting role in the formation of the hair fibre and co-migrates with the developing hair fibre. However, at the level of the sebaceous gland the IRS breaks down and the hair fibre is freed into the pilary canal where it emerges from the follicular opening at the surface of the skin [1]. There is evidence to suggest that the sebaceous gland may play an important role in the breakdown of the IRS [2].

We have reported on the *in vitro* culture of both isolated human hair follicles (without sebaceous gland) [3] and intact human pilosebaceous units (hair follicle plus sebaceous gland) [4]. We have shown that with isolated hair follicles hair growth occurs over 10 days but is associated with attached root sheaths, whereas cultured pilosebaceous units produce a hair fibre generally free of IRS [3, 4]. This suggests that the sebaceous gland may play a role in separation of the root sheaths from the hair fibre.

In this study we have taken pilosebaceous units and carefully removed by microdissection either:
a) the epidermis
b) the sebaceous gland
c) the epidermis plus sebaceous gland.

These follicles were then maintained for 7 days and hair fibre formation observed. Control experiments were carried out using intact pilosebaceous units.

Materials and methods

Isolation and culture of intact human pilosebaceous units

Human pilosebaceous units were isolated from facelift skin by microdissection as previously described [4]. Briefly, skin was cut into 3x10 mm strips and placed in Earles balanced salt solution: PBS (1:1). Pilosebaceous units were then carefully isolated by microdissection using watchmakers forceps and a fine scalpel blade (N° 15). Considerable care was taken to remove fat and connective tissue surrounding the follicle but not to damage the follicle itself.

Further dissection to remove sebaceous glands and/or epidermis was carried out under a dissecting microscope. Isolated pilosebaceous units were maintained in Williams E medium supplemented with 2 mM L-glutamine, 10 µg/ml insulin, 10 ng/ml hydrocortisone, 100 U/ml penicillin and 100 µg/ml streptomycin.

Morphology and histology

The morphology of pilosebaceous units in culture was examined using a Nikon Diaphot inverted microscope. Photographs were taken using Ilford FP4 film. Pilosebaceous units were processed for histology by fixing overnight in 3.5% phosphate buffered formaldehyde and then mounted into 3% agar blocks, which facilitated the subsequent handling of the follicles during sectioning. Agar blocks, containing follicles, were then fixed overnight in 3.5% phosphate buffered formaldehyde and then embedded in wax. 5 mm sections were cut and stained using hematoxylin and eosin.

Results

The effects of removing the sebaceous gland from isolated human pilosebaceous units are shown in table 1. In controls 36% of pilosebaceous units produce a fibre with IRS attached; when the sebaceous gland was removed this increased to 79%. If the upper epidermis was removed from controls, but the sebaceous gland left intact, only 25% of pilosebaceous units produce a fibre with IRS attached. However, when the sebaceous gland was also removed, 95% of pilosebaceous units produced fibres with IRS attached.

Histology showed that, in the absence of the sebaceous gland, breakdown of the root sheaths may not be completed and that this was also associated with an apparent hypercornification of the root sheaths. This suggests that the sebaceous gland may play an important role in breakdown or separation of the hair follicle IRS from the hair fibre, which may be cytolytic, and that the epidermis plays a secondary, co-operative role which may be physical.

Table 1.

The effects of removing the sebaceous gland on hair fibre formation in isolated human pilosebaceous units

Condition	Fibres with IRS
plus epidermis plus sebaceous gland	8/22 (36%)
plus epidermis minus sebaceous gland	19/24 (79%)
minus epidermis plus sebaceous gland	6/24 (25%)
minus epidermis minus sebaceous gland	19/20 (95%)

Results are from n=5 skin biopsies using 4 or 5 pilosebaceous units from each biopsy

Conclusions

Previous studies have shown that transection of isolated sheep pilosebaceous units either above, or below, the sebaceous gland gave rise to different patterns of hair follicle sheath growth *in vitro* [5]. In this study we have carefully isolated human pilosebaceous units and microdissected the sebaceous gland. Our data suggest that the sebaceous gland may play an important role in either the breakdown or separation of the IRS from the hair fibre and that, in the absence of the sebaceous gland, hypercornification of the IRS and ORS may occur. We suggest that the epidermis plays a secondary, co-operative role in the separation which may be physical and *in vitro* culture of the human pilosebaceous unit represents an excellent model for studying the role of the sebaceous gland in hair follicle biology.

References

1   Gemmell RT, Chapman RE. J Ultrastruc Res. 1971; 36: 355-366
2   Trigg MJ. J Zool Lond. 1972; 168: 165-198
3   Philpott MP, Green MR, Kealey T. J Cell Sci. 1990; 97: 463-471
4   Sanders DA, Philpott MP, Nicolle FV, Kealey T. Br J Dermatol. 1994; 131: 166-176
5   Williams D, Stenn KS. Dev Biol. 1994; 165: 469-479

Paracrine factors in the hair follicle

Immunocytochemical studies on hair-follicular stem cells and their intracytoplasmic neuronal factors

M. Takahama[1] and H. Kamoda[2]

[1]Department of Pathology, Saitama Medical School, Morohongo 38, Saitama 350-04, Japan
[2]Institute for Advanced Skin Research Inc., Fukuura 2-12-1, Kanazawa-ku, Yokohama 236, Japan

Introduction

In hair follicles of animals and human scalps, hair-follicular stem cells (HFSC) are assumed to locate at the level involving the arrector pili muscle attachment site (bulge area) [1, 2]. It is obvious HFSC play an important role in reproduction of a new anagen hair follicle after the end of telogen phase of the hair cycle, however it has not been clarified what cellular mechanism evokes HFSC replication and activates a telogen follicle to reproduce a new anagen follicle. We have already found that immunostaining techniques using a monoclonal antibody for cytokeratin RCK102 (cytokeratin 5 and 8) specifically stain basal cells of the outer root sheath at the level between the acinus of the sebaceous gland and the distal portion of the arrector pili muscle attachment site [3], which corresponds to the level where HFSC were presented in references. Recently, integrin β_1 was revealed to be expressed in stem cells of the skin epidermis and also of hair follicles [4, 5]. In the present study, we demonstrated HFSC by immunocytochemical technique by avidin-biotin complex (ABC) method using antibodies for RCK102 and integrin β_1 on formalin-fixed paraffin-embedded sections of human scalp tissue, and also we looked for a biosensor mechanism of the HFSC by fluorescence immunocytochemical staining method using antibodies for neuronal factors as observed with a confocal laser scanning microscope (CLSM).

Materials and methods

Tissue specimens of the human scalp were obtained from 75 autopsy cases and 12 biopsy cases, fixed either in 10% formalin solution in PBS or in 4% paraform-40% ethanol-phosphate buffer solution and embedded in paraffin. Tissue sections were studied after staining by hematoxylin-eosin (HE) and immunostaining by ABC method using the following antibodies: anti-cytokeratin mAb RCK102, (SANBIO, antibody for cytokeratin 5, 8, obtained from squamous cell carcinoma of lung); anti-integrin β_1 mAb (BIOHIT OY, antibody for stem cells and progenitors); anti-S100, polyclonal Ab (IMMUNOTECH S.A., antibody for Schwann cell and other cells of neural crest origin); anti-synaptophysin mAb (BioMakor bm., antibody for synaptosome preparation of rat retina); anti-NSE mAb (Cambridge Research Biochemicals, antibody for neuron specific enolase); anti-Ki67 mAb (IMMUNOTECH S.A., antibody for MIB1; nuclear marker protein of cyclic cells - G_1, S, G_2M).

Results

On HE-stained histological sections of the scalp, basal cells of the outer root sheath at the level involving the arrector pili muscle attachment site (BCORS-APMA) are characteristically small cuboidal cells regularly arranged on the basement membrane of hair follicles.

On ABC immunostained sections, the BCORS-APMA showed their cytoplasm RCK102$^+$ (Fig. 1), their cell membrane integrin β_1^+, nuclei Ki67$^-$. On fluorescence immunostaining and CLSM observation, infranuclear cytoplasm of every BCORS-APMA showed S100$^+$, NSE$^+$, synaptophysin$^+$ (Fig. 2). On electron microscopy, no neurosecretory granules were identified in BCORS-APMA.

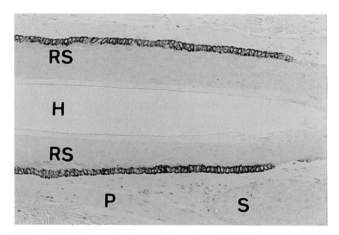

Figure 1. Microscopic picture of cytokeratin RCK102 immunostaining. Cytoplasm of BCORS-APMA (HFSC) are specifically strong-positively stained. P: arrector pili muscle; S: sebaceous gland; RS: root sheath; H: hair. 120x.

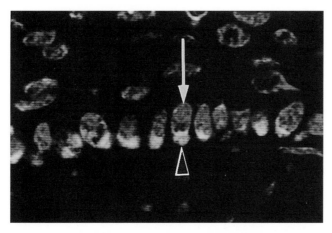

Figure 2. CLSM high-power view of synaptophysin fluorescence-immunostaining. Infranuclear cytoplasm (open arrowhead) of BCORS-APMA show a strong positive staining reaction. Arrow: nucleus of BCORS-APMA. 1200x.

Conclusion

BCORS-APMA showing their unique location and the exclusive immunostaining results as RCK 102[+], integrin β_1[+], Ki67[-] could be recognized as stem cells of human scalp hair follicle. Concerning the staining results with S100[+], synaptophysin[+], NSE[+] of the infranuclear cytoplasm of BCORS-APMA on CLSM observation, we presume those neuronal proteins might act as an intracytoplasmic biosensor and they modulate the internal stress pressure in a telogen follicle produced by a synthesized hair to the reactivation of BCORS-APMA.

References

1   Cotsarelis G, Sun T-T, Lavker RM. Cell. 1990; 61: 1329-1337
2   Sun T-T, Cotsarelis G, Lavker RM. J Invest Dermatol. 1991; 96 (suppl): 77s-78S
3   Takahama M. Hifubyou-Shinryoh (Japanese). 1993; 15: 755-758
4   Moll L. J Invest Dermatol. 1995; 105: 14-21
5   Jones PH, Watt FM. Cell. 1993; 73: 713-724

Involvement of vasoactive intestinal peptide (VIP) and VIP-receptor in hair follicle growth?

U. Wollina[1], D. Lange[1], K. Funa[2] and R. Paus[3]

[1]Department of Dermatology, Friedrich-Shiller-University, Erfurter Straße 35, 07740 Jena, Germany
[2]Ludwig Institute for Cancer Research, Uppsala Branch, Box 595, 75124 Uppsala, Sweden
[3]Department of Dermatology, R.-Virchow-Krankenhaus, Alexander-von-Humboldt-University, Augustenburger Platz 1, 13353 Berlin, Germany

Introduction

The hair follicle is characterized by specialized nerve endings including Merkel cell neurite complexes and an intense innervation. Neuroendocrine cells are found in the dermis surrounding follicles-especially mast cells. Neuroendocrine cells have been implicated in growth control of hair follicles [1-3]. Neuropeptides released by cutaneous nerve endings or neuroendocrine cells like vasoactive intestinal peptide (VIP) have been shown to act as growth factors for keratinocytes *in vitro* [4-6]. We wanted to investigate whether VIP and VIP-receptor are involved in growth control of hair follicle epithelium or not. In the present paper we demonstrate immunohistochemical stainings and in situ hybridization for VIP and VIP-receptor.

Materials and methods

Animals

Female syngenic C57 BL/6 mice of an age between 6 to 9 weeks were purchased from Charles River (Hannover, Germany). They were housed in community cages with 12 hours light periods and fed *ad libitum* with water and rat/mouse chow (Agway, Syracuse, NY/USA). Telogen mice were anaesthesized with 30 mg sodium pentobarbital per kg body weight and hair was stripped with a mixture of beeswax and resin to induce anagen [7]. The technique generates mature anagen hair follicles indistinguishable from spontaneously developing ones. Animals were sacrified by an ethyl ether overdose. Different hair cycle stages were investigated: spontaneous telogen (day 0), anagen I to VI (days 1 to 18), post-epilation catagen (day 19), and post-epilation telogen (day 25). For each cycle stage five mice were studied.

Antibodies

Monoclonal antibody 109.10 against VIP-receptor protein [8], polyclonal anti-VIP [9], monoclonal PT-66 against phosphotyrosinase [10], CALD-8 against caldesmon and isoform specific antibodies against glutathione-S-transferase (GST α, μ, π) (Sigma, Deisenhofen, Germany) have been used.

Immunohistochemistry

The antibodies except anti-VIP were used at 4°C overnight on snap frozen skin samples, cut at 4 μm and fixed with acetone. Antibody binding was visualized by the unlabeled immunoperoxidase technique with 3-amino-9-ethylcarbazole (EGA-Chemie, Steinheim, Germany). Anti-VIP has been employed on formalin-fixed, deparaffinized 4 μm sections in combination with an ABC immunoperoxidase technique developed with 3-amino-9-ethylcarbazole.

In-situ hybridization (ISH)

The VIP/PHI-insert (380 bp) was ligated from the unidirectional plasmid pSP64 [11] to the bidirectional transcription vector pGEM. It was linearized with the restriction enzymes NdeI (antisense) and HindIII (sense). The *in vitro* transcription was performed with [^{35}S]-UTP using RNA polymerases Sp6 (antisense) and T7 (sense). The plasmid carrying the bases 711 to 1192 of VIPII-receptor [12] was linearized with EcoRI (antisense) and BamHI (sense) and transcribed with T7- (antisense) and T3-RNA polymerase (sense) using [^{35}S]-UTP. We used oligonucleotide ISH for detecting VIP and VIP-receptor type I and II. Two different oligonucleotides with 26 bp for VIP [13], with 24 bp for VIPI-receptor [14] and with 24 and 25 bp for VIPII-receptor [12] have been synthesized. We used a 3'-labeling with [^{35}S]-ATP. Snap frozen tissue sections were pretreated with 100 μg proteinase K/ml, 0.2% glycine/PBS, 0.1M triethanolamine and acidic acid anhydrite/0.1M triethanolamine. Radioactive cRNA oligonucleotides were added in hybridization buffer for 16 hours at 55°C. Thereafter slides were washed with high stringency in SSC. The RNA-probe was treated with RNAse (20 μg/ml) and washed again with SSC. The dried sections were overlaid with Hypercoat emulsion LM-1 (Amersham), stored at 4°C for three weeks and developed with Dektol/Unifix (Kodak). Sections were counterstained with haematoxylin.

Results

VIP-receptor was demonstrated between day 12 and day 17. Immunoreactivity was found in the bulge area of hair follicles and in endothelial dermal cells. The bulbs and the sebaceous glands remained negative. VIP was absent in hair follicles but shown in sebocytes of hair follicles between days 0 to 8 and 19 to 21. VIP could not be demonstrated in endothelial cells. Anti-phosphotyrosinase labeled the bulge region of hair follicles from day 0 to 8, was negative at day 12 and weakly bound during days 18 to 25. Caldesmon immunoreactivity was found in bulge region during anagen I to IV, GST isoformes were expressed in the bulge region and inner hair root sheath during anagen (GST μ, π) or anagen and telogen (GST α). ISH with

RNA probes and oligonucleotides remained negative for VIP, VIPI-and VIPII-receptor mRNA.

Table 1.
Expression of VIP, VIP-receptor and phosphotyrosinase (PT) in hair follicle stages.

	VIP	VIP-receptor	PT
Telogen	+	-	+
Anagen I	+	-	+
Anagen II	+	-	+
Anagen III	+	-	+
Anagen IV	+	-	(+)
Anagen V	-	+	-
Anagen VI	-	-	-
Post-epilation catagen	+	-	-
Post-epilation telogen	-	-	+

Discussion

VIP is an important cutaneous neuropeptide which has been localized in nerve endings, Merkel and mast cells. It acts by binding to its receptor, which shows functional and genetic heterogeneity [14,15]. Signal transduction may be realized on different pathways including adenylate cyclase activation [4,5]. In vitro VIP facilitates growth and survival of keratinocytes [4-6]. The involvement of VIP/VIP-receptor in hair follicle growth control has not been investigated yet. Only recently, VIP-receptor has been immunolocalized in the bulge region of murine anagen follicles [16]. In the present study we were able to extend our knowledge by the additional investigation of VIP expression. It was shown that VIP and its receptor disclose a sequential expression in hair follicle and sebaceous gland epithelium on the protein level. VIP was found in sebocytes during telogen, anagen I to IV and at the anagen/catagen switch. VIP-receptor has been demonstrated in the bulge region only in anagen V. On the other hand we could not succeed to demonstrate mRNA for VIP and type I and II VIP-receptors. ISH and immunohistochemistry of VIP-receptor are not directly comparable, because antibody 109.10 is known to detect a receptor associated protein [8]. There is no evidence that it may differentiate between the two receptor types. ISH with oligonucleotides is a sophisticated procedure. False negative results are possible. From our data, it seems reasonable that VIPII-receptor mRNA is lacking in murine hair follicle apparatus. For type I, negative findings should be interpreted more cautiously since there was no plasmid available. Since the bulge region serves as stem cell reservoir of hair follicle epithelium [17], a limited expression of this neuropeptide receptor may be involved in timing of hair growth stages. Anagen V represents the end of extensive follicle growth and enlargement. Therefore, we assumed VIP-receptor expression may be involved in terminating the anagen growth and initiating the differentiation. This view gains further support by the relationship of VIP-receptor expression to phosphotyrosinase and other proteins [16]. Surprisingly enough, the follicle epithelium did not express VIP as far as demonstrated by immunohistochemistry and ISH. On the other hand, we found a remarkable expression in sebocytes of different hair follicle stages on the protein level. There was a clear cut of VIP expression during anagen, when its receptor could be detected in the bulge region. ISH with plasmids and oligonucleotides could not demonstrate mRNA for VIP. The origin of the protein remains to be detected. An autocrine mechanism of sebaceous gland growth could not be substantiated, but mast cell numbers and activity has been related to hair follicle phases [1-3]. Mast cells may secrete VIP. Our findings suggest a regulatory involvement of sebocytes in the hair cycle and a growth inhibitory role for neuropeptides acting via VIP-receptors in the bulge area.

Acknowledgements

Parts of this study have been supported by a DAAD grant to D. Lange and the project «clinically oriented neurosciences» (German Ministry of Science and Technology).

References

1 Paus R, Mauer M, Slominski A, Czarnetzki BM. Dev Biol. 1994; 63: 230-240
2 Botchkarev VA, Paus R, Czarnetzki BM, Kukriyanov VS, et al. Arch Dermatol Res. 1995; 287: 683-686
3 Wollina U. Acta Histochem. 1992; 92: 171-178
4 Haegerstrand A, Jonzon B, Dalsgaard C-J, Nilsson J. Proc Natl Acad Sci. USA. 1989; 86: 5993-5996
5 Wollina U, Bonnekoh B, Klinger R, Wetzker R, Mahrle G. Neuroendocrinol Lett. 1992; 14: 21-31
6 Wollina U, Bonnekoh B, Mahrle G. Int J Oncol. 1992; 1: 17-24
7 Slominski A, Paus R, Constantino R. J Invest Dermatol. 1991; 75: 122-127
8 Pichon J, Hirn M, Muller JM, Mangeat A, et al. EMBO J. 1983; 2: 1017-1022
9 Ekblad E, Ekman R, Hakasson R, Sundler F. Neuroscience. 1988; 27: 655-674
10 Kodate C, Fukushi A, Karita T, Kudo H, et al. Jpn J Cancer Res. 1986; 77: 226-229
11 Donaldson LF, Hamar AJ, McQueen DS, Seckl IR. Brain Res Mol Res. 1992; 16: 143-149
12 Lutz EM, Sheward WJ, West KM, Morrow JA, et al. FEBS Lett. 1993; 334: 3-8
13 Nishizawa M, Hayakawa Y, Yanaihara N, Okamoto H. FEBS Lett. 1985; 183: 55-59
14 Sreedharan SP, Patel DR, Huang JX, Goetzl EJ. Biochem Biophys Res Commun. 1993; 193: 546-553
15 Robberecht P, Cauvin A, Gourlet P, Christophe J. Arch Int Pharmacodyn. 1990; 303: 51-66
16 Wollina U, Paus R, Feldrappe S. Histol Histopathol. 1995; 10: 39-45
17 Cotsarelis G, Sun T-T, Lavker R. Cell. 1990; 61: 1329-1337

VEGF mRNA expression in different stages of the human hair cycle: analysis by confocal laser microscopy

S. Lachgar[1, 2], M. Charvéron[1, 2], I. Ceruti[2], J.M. Lagarde[2], Y. Gall[2] and J.L. Bonafé[1]

[1]Clinical and Bio-Clinical Research Group in Dermatology, Laboratoire Culture de Peau, C.H.U. Rangueil, Toulouse, France
[2]Pierre Fabre Research Institute, Vigoulet-Auzil, Castanet-Tolosan, France

Introduction

Hair growth during anagen is associated with a pronounced vascularisation of the hair bulb. In contrast to this, the vascular network is reabsorbed when the hair follicle enters into the catagen phase, and almost completely disappears in the telogen phase. Multiple growth factors or their receptors (e.g. bFGF, TGF-β1, TGF-β2, EGF ...) have been localized to the active follicle [1-3]. Since the expression of these factors changes during the hair cycle, they are implicated in the processes involved. Since vascular endothelial growth factor (VEGF) receptors are present in cultured dermal papilla cells of anagen hair follicles, and VEGF acts chemotactically and mitogenically on these cells [4], we hypothesise that VEGF may be involved in the initiation and/or development of the vascularization of the dermal papilla at the beginning of the anagen stage of the hair cycle. We suggest that VEGF secretion by the dermal papilla cells could support neovascularization of the hair bulb.

VEGF is involved in numerous vascular functions. It induces increased vascular permeability and tumour angiogenesis [5-7] and it is also a potent mitogenic agent for vascular endothelial cells [8-11]. VEGF is expressed by many types of normal [11] and tumour cells [5, 12, 13, 7]. Brown et al. [14] have shown that rat and guinea pig keratinocytes express VEGF mRNA during wound healing and secrete VEGF in primary culture. Others have characterized the different forms of VEGF produced by human keratinocytes in primary culture [15]. Elsewhere, VEGF has been examined for a pathogenic role in skin diseases characterized by neoangiogenesis and alterations of the epidermis. An overexpression of VEGF mRNA and its receptors flt-1 and KDR has been observed in psoriasis [16] and in epidermal lesions of patients affected by bullous pemphigoid, dermatitis herpetiformis, and erythema multiforme [17]. In all these diseases VEGF has been ascribed a role in the induction and maintenance of neovascularization. These factors led us to suppose that, during the hair cycle, VEGF may have a paracrine role in the induction of hair bulb vascularization and possibly a determinant role in hair growth. Therefore, we have investigated the expression of VEGF mRNA during different stages of the hair cycle using in situ hybridization on scalp biopsies of normal subjects.

Materials and methods

In order to detect cells synthesizing VEGF-specific mRNA, we performed fluorescent *in situ* hybridization on frozen sections (5 μm) obtained from normal human scalp skin. The hybridization technique used was a modification of a procedure previously described. We used fluorescein labelled sense and antisense purified probes. The antisense probe hybridizes specifically with a region of VEGF mRNA common to all four VEGF splicing variants. Slides were fixed in 4% paraformaldehyde in phosphate buffered saline (PBS), rinsed twice in PBS, then incubated for 10 min in PBS, dehydrated in serial alcohols and air dried for 30min. They were then overlaid with the hybridization buffer containing the antisense or sense probes (1 μg/ml). After mounting and sealing with rubber cement, the slides were incubated overnight. The sections were washed three times with Standard Sodium Citrate (SSC) 2x, blocked and incubated for 1h with anti-fluorescein diluted 1:100 in blocking solution. Finally, after several washings, the slides were mounted with a Vectashield mounting medium, before observation with a confocal laser scanning microscope (Zeiss). All slides were serially measured with the same voltage gain and sensitivity in any given series. Microscopic images were transferred to an image analysis dedicated work station (SUN IPC), where a specially developed software routine evaluated the number of fluorescent grains present in the follicle.

Results

As shown in Table 1, VEGF mRNA expression in the dermal papilla varied with the stage of the hair cycle, with the percentage of fluorescent spots being greatly reduced in catagen and telogen stages.

Table 1.
Quantification of VEGF transcripts in dermal papilla by confocal laser microscopy combined with image analysis.

	Number of spots	Spot surface area (μm^2)	Derma papilla surface area	% Surface area Hybridized
Anagen stage	2922	521	2900	18
Catagen stage	243	37	658	6
Telogen stage	175	34	854	4

Dermal papillae (DP) from anagen follicles (Fig. 1B) revealed a considerable amount of VEGF mRNA, particularly at the base of the papillae. Weak fluorescence was seen in bulb matrix cells.

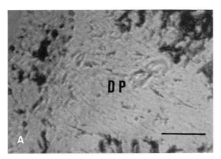

Figure 1. VEGF mRNA expression in anagen follicles. Bright-field (A) and corresponding dark-field (B) photomicrographs of in situ hybridization. Bar, 25 μm

In catagen (Fig. 2B) and telogen stages (Fig. 3B), very, few or no grains of fluorescence were detected in dermal papillae, but the keratogenous zone was strongly positive. Controls which included sense transcripts were found to be negative. No specific labelling was seen with control sense probes in any hair follicle stage (data not shown).

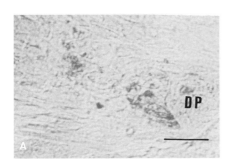
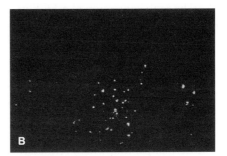

Figure 2. VEGF mRNA expression in catagen. Bright-field (A) and corresponding dark-field (B) photomicrographs of in situ hybridization. Bar, 25 μm

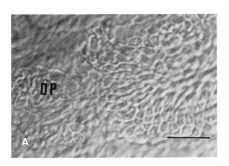
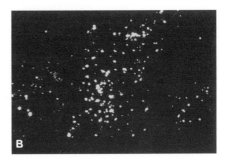

Figure 3. VEGF mRNA expression in telogen. Bright-field (A) and corresponding dark-field (B) photomicrographs of in situ hybridization. Bar, 25 μm

Discussion

The formation of blood vessels in the hair bulb is of prime importance for hair growth. These processes involve the proliferation of endothelial cells and are likely to be regulated by angiogenic growth factors. We chose to study VEGF because it is the only known secreted mitogenic polypeptide factor [9] that acts exclusively on vascular endothelial cells [7, 11]. *In situ* hybridization studies confirmed our immunohistochemical observations (unpublished data) with detection of VEGF in both dermal papillae and outer root sheath keratinocytes of anagen follicles. VEGF mRNA was strongly expressed in dermal papillae, particularly at the base. In contrast, dermal papillae from catagen and telogen follicles expressed little, or no, VEGF mRNA, while VEGF transcripts were highly expressed in matrix cells surrounding dermal papillae. This indicates that VEGF mRNA expression varies with the different hair cycle stages, with the greatest abundance being within the dermal papilla in anagen, more than in any other compartment of the hair follicle, and implies an important role of VEGF in the hair cycle. The reduced amounts of VEGF mRNA in dermal papillae during catagen and telogen are not surprising, because a low vascularization of the hair bulb is observed in these stages.

The high expression of VEGF in anagen dermal papillae may explain some of the characteristics of this richly vascularized follicle. This hypothesis is supported by the finding of Goldman *et al.* [19] that VEGF is absent from hair follicles in alopecia areata and, to a lesser extent, in androgenetic alopecia. We suggest that the reduction of VEGF production may affect the maintenance of hair vascularization during the hair cycle. So that follicle cell function and, subsequently, hair growth may be regulated by VEGF.

In summary, the expression of VEGF mRNA only in dermal papilla at the anagen phase of the hair cycle appears to be linked to the induction function of the dermal papilla, which stimulates hair growth [2]. It would be interesting to know if this pattern of expression is modified in dermal papilla from catagen and telogen stages and in all the compartments of hair follicle after treatment with different drugs.

References

1   Lehnert SA, Akhurst RJ. Development. 1988; 104: 263-273
2   Pelton RW, Nimura S, Moses HL, Hogan BLM. Development. 1989; 106: 759-767
3   Nanney LB, Stoscheck CM, King LE, Underwood Jr RA, Holbrook KA. J Invest Dermatol. 1990; 94: 742-748
4   Lachgar S, Charvéron M, Plouët J, Gall Y, Bonafé JL. (abstract). J Invest Dermatol. 1995; 104: 158
5   Connolly DT, Olander JV, Heuvelman D, Nelson R, Monsell R, Siegel N, Haymore BL, Leimgruber R, Feder J. J Biol Chem. 1989; 264: 20017-20024
6   Connolly DT, Heuvelman D, Nelson R, Olander JV, Monsell R, Eppley BL, Siegel NR, Leimgruber RM, Feder J. J Clin Invest. 1989; 84: 1470-1478

7   Ferrara N, Houck K, Jakeman L, Leung DW. Endocr Rev. 1992; 13: 18-32
8   Keck PJ, Hauser SD, Krivi G, Sanzo K, Warren T, Feder J, Connolly DT. Science. 1989; 246: 1309
9   Leung DW, Cachianes G, Kuang W-J, Goeddel DV, Ferrara N. Science. 1989; 246: 1306-1309
10   Gospodarowicz D, Abraham JA, Shilling G. Proc Natl Acad Sci USA. 1989; 86: 7311-7315
11   Ferrara N, Henzel WJ. Biochem Biophys Res Commun. 1989; 161: 851-858
12   Plouët J, Shilling J, Gospodarowicz D. EMBO J. 1989; 8: 3801-3806
13   Conn G, Soderman D, Schaffe MT, Wile M, Hatcher V, Thomas K. Proc Natl Acad Sci USA. 1990; 87: 1323-1327
14   Brown LF, Yeo K-T, Berse B, Yeo T-K Senger DR, Dvorak HF, Van de Water L. J Exp Med. 1992; 176: 1375-1379
15   Ballaun C, Weninger W, Uthman A, Weich H, Tschachler E. J Invest Dermatol. 1995; 104: 7-10
16   Detmar M, Brown LF, Claffey KP, Yeo K-T, Kocher O, Jackman RW, Berse B, Dvorak HF. J Exp Med. 1994; 180: 1141-1146
17   Brown LF, Harrist TJ, Yeo KT, Stahle-Bäckdahl M, Jackman RW, Berse B, Tognazzi K, Dvorak HF, Detmar M. J Invest Dermatol. 1995; 104: 744- 749
18   Yarov YB, Mitkevich SP, Alexandrov IA. Human Genet. 1987; 76: 157
19   Goldman CK, Tsai JC, Soroceanu L, Gillespie Y. J Invest Dermatol. 1995; 104S: 18-20
20   Jahoda CAB and Oliver RF. In: Orfanos CE and Happle R, eds. Hair and Hair Diseases. Berlin: Springer Verlag. 1990; 19-44

©1996 Elsevier Science B.V. All rights reserved.
Hair research for the next millenium
D.J.J. Van Neste and V.A. Randall (Eds)

HMG-CoA reductase activity and regulation in the isolated human hair follicle

C.D.W. Smythe and T. Kealey

Department of Clinical Biochemistry, Cambridge University, Addenbrookes Hospital, Hills Road, Cambridge, CB2 2QR, UK

Introduction

HMG-CoA reductase catalyses the important regulatory step of cholesterol biosynthesis, the conversion of HMG-CoA to mevalonate, and is subject to complex control mechanisms [1]. Regulation of enzyme activity is mediated by alteration of protein content and by reversible phosphorylation. Exogenous cholesterol in the form of low density lipoprotein (LDL) may be delivered to cells via the LDL receptor. In such cases transcription of HMG-CoA reductase decreases, degradation increases, and the enzyme is phosphorylated and thereby inactivated.

Cholesterol metabolism and its regulation in the skin is being increasingly understood, with the trans-epidermal water barrier being found to play an important role in determining the amount of HMG-CoA reductase present and its phosphorylation status [2]. Few studies however have concentrated on HMG-CoA reductase within skin appendages. We have carried out experiments to determine whether HMG-CoA reductase is present and active in isolated human hair follicles, and to investigate its regulation by LDL and 25-hydroxycholesterol.

Materials and methods

Isolation of human hair follicles

Human anagen hair follicles were isolated from scalp skin from females undergoing facelift surgery using the method previously described by Philpott et al. [3]. Follicles were maintained overnight in supplemented William's E medium at 37°C in a humidified 5% CO_2/95% air atmosphere, and then individually snap frozen in liquid nitrogen.

RT-PCR

Single stranded cDNA was prepared from hair follicle total RNA [4]. HMG-CoA reductase cDNA was amplified as previously described by Wang et al. [5]. Digestion of the PCR products with the restriction enzyme Sty was carried out at 37°C for 2 hours in buffer containing 100mM NaCl, 50mM Tris-HCl, 10mM $MgCl_2$, 1mM DTT and 100 µg/ml BSA. PCR products were visualised using ethidium bromide staining on an SDS PAGE gel.

HMG-CoA reductase assay

Follicles were homogenized and assayed for HMG-CoA reductase activity using a radiochemical method [6, 7] where [^{14}C]HMG-CoA was converted to [^{14}C]mevalonolactone. Following completion an aliquot of the reaction mixture was applied to a silica gel LK5D thin layer chromatography plate, and chromatographed in toluene/acetone (1:1). The product was visualised upon contact with iodine, and the stained area scraped from the plate into a scintillation vial and counted. Recovery of a [^{3}H]mevalonolactone marker was used to correct the value of [^{14}C]mevalonolactone product.

Results

RT-PCR

HMG-CoA reductase is expressed in hair follicles, as shown by RT-PCR. A 247 base pair segment of the RNA message encoding HMG-CoA reductase was amplified from hair follicle cDNA using RT-PCR. Restriction digest yielded product lengths of 142 and 105 base pairs, consistent with those predicted from the published human sequence [8].

HMG-CoA reductase activity

HMG-CoA reductase activity was measured in hair follicles which had been maintained overnight in supplemented William's E medium. In order to maintain the phosphorylation status of the enzyme before assaying, follicles were snap frozen in liquid nitrogen. Follicles homogenized in the presence or absence of fluoride, and incubated for 1 hour at 37°C, gave rise to «expressed» and «total» activities respectively, from which an activation ratio of 0.34 was calculated. Reduced activity upon homogenization in the presence of fluoride indicates that enzyme inactivation is modulated by phosphorylation. Enzyme activity was measured with increasing HMG-CoA concentration and a double reciprocal plot of the data drawn. The enzyme exhibited a V_{max} of 75.5 ± 8.3 pmol/min/mg and a K_m for HMG-CoA of 4.6 ± 1.0µM.

Effect of LDL and 25-Hydroxycholesterol on HMG-CoA reductase activity

Overnight maintenance in the presence of 5 µg/ml LDL had no effect on HMG-CoA reductase activity (Table 1). However incubation with 5 µg/ml 25-hydroxycholesterol significantly reduced HMG-CoA reductase activity to 88% of the control ($p < 0.01$).

Table 1.
Effect of LDL and 25-Hydroxycholesterol on HMG-CoA reductase activity

	Reductase Activity (% of control ± SE)
5μg/ml LDL	116.19 ± 12.24
5μg/ml 25-HC	87.86 ± 2.17*

significantly different from control containing 0.1% ethanol (p<0.01)

Discussion

The skin and its appendages have been shown to be important sites of *de novo* lipid synthesis. In 1974, Goldstein and Brown assayed plucked scalp hairs and found HMG-CoA reductase activity [9]. In this study we have identified mRNA expression for the enzyme, measured activity in maintained whole human hair follicles and estimated its activation state *in vivo*. We have not localized HMG-CoA reductase activity to any particular compartment within the hair follicle.

Following maintenance the follicles were snap frozen and stored prior to assay. Enzyme activity measured following rapid freezing of the material once isolated, and homogenization in the presence of phosphatase inhibitors, is considered to represent the enzyme activity expressed *in vivo* [10]. «Total» activity can be measured in the absence of phosphatase inhibitors. Under these conditions the enzyme is dephosphorylated by endogenous phosphatases. Follicles were therefore homogenized in the presence or absence of fluoride, a phosphatase inhibitor, incubated for 1 hour at 37°C, and gave rise to «expressed» and «total» activities respectively. Reduced activity upon homogenization in the presence of fluoride, an inhibitor of dephosphorylation, indicates that phosphorylation is the mechanism for enzyme inactivation within the follicle. Approximately 34% of the hair follicle enzyme is in the activated form.

The enzyme exhibited a K_m for HMG-CoA of 4.6 μM, a value similar to that reported for rat liver and mammary gland enzymes [11, 12].

The hair follicle enzyme does not appear to be regulated by low density lipoproteins (LDL). 25-Hydroxycholesterol, an oxysterol that bypasses the LDL receptor and is therefore capable of introducing cholesterol in the absence of LDL receptors, significantly reduced HMG-CoA reductase activity. This implies that the intracellular feedback control mechanisms are present. An absence of functional LDL receptors on the hair follicle would explain the lack of response to exogenous LDL.

References

1   Goldstein J L, Brown M S. Regulation of the mevalonate pathway. Nature. 1990; 343: 425-430

2   Proksch E, Holleran W M, Menon G K, Elias P M, Feingold K R. Barrier function regulates epidermal lipid and DNA synthesis. Br J Dermatol. 1993; 128: 473-482

3   Philpott M P, Green M R and Kealey T. Human hair growth *in vitro*. J Cell Sci. 1990; 97: 463-471

4   Chomczynski P, Sacchi N. Single-step method of RNA isolation by acid guanidium thiocyanate-phenol-chlorofom extraction. Analytical Biochem. 1987; 162: 156-159

5   Wang A M, Doyle M V, Mark D F. Quantitation of mRNA by the polymerase chain reaction. Proc Natl Acad Sci. 1989; 86: 9717-9721

6   Shapiro D J, Nordstrom J L, Mitschellen T J, Rodwell W, Schimke R T. Micro assay for 3-hydroxy-3-methylglutaryl-CoA reductase in rat liver and in L-cell fibroblasts. Biochim Biophys Acta. 1974; 370: 369-377

7   Easom R A, Zammit V A. Diurnal changes in the fraction of 3-hydroxy-3-methylglutaryl-CoA reductase in the active form in rat liver microsomal fractions. Biochem J. 1984; 220: 739-745

8   Luskey K L, Stevens B. Human 3-hydroxy-3-methylglutaryl coenzyme A reductase conserved domains responsible for catalytic activity and sterol-regulated degradation. J Biol Chem. 1985; 260: 10271-10277

9   Brannan P G, Goldstein J L, Brown M S. 3-hydroxy-3-methylglutaryl-CoA reductase in human hair roots. J Lipid Res. 1974; 16: 7-11

10 Easom R A, Zammit V A. A cold clamping technique for the rapid sampling of rat liver for studies on enzymes regulated by reversible phosphorylation-dephosphorylation. Biochem J. 1984; 220: 733-738.

11 Ness G C, Sample C E, Smith M, Pendleton L C, Eichler D C. Characteristics of rat liver microsomal 3-hydroxy-3-methylglutaryl-CoA reductase. Biochem J. 1986; 233: 167-172

12 Smith R A W, Middleton B, West D W. Diurnal variation in the fraction of 3-hydroxy-3-methylglutaryl-CoA reductase in the active form in the mammary gland of the lactating rat. Biochem J. 1986; 239: 285-293

©1996 Elsevier Science B.V. All rights reserved.
Hair research for the next millenium
D.J.J. Van Neste and V.A. Randall (Eds)

Characterization of expression and modulation of cell-surface antigens on cultured human dermal papilla cells

Y. Kubota, Y. Kawa, Y. Nakamura, T. Kushimoto and M. Mizoguchi

Department of Dermatology, St. Marianna University School of Medicine, 2-16-1, Sugao, Miyamae-ku, Kawasaki, Japan 216

Introduction

The dermal component of the human hair follicle is believed to play a crucial role in hair growth and some hair diseases, such as alopecia areata [1]. It has been shown that the human dermal papilla cells are embedded in a dense extracellular matrix *in vivo* and a functionally unique population of fibroblast-like cells. A method for culturing cells from human dermal papillae has been described [2] and the *in vitro* properties of cultured dermal papilla cells have been studied [3], however, very little is known about the precise cell surface antigens including cell adhesion molecules (CAM), expressed by human dermal papilla cells or cultured human dermal papilla cells and their immunological attributes [4]. In this study, we examined the expression of a variety of cell surface antigens and their regulation by including MHC class antigens, integrin receptors, and cell adhesion molecules by selected relevant cytokines using immunohistochemical staining or ELISA. Parallel studies were carried out on human dermal fibroblasts for comparison.

Materials and methods

Isolation and culture of human dermal papilla cells [2]

Full-thickness biopsies were obtained from the hairy region of the scalp of healthy men. All microsurgical procedures were performed under a binocular dissecting microscope. The bulbs were cut off and, using a 23G needle attached to a 5 ml syringe, the papilla was gently teased out, its basal stalk cut off and discarded. The papillae were finally transferred into 35 mm fibronectin-coated plastic culture dishes containing the culture medium, M-199 supplemented with fetal calf serum 20% (FCS). Within 48 hours of attachment cells began to migrate from the explant and proliferative activity became apparent after one to three weeks (Figs. 1a and 1b). The medium was changed every third day after the culture was established. Nearly confluent dermal papilla cells were removed and subcultured with 0.25% trypsin-EDTA solution. Cells in the early passages appeared to retain the morphology and growth characteristics that were seen in primary culture.

418

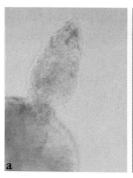

Figure 1a. Freshly isolated dermal papilla from human hair follicule 1b. Cultured dermal papilla cells (phase contrast, x100)

a   b

Monoclonal antibodies and biologic response modifiers

CDw49b (Gi9, Immunotech.), CDw49c (M-KID 2, Cosmo bio.), CDw49d (HP2/1, Immunotech.), CDw49e (SAM1, Immunotech.), CDw49f (GoH3, Immunotech), CD29 (K20, Immunotech), CD44 (BU52, Birmingham,UK), CD45 (T29/33, DAKO), CD51 (AMF7, Serotec.), CD61 (BB10, Biohit.), CD18 (BL5, Cosmo bio.), CD11a (YTH81.5, Serotec.), CD11b (D12, Becton Dickinson.), CD11c (S-HCL-3, BD.), VCAM-1 (E1/6, BD.), ICAM-1 (84H10, Immunotech.), Sialyl-Lew^x (CSLEX1, BD.), ELAM-1 (BBA2, British Bioteck.), HLA-DR (L243, BD.), HLA-ABC (SPV-L7, Monosan.), c-Kit (95C3, Serotec., 17F11, Immunotech.), Endoglin (1G2, Cosmo bio.), E-cadherin (HECD-1, Takara.). rIL-1 α (human, Ohtuka Pharmacy co.), rTNF-α (human, Collaborative Research), γ-IFN (human, Genzyme), rIL-6 (human, Kirin co.).

Immuno-histochemical staining

Cytospin preparations of dermal papilla cells at passages were fixed in cold acetone for 5 min before staining by a ZYMED LAB-SA SYSTEM (Streptavidin-Biotin Amplification Method), using the panel of monoclonal antibodies. All monoclonal antibodies were diluted 1:100. After processing, all specimens were examined by light microscopy and the staining intensities of peroxidase reaction products (AEC) classified on a four-point scale; (-): negative, (+): weakly positive, (+): fairly positive, and (++): strongly positive. An appropriate isotype-matched, irrelevant monoclonal antibody was used as a control.

ELISA assay [5]

Dermal papilla cells at passage 3-5 were plated in 96-well tissue culture plates at a concentration of 10^4 cells/well 24~48 h prior to the assay. They were then stimulated with biologic response modifiers as described above for varying periods of time and at a range of concentrations. After stimulation, dermal papilla cells were fixed in 2% paraformaldehyde for 15 min at room temperature. They were then washed in the Hanks balanced salt solution (HBSS) and incubated with 2% bovine serum albumine (BSA) in HBSS for 1h at 37°C. Fifty microliters of an antibody to the relevant antigen or an irrelevant control antigen at a concentration of 1 µg/ml in HBSS with 2% BSA was added to each well and incubated for further hour.

The cells were then washed and incubated for 1h with peroxidase-conjugated goat anti-mouse IgG diluted 1:1000 in HBSS with 2% BSA. The wells were then washed and antibody binding detected by the addition of 100 μl 0.05% o-phenylendiamine dihydrochloride. The reaction was stopped by the addition of 25 μl of 2N H_2SO_4. Plates were read on a Labsystems Multiscan ELISA reader at O.D. 492 after blanking on rows stained with irrelevant monoclonal antibody.

Results

Human dermal papilla cells were strongly stained by antibodies to HLA-class I, CD29, CD44, and CDw49c and fairly positively stained by those to CDw49e, CD51, and ICAM-1. On the other hand, CDw49b, 49d, endoglin and VCAM-1 were only weakly positive and HLA-DR, CD11a,b /18, CDw49f, CD61, ELAM-1, c-kit and E-cadherin were all negative (Table 1).

Stimulation of human dermal papilla cells with IL-1 α and TNF-α induced dose- and time-dependent increases in ICAM-1 and VCAM-1 expressions. ICAM-1 and VCAM-1 upregulation peaked at 6~12 hours and 48 hours, respectively and doses as low as 0.1 U/ml elicited a response (Figs. 2 and 3). IFN-γ also induced HLA-DR and ICAM-1 expression in a dose- and time-dependent manner, but not VCAM-1 expression, these increases occurred as early as 48 hours and 3-6 hours respectively, and with doses as low as 10 U/ml. IL-6 stimulation had no effect on these three molecules. IL-1 α, TNF-α, and IFN-γ had no effect on CDw49b, CD51, and CD61 expression. Stimulation of human dermal fibroblasts with IL-1 α and TNF-α also induced dose and time increases in ICAM-1, but, in contrast the dermal papilla cells did not alter VCAM-1 expression.

Table 1.
Detection for cell surface antigen of DPC

Antigen	Result	Antigen	Result
CDw49b	±	CD18	-
DDw49c	+ +	ICAM-1	+
CDw49d	±	VCAM-1	±
CDw49e	+	ELAM-1	-
CDw49f	-	s-LewX	-
CD29	+ +	β 7	-
CD44	+ +	endoglin	±
CD45	-	c-kit	-
CD51	+	HLA-DR	-
CD61	-	HLA-ABC	+

420

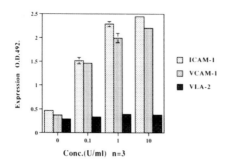

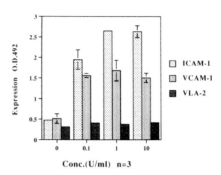

Figure 2. The effect of TNF-α on the expression of CAM's of human DPC

Figure 3. The effect of IL-1 on the expression of CAM's of human DPC

Discussion

We have examined cultured human dermal papilla cells for the expression and regulation of a variety of cell surface antigens by selective cytokine using immunohistochemical staining and ELISA. IL-1 α, TNF-α, and IFN γ increased the expression of ICAM-1, VCAM-1, and MHC protein by human dermal papilla cells in a dose- and time-dependent manner. Although the expression and regulation of these proteins appeared to be generally similar to what has been reported on human dermal fibroblasts [6], human dermal papilla cells are distinctly different in their response to TNF-α on VCAM-1 expression.

These data demonstrate the complexity of cytokine-modulated regulation of human dermal papilla cells cell surface antigens and dermal papilla cells compared to dermal fibroblasts demonstrate an unique immunophenotypic characteristic of human dermal papilla cells. The expressions of these antigens and their regulation may play a role in the pathophysiology of human hair growth and hair diseases.

References

1   MacDonald Hull SP, Nutbrown M, Pepall L, *et al*. J Invest Dermatol. 1991; 96: 673-681
2   Messenger AG. Br J Dermatol. 1984; 110: 685-698
3   Jahoda C, Reynolds A. J Invest Dermatol. 1993; 101: 33S-38S
4   Mcdonagh AJG, Snowden JA, Stierle C *et al*. Br J Dermatol. 1993; 129: 250-256
5   Swerlick RA, Garcia-Gonzalez E, Kubota Y *et al*. J Invest Dermatol. 1991; 97: 190-196
6   Needleman BW. Arthritis Rheum. 1990; 33: 1842-1851

Hair research for the next millenium
D.J.J. Van Neste and V.A. Randall (Eds)

Sequential expression of TGF-β and its receptors during hair growth phases in mice

D. Lange[1], K. Funa[2], U. Wollina[1] and R. Paus[3]

[1]Department Dermatology, Friedrich-Schiller-University, Erfurter Straße. 35, 07740 Jena, Germany
[2]Ludwig Institute for Cancer Research, Uppsala Branch, Box 595, 75124 Uppsala, Sweden
[3]Department Dermatology, R.-Virchow-Krankenhaus, Alexander-von-Humboldt University of Berlin, Augustenburger Platz 1, 13353 Berlin, Germany

Introduction

TGF-βs belong to a large superfamily (TGF-β superfamily). TGF-β was found to be a potent growth inhibitor on most cell types, possessing a number of other biological effects on different cell types, i.e. regulation of cellular differentiation, migration, production of extracellular matrix and adhesiveness to the matrices, and modulation of immune functions [1, 2]. The growth inhibitory activity of TGF-β makes it a candidate molecule for induction of regression and apoptosis. We used the hair follicle as a model since it shows regressive cycle phases in catagen and telogen. Various TGF-β-receptors and -binding proteins on the cell surface are known [3-5]. Type I receptor (TβR-I) , type II receptor (TβR-II) and type III receptor (TβR-III) have been characterized. TβR-I and TβR-II are widely expressed on many different cell types and both are necessary for signal transduction [6, 7]. TGF-β acts as a growth inhibitor on proliferating basal cells in the skin [8], and TGF-β2 has been shown to be expressed in the stratifying keratinocytes in developing mouse epidermis [9], and by keratinocytes during the terminal differentiation process [10, 11].

Materials and methods

Animals

In C57 BL-6 mice anagen was induced as described by Paus et al. [12]. Nine different hair cycle stages were investigated [13]: spontaneous telogen (day 0), anagen I-VI (day 1-18), post-epilation catagen (day 19) and post-epilation telogen (day 25).

Antibodies

The rabbit polyclonal antibodies Ab 96, Ab 94 and Ab 95, directed against synthetic peptides corresponding to specific amino acid sequences of the latency associated peptide (LAP) portions of the TGF-β1, -β2, -β3 precursors [14] as well as against synthetic peptides corresponding to the intracellular juxtamembrane parts of the receptor, TβR-I and TβR-II, were used [15, 16]. Antisera were affinity purified using CNBr-activated Sepaharose CL-4B (Pharmacia-LKB) columns with immobilized peptides as described before [17]. An antiserum Ab 39 against latent LTBP was used [18].

Immunohistochemistry

ABC peroxidase immunohistochemistry was performed as described before [19].

Results

General immunoreactivity

The mouse skin remained completely negative for antibodies Ab 94. Antibodies Ab 96, Ab 95, Ab 39 and anti-TβR-I produced a variable staining dependent on hair cycle phases. Anti-TβR-II gave positive signals throughout the hair cycle.

Expression of TGF-β1 and -β3

TGF-β1 was expressed in the inner hair root sheath (IRS) during day 5-7 (anagen) and 19-21 (anagen/catagen switch). Dermal connective tissue cells (CT) expressed TGF-β3 with moderate intensity during early anagen (day 0-3) and post-epilation catagen and telogen.

Expression of TβR-I and -II

Antibody against TβR-I stained sebocytes (SC) during early anagen (day 3-8). The outer hair root sheath (ORS) was labeled at the anagen/catagen switch, i.e. day 17-19, in the infraseboglandular but not suprabulbar region. During telogen the dermal tissue disclosed a weak staining intensity for TβR-I. Anti-TβR-II gave positive signals for sebocytes throughout the hair cycle. A moderate connective tissue staining was also seen.

Expression of LTBP

Antibody Ab 39 was fixed by different skin cells. Sebocytes gave an immunostaining during day 5-8 (anagen). During telogen a LTBP-positivity was seen in the connective tissue of the dermis (day 25-34).

Table 1.
Location of TGF-β's, TGF-receptors and LTBP

	TGF-β			TβR		LTBP
	β-1	β-2	β-3	R-I	R-II	
Telogen			CT	CT	SC, CT	
Anagen I			CT		SC, CT	
Anagen II			CT		SC, CT	
Anagen III			CT	SC	SC, CT	
Anagen IV	IRS			SC	SC, CT	SC
Anagen V	IRS			SC	SC, CT	SC
Anagen VI				ORS	SC, CT	SC
Post-epilation catagen	IRS		CT	ORS	SC, CT	
Post-epilation telogen			CT	CT	SC, CT	CT

Discussion

We report the first profile of TGF-β isoforms as well as receptor expression and their relationship in murine hair follicles.

TGF-β1 was expressed in the early anagen and along the anagen/catagen switch in the epithelium of the inner hair root sheath. Expression of LTBP has been observed in sebocytes during anagen. The coexpression of LTBP and TGF-β1 therefore may be related to the abrogation of hair follicle growth, because LTBP is necessary for the activation of the native TGF-β. A binding to TβR-II and/or TβR-I, expressed by sebocytes, seems to be possible.

At the anagen/catagen switch (day 17-19) TβR-I is expressed in the outer hair root sheath. TGF-β1 shows a reactive pattern in the inner hair root sheath in nearly the same time (day 19-21). Though we failed to demonstrate TβR-II, others could detect TβR-II in late anagen using different antibodies [20, 21]. These results suggest that:

a) TGF-β1 may be a candidate peptide for interactions between epithelial cell layers of the hair follicle,

b) the different cell layers are regulated separately,

c) TGF-β1 could be involved in the initiation of catagen and

d) TGF-β1 may regulate the downward movement of transient amplifying cells from the bulge to the bulb, which is a critical step in growth control of the hair follicle concerning the bulge activation thesis [22]. TGF-β1 produced by inner hair root sheath cells could act on TβR-I expressing outer hair root sheath, thereby probably regulating the flow of transient amplifying cells.

Our results suggest that the study of TGF-β and its receptors in hair research promises insight into the interactivity of the epithelial cell layers and sebocytes.

424

Acknowledgements

This study was supported by the DAAD.

References

1   Roberts AB, Sporn MB. In: Sporn MB, Roberts AB, eds. Handbook of Experimental
     Pharmacology. Berlin: Springer-Verlag. 1990; 419-472
2   Sporn MB, Roberts AB. J Cell Biol. 1992; 119: 1017-1021
3   Massague J. Cell. 1992; 69: 1067-1070
4   ten Dijke P, Yamashita H, Ichijo H, Franzen P, Laiho M, Miyazono K, Heldin C-H. Science
     (Wash. DC). 1994; 264: 101-104
5   Kingsley DM. Genes and Dev. 1994; 8: 133-146
6   Lin HY, Wang X-F, Ng-Eaton E, Weinberg RA, Lodish HF. Cell. 1992; 68: 775-785
7   Wrana JL, Attisano L, Carcamo J, Zentella A, Doody J, Laiho M, Wang X-F, Massagué J. Cell.
     1992; 71: 1003-1014
8   Choi Y, Fuchs E. Cell Regul. 1990; 1: 791-809
9   Lyons KM, Pelton RW, Hogan BLM. Genes and Dev. 1989; 3: 1657-1688
10   Glick AB, Flanders KC, Danielpour D, Yuspa SH, Sporn M B. Cell Regul. 1989; 1: 87-97
11   Glick AB, Danielpour D, Morgan D, Sporn MB, Yuspa SH. Mol Endocrinol. 1990; 4: 46-52
12   Paus R, Hofmann U, Eichmüller S, Czarnetzki BM. Br J Dermatol. 1994; 130: 281-289
13   Chase HB, Rauch H, Smith VW. Physiol Zool. 1951; 24: 1-8
14   Olofsson A, Miyazono K, Kanzaki T, Colosetti P, Engström U, Heldin C-H. J Biol Chem.
     1992; 267: 19482-19488
15   Franzen P, ten Dijke P, Ichijo H, Yamashita H, Schulz P, Heldin C-H, Miyazono K. Cell.
     1993; 75: 681-692
16   Yamashita H, Ichijo H, Grimsby S, Morén A, ten Dijke P, Miyazono K. J Biol Chem.
     1994; 269: 1995-2001
17   Waltenberger J, Lundin L, Öberg K, Wilander E, Miyazono K, Heldin C-H, Funa K.
     Am J Pathol. 1993; 142: 71-74
18   Eklöv S, Funa K, Nordgren H, Olofsson A, Kanzaki T, Miyazono K, Nillson S. Cancer Res.
     1993; 53: 3193-3197
19   Waltenberger J, Wanders A, Fellström B, Miyazono K, Heldin CH, Funa K. J Immunol.
     1993; 151: 1147-1157
20   Maurer M, Foitzik K, Eichmüller B, Handjiski B, Czarnetzki BM, Paus R. J Invest Dermatol.
     (in press)
21   Foitzik K, Eichmüller S, Czarnetzki BM, Paus R. Arch Dermatol Res. 1995; 287: 373
22   Cotsarelis G, Sun TT, Lavker RM. Cell. 1990; 61: 1329-1337

1996 Elsevier Science B.V.
Hair research for the next millenium
D.J.J. Van Neste and V.A. Randall (Eds)

Altered hair follicle morphogenesis in epidermal growth factor receptor deficient mice

L.A. Hansen[1], U. Lichti[1], T. Tennenbaum[1], A.A. Dlugosz[1], D.W. Threadgill[2], T. Magnuson[2] and S.H. Yuspa[1]

[1]Laboratory of Cellular Carcinogenesis and Tumor Promotion, NCI, Bethesda, MD
[2]Department of Genetics, Case Western Reserve University, Cleveland, OH

Introduction

Epidermal growth factor (EGF) was the first growth factor to be implicated in the normal development of the skin, as its administration to newborn mice delays hair follicle development [1, 2], and results in epidermal hyperproliferation [2, 3], increased keratinization, and skin thickening [4]. Not only does EGF injection delay the development of the follicle [1, 2], it also decreases the rate of hair growth and hair diameter [5]. Multiple actions of EGF in the skin are also suggested by *in vitro* studies utilizing primary keratinocytes which have shown that EGF acts as a mitogen for keratinocytes [6], promotes cell migration [7], and is effective at auto- and cross-induction of other growth factors [8]. Abrogation of EGFR signalling in spontaneously arising mutants of EGFR (waved-2) and TGF-α (waved-1) or as a result of disruption of the TGF-α gene by homologous recombination experiments suggests a role for EGFR signalling in the organization and function of the hair follicle [9, 14]. The mutant and TGF-α null mice exhibit a wavy hair follicle and curly whisker phenotype as a result of disorganization of the hair follicles which decreases in severity with increasing age [9-14].

Recent studies in mice harboring a targeted disruption of the EGFR have reported much more severe effects [15-17]. EGFR null homozygosity is lethal at different stages of embryogenesis or postnatally depending on the genetic background of the mice [15, 16]. EGFR null mice on a CD-1 background, which survive as long as 18 d [15], exhibit a dramatic skin phenotype as well as neurological deficits, and kidney, liver, and colon abnormalities [15]. Vibrissae of homozygous mice are curled and fragile at birth, while follicular disorganization appears histologically as early as 5 d [15]. These mice develop a delayed and defective fuzzy coat between 10 and 14 d [15].

In order to understand the role of EGFR in the skin we have further characterized the epidermal and hair follicle defects in EGFR null mouse skin. We report aberrant and premature differentiation of EGFR null hair follicles. In contrast to the rather dramatic hair follicle phenotype, the differentiation of the interfollicular epidermis was relatively less affected by the loss of EGFR signalling. However, interfollicular epidermal cell proliferation appeared to be dependent on the EGFR while follicular cell proliferation continued relatively unaffected in the EGFR null mice. Taken together, these results suggest that signalling through the EGFR is important in the differentiation and maturation of the hair follicle and maintenance of cell proliferation in the interfollicular epidermis.

Materials and methods

Animals

Homozygous or heterozygous EGFR null mice and wild type siblings on a CD-1 background were developed using homologous recombination in 129/Sv-derived D3 embryonic stem cells [15]. Mice were genotyped using PCR, as described elsewhere [15].

BrDU labelling and immunohistochemistry

Dorsal skin from mice that were injected i.p. with 250 µg/g BrDU were fixed in 70% ethanol, processed and embedded in paraffin. Sections were immunohistochemically stained for BrDU as described elsewhere [18] using anti-BrDU antibody (Becton-Dickinson), a horseradish peroxidase conjugated secondary antibody (Jackson ImmunoResearch), with diaminobenzidine as the substrate (Sigma Chemical Corp.) and a haematoxylin counterstain. Interfollicular epidermal BrDU incorporation was quantitated by counting BrDU-labelled nuclei in 100 basal interfollicular epidermal cells from 3 randomly chosen areas in BrDU-stained sections of skin.

Immunohistochemistry

Dorsal skin from EGFR +/+, +/-, and -/- mice was fixed in 70% ethanol, processed and embedded in paraffin. For immunohistochemistry of differentiation markers, rabbit antiserum produced against keratin 6 [19], keratin 1 [19], keratin 10 [19], keratin 14 [19], loricrin, or filaggrin was incubated with skin sections, followed by incubation with anti-rabbit biotinylated secondary antibody (Vector Laboratories, Burlingame, CA), an ABC reagent (Vector Laboratories, Burlingame, CA), diaminobenzidine substrate and contrast green counterstain.

Immunofluorescence

For immunofluorescence localization of integrins, acetone fixed frozen sections were incubated with rabbit antiserum to $\alpha 3$ (Chemicon) or rat monoclonal antibody to $\alpha 6$ (GOH3, Amac). Fluorescence was detected by incubation with biotinylated secondary antibodies followed by streptavidin-Texas red (BRL) as described elsewhere [20].

Results

Histopathology of the skin of EGFR deficient mice

Previous work has shown that major phenotypic abnormalities occur in the skin of mice deficient for TGF-α [9, 10]. Specifically, disorientation of hair follicles was described where misalignment, crowding, and angling was associated with the emergence of a waved hair. Hair bulbs extended deeper into the dermis of mutant mice, and septulation of the hair medulla and reduced dermal adipose tissue were additional pathological findings. In EGFR null mice, these microscopic changes were also noted, but were more exaggerated, and the animals failed to develop a hairy coat during the first two weeks of postnatal life. Around 14 d the EGFR null mice began to show a severely defective 'fuzzy coat'. In addition, histological analysis of mutant skin over an 18 d postnatal period revealed abundant primordial follicles at birth, indicating that EGFR is not required for early stages of hair follicle development. From 5 to 12 d, hair follicles of varying size developed showing remarkable disorientation, some penetrating to maximum depth, then growing horizontally above the skeletal muscle and, occasionally, reversing direction of growth (Fig. 1A). In EGFR null mice, hair shaft abnormalities were also observed along with premature separation of the hair shaft from the inner root sheath (Fig. 1C). The medulla frequently contained multiple columns of cells, sometimes out of register, and hair keratinization in the matrix region appeared to occur prematurely (Fig. 1C). These maturation defects suggest that EGFR-ligand interactions are important for hair integrity and predict that fragility of emerging hair is responsible for the hairless appearance of EGFR null mice. In contrast to the remarkable changes in hair follicle morphology, the epidermis of EGFR null mice appeared relatively normal until 18 d when it was thinner and the basal cells appeared flattened (Fig. 1B). Thus, loss of EGFR resulted in a dramatically disorganized hair follicle phenotype with apparently less severe effects on epidermal morphology.

Follicular proliferation is independent of EGFR signalling

Because of the strong body of evidence showing that EGF is a potent mitogen in skin cells in culture, we examined cell proliferation in EGFR null skin. Proliferation was monitored by injecting 5-bromodeoxyuridine (BrDU) into neonatal mice prior to sacrifice and immunohistochemically staining skin sections using an anti-BrDU antibody. In the interfollicular epidermis, no significant differences in BrDU labeling were noted at birth, but by 2 days and thereafter, EGFR null mice had progressively decreasing epidermal labeling so that by 8 d few proliferating cells were detected. In contrast, BrDU labeling in the infundibular region of the hair follicles was similar in mutant and wild-type genotypes. This labeling pattern is consistent with the central role proposed for the EGFR ligand family in epidermal proliferation from studies of cultured keratinocytes, as well as experiments that targeted overexpression of TGF-α to transgenic epidermis [21, 22]. In the first week of postnatal growth, BrDU

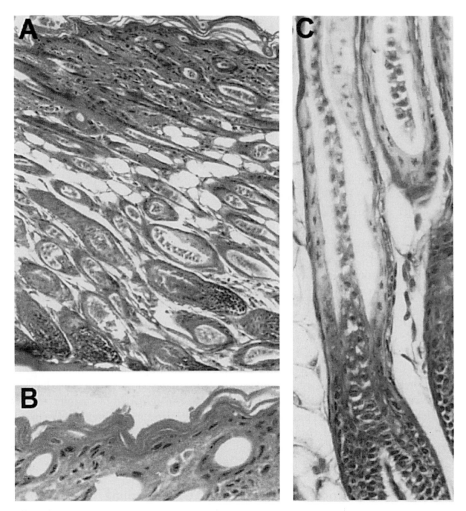

Figure 1. Altered histology in hematoxylin and eosin stained sections from 14 d (panel A) or 18 d (panels B and C) EGFR null skin

labeling in the anagen hair bulbs from all EGFR genotypes was high, consistent with the rapid growth and development of hair follicles in perinatal mice. BrDU labeling persisted in follicle matrix cells at 18 d. Previous immunohistochemical and EGFR-binding studies had determined that the anagen hair follicles are focally deficient in EGFR [23], suggesting that other cytokine-receptor pathways may contribute to the rapid downgrowth of anagen follicles. These results suggest that EGFR-ligand interactions produce specific responses in the epidermal and dermal skin compartments. In the epidermis, this pathway regulates proliferation while follicular proliferation is independent of EGFR signalling.

Altered localization of follicularly expressed gene products

In order to link functional changes in skin compartments to EGFR, a series of specific markers was examined. Immunohistochemical analysis of EGFR null skin revealed aberrant maturation of hair follicles, as well as changes in matrix receptors associated with cell migration. Keratin 6, normally expressed in the upper and middle portions of the inner root sheath of the hair follicle, was expressed prematurely in the region just above the hair bulb in EGFR null animals. The α6β4 integrin, confined normally to the basement membrane zone of the epidermis and upper follicle, was detected along the outer root sheath of growing follicles deep in the dermis of EGFR null mice, but not in normal littermates. Furthermore, the α3β1 integrin, normally confined to epidermis, was also detected along the outer root sheath of a subpopulation of mature follicles in EGFR null mice. However, laminin I, collagen IV, and fibronectin distribution was similar in skin sections from mutant and normal genotypes at several postnatal times. In further studies, no differences in expression of distribution of the basal cell and outer root sheath marker keratin 14, or the suprabasal epidermal markers keratin 1 and keratin 10, loricrin, and filaggrin were detected. However, a significant increase in suprabasal expression of α3β1 integrin in the epidermis was detected in EGFR null mice as early as 2 days. Since EGFR ligands have been shown to influence integrin expression and cell migration *in vitro* [24, 25], aberrant expression of α3β1 or α6β4 in EGFR null mice could be responsible for the abnormal migratory properties of skin cells.

Discussion

In this study, we have shown that a null mutation in the EGFR gene results in dramatic alterations in the structure of the hair follicle, including misalignment, disorganization, and premature differentiation of follicular cells. We suggest that alterations in the localization of expression of integrin receptors may be responsible for this misalignment of the hair follicles. In contrast to the striking hair follicle phenotype in EGFR null mice, the interfollicular epidermis appeared relatively normal. Cell proliferation, however, was relatively independent of EGFR signalling only in the hair follicles, since loss of EGFR did result in a large decrease in epidermal cell proliferation. Thus, EGFR appears to function to regulate both epidermal proliferation and follicular orientation and differentiation.

Although a similar hair follicle phenotype has been observed in other animals harboring mutations which impair signalling through the EGFR, some minor differences are apparent. A similar disorganization of the hair follicles accompanied by curled or absent vibrissae at birth has been reported in independently generated EGFR null mice [16, 17]. In contrast to our findings, these researchers reported a thinner epidermis at birth with decreased or defective keratinization of the stratum corneum [16] or stratum granulosum [17]. These variations may be due to differences in genetic background of the animals under study, since placing the EGFR null mutation on various genetic backgrounds has been shown to dramatically affect survival of the mice [15].

EGFR null mice might be very useful in clarifying the interactions of multiple EGFR family members in the skin. EGFR family members are believed to form heterodimers and at least two other members, neu [26, 27] and HER-3 [27], and several EGFR ligands [28-30] have been localized to the skin. The EGFR itself has been localized to the outer root sheath and matrix of hair follicles as well as the interfollicular epidermis of rat and human skin with the strongest signal in basal cells [23, 31]. The ligand EGF is expressed in the outer root sheath and the differentiating cells of the sebaceous gland in developing and mature sheep follicles as well as in the upper layers of both adult mouse and fetal sheep epidermis [28, 29], although not in primary keratinocytes [32]. Another EGFR ligand, TGF-α, is expressed in the basal, spinous, and granular layers of the epidermis and in the inner root sheath of hair follicles [9, 30]. Crosses of EGFR null mice with other genetically engineered animals harboring defects in EGFR signalling are now possible. Since overexpression of the EGFR has been detected in a variety of neoplasms, including epithelial squamous cell carcinomas [33, 34], the EGFR null mouse model also has potential value for studying the importance of EGFR in skin tumorigenesis. In particular, the role of EGFR in epithelial versus dermal cell populations in tumor development may be investigated using grafting of isolated cell populations onto nude mice.

In summary, this study clarifies the diverse actions of EGFR in the skin. While cell proliferation in the hair follicles appears to be relatively independent of EGFR signalling, epidermal cell proliferation is not. Conversely, loss of EGFR results in numerous abnormalities in follicular organization, placement, and differentiation. Ongoing experiments are designed to further characterize the hair follicle abnormalities in these mice as well as to define the signalling pathways affected by loss of EGFR.

References

1   Moore GP, Panaretto BA, Robertson D. Anat Rec. 1983; 205: 47-55
2   Moore GPM, Panaretto BA, Robertson D. J Endocrinol. 1981; 88: 293-299
3   Moore GP, Panaretto BA, Carter NB. J Invest Dermatol. 1985; 84: 172-175
4   Cohen S. Dev Biol. 1965; 12: 394-407
5   du Cros D. J Invest Dermatol. 1993; 101: 106S-113S
6   Pisansarakit P, Du Cros DL, Moore GPM. Arch Dermatol Res. 1990; 281: 530-535
7   Barrandon Y, Green H. Cell. 1987; 50: 1131-1137
8   Barnard JA, Graves-Deal R, Pittelkow MR, DuBois R et al. J Biol Chem. 1994; 269: 22817-22822
9   Luetteke NC, Qiu TH, Peiffer RL, Oliver P et al. Cell. 1993; 73: 263-278

10 Mann GB, Fowler KJ, Gabriel A, Nice EC *et al.* Cell. 1993; 73: 249-261

11 Crew FAE. J Genet. 1933; 27: 95-96

12 Butler L, Robertson DA. J Hered. 1992; 44: 13-16

13 Bennett JH, Gresham GA. Nature. 1956; 178: 272-273.

14 Trigg M, Gluecksohn-Waelsch S. J Cell Biol. 1973; 58: 549-563.

15 Threadgill DW, Dlugosz AA, Hansen LA, Tennenbaum T *et al.* Science. 1995; 269: 230-234

16 Sibilia M, Wagner E. Science. 1995; 269: 234-238

17 Miettinen P, Berger J, Meneses J, Phung Y *et al.* Nature. 1995; 376: 337-341

18 Glick AB, Kulkarni AB, Tennenbaum T, Hennings H *et al.* Proc Natl Acad Sci USA. 1993; 90: 6076-6080

19 Roop DR, Huitfeldt H, Kilkenny A, Yuspa SH. Differentiation. 1987; 35: 143-150

20 Tennenbaum T, Weiner AK, Belanger AJ, Glick AB *et al.* Cancer Res. 1993; 53: 4803- 4810

21 Vassar R, Hutton ME, Fuchs E. Mol Cell Biol. 1992; 12: 4643-4653

22 Wang X, Greenhalgh DA, Eckhardt JN, Rothnagel JA *et al.* Mol Carcinog. 1994; 10: 15-22

23 Green MR, Couchman JR. J Invest Dermatol. 1984; 83: 118-123

24 Chen JD, Kim JP, Zhang K, Sarret Y *et al.* Exp Cell Res. 1993; 209: 216-223

25 Carey TE, Laurikainen L, Nair TS, Reinke TS *et al.* Monograph of the National Cancer Institute. 1992; 13: 75-86

26 Kokai Y, Cohen JA, Drebin JA, Greene MI. Proc Natl Acad Sci. 1987; 84: 8498-8501

27 Danilenko DM, Ring BD, Lu JZ, Tarpley JE *et al.* J Clin Invest. 1995; 95: 842-851

28 Du Cros DL, Isaacs K, Moore GPM. J Invest Dermatol. 1992; 98: 109-115

29 Sakai Y, Nelson KG, Snedeker S, Bossert NL *et al.* Cell Growth & Diff. 1994; 5: 527-535

30 Finzi E, Harkins R, Horn T. J Invest Dermatol. 1991; 96: 328-332

31 Nanney LB, Magid M, Stoscheck CM, King LE, Jr. J Invest Dermatol. 1984; 83: 385-393

32 Dlugosz AA, Cheng C, Williams EK, Darwiche N *et al.* Cancer Res. 1995; 55: 1883-1893

33 Yamamoto T, Kamata N, Kawano H, Shimizu S *et al.* Cancer Res. 1986; 46: 414-416

34 Derynck R, Goeddel DV, Ullrich A, Gutterman JU *et al.* Cancer Res. 1987; 47: 707-712

Local injection of hepatocyte growth factor/scatter factor (HGF/SF) promotes hair follicle growth *in vivo*

T. Jindo, R. Tsuboi, K. Takamori and H. Ogawa

Department of Dermatology, Juntendo University School of Medicine, 2-1-1 Hongo, Bunkyo-ku, Tokyo 113, Japan

Introduction

Hepatocyte growth factor/scatter factor (HGF/SF) is a multifunctional polypeptide which acts as a mitogen, motogen or morphogen depending on the biological context [1]. HGF/SF is secreted by mesenchymally-derived cells and acts on neighbouring epithelial or endothelial cells. Hair follicle is composed of epithelial (the matrix and outer root sheath) and mesenchymal (the follicular papilla and connective tissue sheath) elements. Although the cooperative interaction of these two components is thought to be crucial for hair development and growth, the mechanisms regulating these events are not well understood. Recently, we found that HGF/SF stimulated the hair follicle growth of newborn mouse vibrissae and of the human scalp in an organ culture system [2, 3]. HGF/SF mRNA was later found to be expressed in human follicular papilla cells, and DNA synthesis of human hair bulb-derived keratinocytes was stimulated by the addition of HGF/SF. As a continuation to our series of experiments on HGF/SF, we report here data describing the effect of HGF/SF on hair growth *in vivo*.

Materials and methods

Reagents

Recombinant human HGF/SF (Snow brand, Japan) or recombinant human basic fibroblast growth factor (bFGF, R&D system, Minneapolis, USA) was dissolved in sterile and toxin-free phosphate-buffered saline (PBS) containing 0.1% bovine serum albumin (BSA).

Animals and treatment

B6C3F1 mice which were 1-day-old, 29-day-old (anagen phase) or 45-day-old (telogen phase) were used for the experiments.

Experiment 1: The dorsal skin of the newborn mice (1.4~1.5 g) was injected with 1 µg of HGF/SF or bFGF in 50 µl of BSA-PBS once daily for 5 days (total 5 µg). Control animals received 50 µl of BSA-PBS for 5 days. The mice were sacrificed on day 7, and then subjected to histological evaluation.

Experiment 2: Mice at later stages of the second anagen phase (18.1~21.8 g) were injected with the same doses once daily for 7 days, and were then sacrificed on day 10.

Experiment 3: Mice in the second telogen phase (22.2~25.4 g) were injected with the same doses once daily for 7 days, and were then sacrificed on day 10.

Evaluations

Skin color: The skin color of the reverse side of the dorsal skin was measured using a Minolta chromameter (Minolta, Tokyo, Japan).

Skin thickness and hair follicle tissue: histological sections stained with hematoxylin and eosin were analyzed by an image analyzer (Mac scope, Mitani Co., Fukui, Japan). Skin thickness was defined as the distance from the granular cell layer to the edge of the muscle layer. Hair follicle tissue was indicated in mm^2 by integrating the area of individual hair follicles.

Results and discussion

In this study, we examined the hair growth-stimulatory activity of HGF/SF *in vivo*, the results of which are summarized in Table 1. In newborn mice (Experiment 1), bFGF injection caused a slight reduction in skin color on day 7, while HGF/SF did not cause any difference. HGF/SF slightly increased the amount of hair follicle tissue, while bFGF significantly reduced both skin thickness and hair follicle tissue. Observations on the effect of bFGF on hair growth were found to coincide with a previous report [5], thereby supporting the probability of a positive effect by HGF/SF on hair growth. The effect of HGF/SF on hair growth in newborn rats was also found to be significant ($p<0.05$, data not shown), suggesting the species-independent effect of HGF/SF.

Subsequently, the effect of HGF/SF on anagen or telogen was examined. In experiment 2, HGF/SF was injected into the skin at the later stages of the second anagen phase. The dorsal skin of the BSA-PBS-injected mice progressed to the telogen phase, while HGF/SF-injected mice remained in the anagen phase. The dark skin color of the reverse side of the injection site clearly demonstrated the effect of HGF/SF. The bFGF-injected mice had teleangiectasia at the injection site, confirming the angiogenic effect of bFGF *in vivo*. The HGF/SF-injected mice had increases in skin thickness and hair follicle tissue when compared to those of BSA-PBS-injected mice (Table 1). Meanwhile, bFGF-injected mice had an increase in skin thickness with cellular infiltration but no increase in hair follicle tissue.

In experiment 3, the effect of HGF/SF on telogen was examined. As shown in

Table 1, neither HGF/SF nor bFGF induced anagen at the injection site, however, both reagents increased the skin thickness, with a marked cellular infiltration in bFGF-treated mice.

Table 1.

Effect of the HGF/SF or bFGF on skin thickness and hair follicle tissue *in vivo*

	Skin thickness (mm)			Hair follicle tissue (mm^2)		
	PBS	HGF/SF	bFGF	PBS	HGF/SF	bFGF
Exp. 1	0.71±0.07	0.74 ±0.02	0.49*±0.14	103±20	124±10	49*±26
Exp. 2	0.26±0.06	0.33 ±0.15	0.43*±0.15	7±8	17±14	5±9
Exp. 3	0.22±0.06	0.32*±0.05	0.38*±0.06	(-)	(-)	(-)

Mean±SD, n=5, (-): not detected, *: p<0.05 (vs PBS)

Summarizing our previous and present data, HGF/SF was found to increase follicular length and DNA synthesis in organ culture [2, 3], and to stimulate the DNA synthesis of hair bulb-derived keratinocytes [4]. In the *in vivo* studies, HGF/SF application increased hair follicle tissue in newborn animals, and delayed the transition from anagen to telogen phase. These results suggest that HGF/SF promotes hair growth and has a clinical utility in this regard.

References

1   Rubin JS, Bottaro DP, Aaronson SA. Biochim Biophys Acta. 1993; 1155: 357-371
2   Jindo T, Tsuboi R, Imai R, Takamori K, Rubin JS, Ogawa H. J Invest Dermatol. 1994; 103: 306-309
3   Jindo T, Tsuboi R, Imai R, Takamori K, Rubin JS, Ogawa H. J Dermatol Sci. 1995; 10: 229-232
4   Shimaoka S, Tsuboi R, Jindo T, Imai R, Takamori K, Rubin JS, Ogawa H. J Cell Physiol. 1995; 165: 333-338
5   du Cross DL. Dev Biol. 1993; 156: 444-453

Induction of anagen by topical application of potent immunosuppressor FK506 in telogen mouse

S. Yamamoto, H. Jiang and R. Kato

Department of Pharmacology, School of Medicine, Keio University, 35 Shinanomachi, Shinjuku-ku, Tokyo 160, Japan

Introduction

FK506, a macrolide antibiotic, is a T cell-specific immunosuppresor. Recently we have demonstrated that the topical application of FK506 markedly suppresses tumor promotion caused by 12-O-tetradecanoylphorbol-13-acetate in the two-stage carcinogenesis of mouse skin [1]. During this experiment, we observed an obvious stimulation of hair growth by topical application of FK506. Oral administration of FK506 at a dose that induces marked immuno-suppression fails to stimulate hair growth [2], consistent with the fact that FK506 does not induce hypertrichosis in clinical trials. Long-term treatment of mice with FK506, i.e., topical application of 1 µmol FK506 twice a week for 6 months, does not affect body weight gain of mice and the FK506-treated mice look healthy [1]. The hair growth-stimulating effect of FK506 is due at least in part to its direct stimulation of hair follicles [2]. Immunosuppression caused by FK506 seems to be unrelated to the hair growth-stimulating effect of this compound [2]. In this study we investigated whether FK506 induces anagen hair growth in telogen mouse skin.

Results and discussion

When mice in telogen phase were treated with 1µmol FK506 on days 0 and 3, 50% of the treated animals entered anagen by day 9 and 100% by day 16. With 0.1 µmol of FK506, 50% of the treated mice entered anagen by day 13 and 80% by day 19, indicating that the effect of FK506 was dose-related. A spontaneous shift from telogen to anagen started on day 14, and 30% of the non-treated animals were in anagen phase at day 19. Histological data revealed that FK506 treatment markedly thickened skin without inducing an inflammatory reaction. The depth and size of hair follicles were also markedly increased in FK506-treated skin compared to control skin. The results were consistent with the fact that skin thickness increases from a thin telogen skin to a thick anagen skin, and that the size and depth of follicles are markedly increased in anagen phase [3-5]. At the same time, FK506 markedly stimulated hair growth, consistent with our previous observation [2]. The produced hair looked normal, and the hairs were of normal length. Moreover, the hair growth was restricted to the site of application. Our present results indicate that the hair growth-stimulating effect of FK506 is due at least in part to its promoting effect on the hair cycle.

Our present findings have been published recently [6].

References

1   Jiang H, Yamamoto S, Nishikawa K, Kato R. Carcinogenesis. 1993; 14: 67-71
2   Yamamoto S, Jiang H, Kato R. J Invest Dermatol. 1994; 102: 160-164
3   Paus R, Stenn KS, Link RE. Lab Invest. 1989; 60: 365-369
4   Hansen LS, Coggle JE, Wells J, Charles MW. Anat Rec. 1984; 210: 569-573
5   Bogovski P. In: Turusov VS, ed. Pathology in Tumors in Laboratory Animals, Vol II. Tumors of the Mouse. IARC Scientific Publications No 23. Lyon: International Agency for Research on Cancer. 1979; 1-40
6   Jiang H, Yamamoto S, Kato R. J Invest Dermatol. 1995; 104: 523-525

The role of insulin-like growth factor I in hair follicle growth

S.M. Rudman, M.P. Philpott and T. Kealey

Department of Clinical Biochemistry, University of Cambridge, Addenbrookes Hospital, Hills Rd, Cambridge, UK

Introduction

The insulin-like growth factors I and II (IGF-I and II) share a high degree of structural and functional homology with insulin [1]. *In vitro*, they have been shown to be potent mitogens in a large number of tissues and cell types [2]. By Northern blot analysis, IGF-I mRNA has been detected in cultured dermal fibroblasts but not in cultured keratinocytes [3]. IGF-I receptor mRNA has been detected in whole skin, dermal fibroblasts and cultured keratinocytes. IGF-I and II have also been shown to stimulate keratinocyte proliferation *in vitro* [4]. Further, in patients suffering from acromegaly, elevated levels of circulating growth hormone result in a marked thickening of the epidermis and acanthosis nigricans [5]. Therefore, it has been suggested that IGF-I may be an important autocrine/paracrine regulator of cellular proliferation and differentiation in the skin.

In the hair follicle, the role of IGF-I has yet to be defined. We have previously reported that, *in vitro*, growth of isolated human hair follicles is maintained at an *in vivo* rate in the presence of physiological concentrations of IGF-I and II or supraphysiological concentrations of insulin [6]. However, in the absence of these, hair follicles show a premature entry into the catagen stage of the hair growth cycle. We have now undertaken to localize the expression of IGF-I mRNA, protein and IGF-I receptor protein in human hair follicles.

Materials and methods

Reverse transcriptase-PCR

Human anagen hair follicles were isolated from facelift skin according to the method of Philpott *et al.* [7]. Following isolation, follicles were either used for total RNA extraction or microdissected into one of four follicular components - dermal papilla, matrix cells, outer and inner root sheaths and connective tissue sheath, and then used for total RNA extraction [8]. cDNA was generated using random hexamers and AMV reverse transcriptase at 42°C for 1 hour and then 80°C for 10 minutes. To control for contamination of the microdissected follicles with mesenchymal or epithelial cells, PCR was performed using primers corresponding to the vimentin and keratin 5 genes respectively. PCR was then performed using primers corresponding to the human IGF-I/II and IGF-I receptor sequences, and the products were visualised using agarose gel electrophoresis and ethidium bromide. Restriction enzyme digests were performed to confirm PCR product identity.

In situ hybridisation

Isolated hair follicles were immediately fixed in 3% buffered formalin and embedded in paraffin wax. 5 μm sections were then cut and placed on APES coated slides.

In situ hybridisation was performed according to the method of Thomas *et al* [8]. Briefly, sections were dewaxed, rehydrated and incubated with 0.2N HCl followed by proteinase K digestion. Sections were pre-hybridised in hybridisation buffer for 60 mins at 37°C and then incubated overnight at 42°C with a digoxigenin labelled cDNA probe corresponding to the human IGF-I sequence. To remove unbound probe, the slides were washed in 0.1 x SSC and then incubated with an alkaline phosphatase conjugated anti-digoxigenin antibody for 60 minutes at room temperature. Sections were then developed overnight using BCIP and NBT. A calcitonin cDNA oligonucleotide probe, and the absence of probe, were used as negative controls.

Immunocytochemistry

Sections were dewaxed in xylene and rehydrated in graded alcohol. Endogenous peroxidase activity was blocked with 3% H_2O_2 and non-specific antibody binding was blocked with 10% rabbit serum. Sections were then incubated overnight with either a rabbit anti-human IGF-I polyclonal antibody or a mouse anti-human monoclonal IGF-I receptor antibody at 4°C. Following washes, sections were incubated with a horseradish peroxidase conjugated secondary antibody and developed using diaminobenzidine and H_2O_2. Sections were counterstained with haematoxylin, dehydrated and mounted using DEPEX. An anti-human calcitonin polyclonal antibody or an anti-human oestrogen receptor monoclonal antibody were used as negative controls.

Results

IGF-I mRNA and IGF-I receptor mRNA were identified by RT-PCR in whole anagen follicles. The PCR products were digested with specific restriction enzymes to confirm the products specificity.

Microdissected parts of follicles were checked for contamination from mesenchymal or epithelial components by looking at the distribution of the vimentin and keratin 5 mRNA. Only cDNA from microdissected follicles which displayed the correct expression pattern for these two genes were used to localize the IGF-I and receptor mRNA. Keratin 5 expression was seen in the matrix cells and the inner and outer root sheaths only, while vimentin expression was seen in the dermal papilla and fibroblast connective tissue sheath.

Using these hair follicle cases, IGF-I mRNA was detected in all regions of the follicle, while IGF-I receptor mRNA was detected in the follicle bulb (dermal papilla and matrix cells), and weakly in the inner and outer root sheath. The fibroblast sheath surrounding the follicle was negative.

To confirm these observations, *in situ* hybridisation for IGF-I was performed in sectioned anagen follicles, and to confirm this localization at the protein level, immunocytochemistry was performed for both IGF-I and the receptor.

IGF-I mRNA was detected in all regions of the hair follicle by *in situ* hybridisation although the expression in the dermal papilla and the connective tissue sheath was weaker than in the other regions. In approximately half of the cases studied some intense staining was seen in the matrix cells at the apex of the dermal papilla. Negative control slides were clear in all regions of the hair follicle.

IGF-I protein was weakly expressed in the hair follicle bulb and in the basal cells of the outer root sheath and fibroblast sheath. There was strong staining in the upper outer root sheath. Staining was variable in the dermal papilla, with some dermal papillae staining positive for IGF-I and some negative. The negative control slides staining for calcitonin were clear in all regions of the follicle.

IGF-I receptor protein only was investigated. The receptor was expressed only in the dermal papilla, suprabasal matrix cells and the suprabasal cells of the outer root sheath. However, the germinative matrix cells and the basal cells of the outer root sheath were negative. In catagen follicles, the expression pattern was maintained although the dermal papilla was negative for the IGF-I receptor. The negative control oestrogen receptor slides were clear in all regions of the follicle.

Discussion

We have taken single whole anagen hair follicles and have shown that IGF-I and II and the type I receptor genes are expressed in whole anagen hair follicles and have confirmed this result using restriction enzyme analysis. We have localized this gene expression within hair follicles using two methods, RT-PCR and *in situ* hybridisation. Follicles were microdissected to isolate the mesenchymal portions of the follicle - the dermal papilla, and connective tissue sheath-and the epithelial portions-the matrix cells, and inner and outer root sheaths.

IGF-I mRNA was expressed in all regions of the follicle. This expression pattern was confirmed by *in situ* hybridisation. The localization of the IGF-I protein was seen in all areas of the follicle although the expression in the follicle bulb appeared to be weak and the staining in the upper outer root sheath was strongest. The presence of IGF-I in the germinative matrix cells suggested that, unlike the epidermal keratinocytes in the skin which apparently have no mRNA for IGF-I, these cells appear to be able to synthesize their own IGF-I and therefore perhaps IGF-I (which is essential for hair follicle growth) is not sequestered from the dermal papilla but is made by the matrix cells themselves.

The IGF-I receptor was localized only to the dermal papilla and suprabasal matrix cells in the follicle bulb. The highly proliferating germinative matrix cells were negative for the receptor. This suggests that IGF-I may have a role in the differentiation of the matrix cells to form a new hair fibre, rather than as a mitogen as initially suggested [6]. We also observed that the IGF-I receptor is switched off in catagen in the dermal papilla, which also suggests that IGF-I is involved in changes occuring in the human hair growth cycle.

In conclusion these findings support the suggestion that IGF-I is a major hair follicle cytokine, and that perhaps it also has a role as a differentiation regulator as well as a direct mitogen on the matrix cells.

References

1   Humbel RE. Eur J Biochem. 1990; 190: 445-462
2   Daughaday WH, Rotwein P. Endocrine Rev. 1989; 10: 68-91
3   Tavakkal A, Elder JT, Griffiths CEM, Cooper KD, Talwar H, Fisher GJ, Keane KH, Foltin SK, Vorkee JJ. J Invest Dermatol. 1992; 99: 343-349
4   Neely EK, Morhenn VB, Hintz RL, Wilson DM, Rosenfeld RG. J Invest Dermatol. 1991; 96: 104-110
5   Barkan AL, Beitins IZ, Kelch RP. J Clin Endocrinol Metab. 1988; 67: 69-73
6   Philpott MP, Sanders DA, Kealey T. J Invest Dermatol. 1994; 102: 857-861
7   Philpott MP, Green MR, Kealey T. J Cell Sci. 1990; 97: 463-471
8   Chomzynski P, Sacchi N. Anal Biochem. 1987; 162: 156-159
9   Thomas GA, Davies HG, Williams ED. J Clin Pathol. 1993; 46: 171-174
10   Pieper FR, Van de Klundert FA, Raats JM, Henderik JB, Schaart G, Ramaekers HC, Bloemendal H. Eur J Biochem. 1992; 210: 509-519

443

The investigation of insulin-like growth factor-I (IGF-I) receptors on the hair follicles of seasonal and non-seasonal fibre producing goats and deer antler velvet

P. Dicks[1] and L.M. Williams[2]

[1]Macaulay Land Use Research Institute, Aberdeen, Scotland AB9 2QJ
[2]Rowett Research Institute, Aberdeen, Scotland AB2 9SB

Introduction

To determine whether insulin-like growth factor-I (IGF-I) is directly involved in the hair follicle cycles of animals with differing patterns of fibre growth and moulting, we have investigated the possible presence of IGF-I receptors on the dermis and hair follicles of cashmere and Angora goats.

Fibre growth in the cashmere goat is highly seasonal. The individual hair follicle cycles of anagen, telogen and the release of the mature fibre from the follicle, which is coincident with the reactivation of the follicle (early anagen) are synchronized over the animal resulting in the development of the winter pelage and a distinct spring moult [1]. In contrast, fibre growth in the Angora goat is aseasonal with the majority of the follicles actively producing fibre at any one time [2].

IGF-I is a polypeptide with a structural homology to insulin. The transport and availability of systemic IGF-I is regulated by at least six specific binding proteins, but the local action of IGF-I is via binding to specific membrane bound receptors [3].

Systemic IGF-I has been implicated in the development of red deer antler velvet, a structure that uniquely involves the generation of a population of follicles *de novo*, and specific IGF-I receptors have been reported on the cartilaginous zone of the antler. However the presence of high total and non-specific binding has been reported in the dermis and consequently the presence of IGF-I receptors is indeterminate [4]. More recently, *in vitro* studies with human hair follicles have demonstrated that IGF-I may have a role in follicle elongation and in preventing the follicles from entering a catagen-like state, suggesting that IGF-I is directly involved in the control of the hair follicle [5].

In this study, the localization and binding characteristics of IGF-I receptors in and around the primary and secondary hair follicles of cashmere and Angora goats have been investigated using *in vitro* autoradiography to determine whether IGF-I acts directly at the hair follicle in both seasonal and non-seasonal fibre producing animals.

444

Materials and methods

Tissue sampling and preparation

On 3 occasions, 3 February, 12 May and 6 June, dates which were selected as being pre- during- and post the moult after visual assessment of the stage of the coat cycle, skin biopsies were removed under local anaesthetic and frozen in isopentane. Twenty μm horizontal serial sections and 12 μm longitudinal sections were cut and mounted onto gelatin coated slides for the characterization and localization studies respectively.

The growing tips of 4 red deer antlers, with the velvet attached, were removed immediately following slaughter and were frozen, quartered and sectioned as for the skin biopsies.

Localization and characterization of IGF-I receptors

[^{125}I]IGF-I was prepared using a lactoperoxidase method and purified using HPLC. To determine specific binding sections were firstly preincubated in a high salt/low pH buffer, to remove any bound IGF-I, then incubated in Tris-HCl (pH 7.5) with 50 pM [^{125}I]IGF-I alone or in the presence of 1000 fold excess of IGF-I. Sections were then washed, dried and apposed to X AR-OMAT film, or coated with liquid emulsion film for light microscopy. The optical densities of the images were measured using image analysis. For saturation studies, slides were incubated with a range of concentrations of [^{125}I]IGF-I to demonstrate that the binding observed was saturable to a finite number of receptor binding sites. Binding was quantified using a [^{125}I] polymer standard. Saturation isotherms generated were analyzed using a one-site binding model and the data transformed for Scatchard plots using the Enzfitter Computer program [6] giving a dissociation constant (Kd) and a theoretical maximal number of binding sites (Bmax) for each sample analyzed. Slides were also incubated for a range of times, at both 4 and 37°C and in the presence of a range of concentrations of IGF-I, IGF-II, insulin and epidermal growth factor (EGF) to determine whether binding was time and temperature dependent and competitive.

Results

Specific binding was observed in both telogen and anagen follicles and in both the cashmere and Angora goat samples. Specific binding was also confirmed in the cartilaginous zone of the red-deer antler and was identified in the velvet producing region (Fig. 1). The binding observed was demonstrated to be saturable, time and temperature dependent and competitive. Values obtained for Kd's and Bmax are presented in Table 1. From light microscopy studies specific binding was localized to the inner and outer root sheaths, the sebaceous glands, the dermal papilla and interestingly within the dermal papilla region higher binding was observed over the germinal matrix.

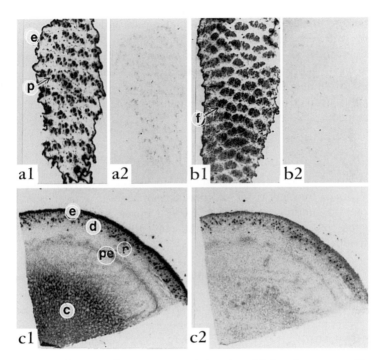

*Figure 1.: Autoradiogram of a transverse serial section of (**a**) cashmere goat skin and (**b**) Angora goat skin cut at the level of the sebaceous gland showing (1) binding with 50 pM [^{125}I]IGF-I alone or (2) in the presence of 50nM IGF-I. The intensely labelled areas correspond to the epidermis (e), the primary follicles (p) and the follicle groups (f).*

*Autoradiogram of a transverse section of (**c**) a growing red-deer antler tip incubated with (1) 50 pM [^{125}I]IGF-I alone or (2) in the presence of 50nM IGF-I. Intense labelling corresponds to the epidermis (e) and the dermis (d), the velvet producing regions, and the cartilaginous zone (c). Other areas marked are the reserve mesenchyme (r) and the perichondrium (p).*

Conclusions

Specific [^{125}I] IGF-I binding was demonstrated to be saturable, time and temperature dependent and competitive thereby satisfying the basic kinetic criteria to be considered representative of an IGF-I receptor. IGF-I receptors were localized around the primary and secondary hair follicles and the sebaceous glands of both the cashmere and Angora goat samples suggesting that IGF-I may be involved in the hair follicle cycle of both seasonal and non-seasonal genotypes. The localization of the receptors was widespread, over the inner and outer root sheaths, the germinal matrix and the dermal papilla and there appeared to be no significant difference due to time of year in any of the pharmacological parameters studied or in the distribution of the binding, indicating that IGF-I may have a potentially wide range of effects on the hair follicle and associated structures throughout the hair follicle cycle. However the specific function of IGF-I in regulating growth and development in the hair follicle cycle remains to be determined.

Table 1.

The dissociation constant (Kd, nM) and the maximal concentration of $[^{125}I]IGF-I$ receptors (Bmax, fmol/mg tissue) calculated from analysis of saturation isotherms using a one-site binding model, of $[^{125}I]IGF-I$ binding to cashmere and Angora goat hair follicles sampled in February, May and June. (Data represent the values from individual animals).

	Kd (nM)		Bmax (fmol/mg)	
Sampling date	Cashmere	Angora	Cashmere	Angora
February (telogen)	0.43	0.15	28.2	28.9
	0.25	0.38	25.7	28.9
May (onset of anagen)	0.34	0.66	29.4	45.6
	0.43	0.61	29.4	37.3
June (anagen)	0.88	0.27	32.6	26.8
	0.50	0.34	34.6	21.4

References

1 Dicks P, Russel AJF, Lincoln GA. J Endocrinology. 1994; 143: 441-448
2 Russel AJF. Progress in sheep and goat research (ed. AW Speedy.). CAB International Oxford. 1992; chapter 11: 235-256
3 Judson J, Van Wyk, Kay Lind P. Molecular and cellular biology of insulin-like growth factors and their receptors. eds. LeRoith D and Raizada MK. Plenum Press. NY, London. 1989
4 Elliott JL, Oldham JM, Ambler GR, Bass JJ, et al. Endocrinology. 1992; 130(5): 2513-2520
5 Philpott MP, Sanders DA, Kealey T. J Investigative Dermatology. 1994; 102(6): 857-861
6 Leatherbarrow RJ. Enzfitter, a non-linear regression data analysis program. Elsevier, Amsterdam. 1987

Hair induction by dermal papilla cells cultured with conditioned medium of keratinocytes

T. Matsuzaki, M. Inamatsu and K. Yoshizato

Yoshizato MorphoMatrix Project, ERATO, JRDC, 242-37 Misonou, Saijyo, Higashihiroshima, Hiroshima 739, Japan

Introduction

The dermal papilla is believed to play a fundamental role in the induction and differentiation of hair follicle. In rat vibrissa follicles, whisker growth permanently ceases when more than the lower third of the follicle base is removed [1]. Hair production resumes if dermal papillae are implanted into follicles whose lower halves have been amputated [2]. The induction of hair follicle was demonstrated by associating glabrous ear and scrotal sac epidermis with dermal papillae [3]. Thus, the dermal papilla is of prime importance in the formation of hair follicles.

The culture of dermal papilla cells was established first from rat vibrissa follicles [4], then from human hair follicles [5]. The cultured papilla cells exhibit unique properties distinguishing them from dermal fibroblasts, that is a low proliferative activity and the formation of cell aggregates at confluence of the culture. Hair inducing capacity of the cultured papilla cells has been demonstrated by Jahoda et al. [6] which, however, reduced as the passage number of the culture increased.

We here report a novel cell culture method which enables the papilla cells to rapidly proliferate and retain their inductive ability for long term.

Materials and methods

Culture of papilla cells

Dermal papillae were removed from F344 rat vibrissae follicles and placed in 35 mm diameter dishes (8 papillae/dish) in three different manners:

1) in Dulbecco's modified Eagle Medium with 10% FBS (DMEM/10);
2) in DMEM/10 with 4×10^5 keratinocytes (co-culture);
3) in 1:1 mixture of DMEM/10 and keratinocytes conditioned medium (CM5 or CM8). CM5 was obtained from the primary culture of keratinocytes which had been cultured with DMEM/10 for 5 days. The cells were refed with fresh DMEM/10 and cultured for an additional 3 days, and the culture medium was collected as CM8. CM5 and CM8 were filtrated through 0.22 μm filters and

stored at 4°C. Keratinocytes were isolated from the epidermis which had been pealed from sole skin after digestion with 1000 U/ml dispase at 4°C overnight and treated with 0.25% trypsin in phosphate buffered saline at 37°C for 10 min. The subculture of the papilla cells was carried out every other week.

Growth analysis

The papilla cells cultured in DMEM/10 of 3-5 passages were inoculated in 96-well plates at 1×10^4 cells per well and cultured for 24 hr to ensure cell attachment. Then the cells were starved in DMEM with 0.1% FBS (DMEM/0.1) for 24 hr and the culture medium was replaced with 100 µl of DMEM/0.1 supplemented with 1µg/ml of FGF1 (aFGF), 5 ng/ml of FGF2 (bFGF), 50 ng/ml of TGFα, 0.5 ng/ml of TGFβ or 10 ng/ml of EGF. The effects of FGF1 and FGF2 were also examined in DMEM containing 1% or 10% FBS. After 16 hr of incubation, BrdU was added in each well (1mM at the final concentration) for 4 hr. The amount of DNA synthesized was estimated using anti-BrdU antibody, alkaline phosphatase conjugated second antibody, and fluorescent substrate AttoPhos. Fluorescence was measured at 590 nm with excitation at 460 nm by CytoFluor 2350.

Assay of inductive ability of cultured papilla cells

Sole skin of adult rats was cut into pieces of about 3 mm square and treated with 500 U/ml dispase in DMEM/10 at 37°C for 3 min to make a space between the epidermis and dermis. Cultured papilla cells were scraped off gently with a rubber policeman and incubated in non-adhesive dishes for one day. The cell aggregates (spheroids) thus obtained were inserted into the space of the skin pieces. Intact dermal papillae and spheroids of Swiss 3T3 were also crammed into the space of the different sole skin. The skin pieces were implanted under kidney capsule of 8-week-old female rats according to the method described by Kobayashi and Nishimura [7]. The implants were recovered from the animal after 8 weeks and subjected to immunohistological examination. Unfixed frozen sections of the implants were incubated with monoclonal antibodies (mABs) which react to inner root sheath (K1318), to hair matrix, outer rooth sheath and basal cells (K1310) and to dermal papilla (K1311). These mABs were produced by immunizing mice with whole hair bulbs and selected based upon specific immunohistochemical reactivity. Bound mABs were visualized with peroxidase-conjugated second antibodies and diamino-benzidine. The sections were counterstained with haematoxylin.

Results

Growth of vibrissae papilla cells was remarkably enhanced when they were cultured with keratinocytes. The area occupied by papilla cells in the co-culture was about 15-fold larger than that in the culture without keratinocytes at day 8.

Conditioned media of keratinocyte culture were also effective on growth stimulation of papilla cells to an extent comparable to the keratinocytes themselves. This fact suggests that the feeder effect of keratinocytes is able to be replaced with conditioned medium. The outgrowth area of papilla cells in the culture with CM5 or CM8 was about 9-fold larger than that without conditioned medium at day 8.

The papilla cells could be subcultured repeatedly more than 90 generations without affecting their replicative potential when they were cultured in the medium containing CM5 or CM8. Population doubling time (PDT) of the cells varied at an early phase of the passages and approached a constant value between 25 and 35 hr which was comparable to the value of normal fibroblasts. However, the papilla cells cultured in normal medium (DMEM/10) showed poor growth activity and ceased proliferation after the 4th passage. Proliferation of papilla cells was also stimulated by supplementing the normal medium with FGF1 or FGF2, but not with TGFα, TGFβ or EGF. However, stimulatory effects of FGFs were reduced as the concentration of FBS was decreased (Fig. 1). Thus both FGFs and FBS were essential for maximal proliferation.

We asked if long-term cultured papilla cells retained the ability to induce hair follicle in the afollicular sole skin. The papilla cells cultured with CM5 (named PCM5) were assayed at 33, 36 and 70 passages and the cells cultured with CM8 (PCM8) at 37 and 56 passages. Those cells were inserted in the space between the epidermis and dermis of the skin pieces, which were then implanted under the kidney capsule. Hair formation was examined immunohistochemically by identifying bulb structure, i.e. dermal papilla, hair matrix, inner and outer root

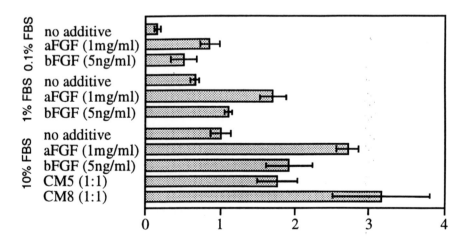

Figure 1. BrdU incorporation in papilla cells. FGF1 and FGF2 stimulated the growth of papilla cells with increasing the amount of FBS in the medium

sheath, and hair shaft. Hair follicles were observed in the almost all implants which had been inserted with PCM5 or PCM8 (Fig. 2), 6 out of 7, 8 out of 9 implants, respectively, as well as the implants with intact papillae. While hair formation was rare in the Swiss 3T3-stuffed or no cell-stuffed implants: 1 out of 6 and 2 out of 5, which might be induced spontaneously.

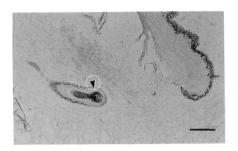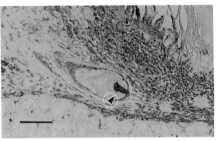

Figure 2. Hair induction in sole skin by PCM8 cells. Hair matrix (left) and a papilla (right) were visualized with mABs K1310 and K1311, repectively. Bar = 100 μm

Discussion

Culture of dermal papilla cells is useful to understand the nature of induction and differentiation of hair follicle and hair cycle. Although several authors reported the culture method, there have been two major problems. First, the cells show low proliferative activity and the second is a reduction of the hair-inducing ability with progress of the passage number of the culture. We solved these problems by culturing papilla cells with conditioned medium of keratinocytes.

Population doubling time was greatly shortened in the papilla cells cultured with the conditioned medium as compared to the cells without it, suggesting that the factor(s) secreted from the keratinocytes can improve proliferative activity of the papilla cells. Growth stimulatory effects were also found in the medium supplemented with FGF1 or FGF2 which had been known to be secreted from keratinocytes. Although FGFs are likely to be most probable candidates as the growth stimulator in the conditioned medium, their effects depend on the amount of FBS. Therefore, some factors in FBS must be required for the growth of the papilla cells in addition to FGFs.

The papilla cells could be maintained over 90 passages when they were cultured with the conditioned medium of keratinocytes. They retained hair-inducing ability for more than 70 generations. Jahoda *et al.* [6] demonstrated that the papilla cells cultured in normal medium lose their inductive ability before 10 generations. The factor(s) in the conditioned medium appeared to allow the papilla cells sustain their original properties including the inductive ability. FGFs and FBS might replace the growth stimulatory effects of the conditioned medium. However, it is not known whether they are also effective in retaining the inductive ability of the papilla cells during long-term cultivation.

In conclusion

1) Growth of rat vibrissae papilla cells was remarkably promoted by culturing them with keratinocytes from sole skin or with conditioned medium of keratinocytes.

2) The papilla cells continuously proliferated over 90 passages with rapid growth by culturing them with the conditioned medium.

3) FGF1 or FGF2 could stimulate the proliferation of the papilla cells to an extent comparable to the conditioned medium of keratinocytes.

4) The papilla cells cultured with the conditioned medium for more than 70 passages of subculture retained their ability to induce hair follicle.

References

1   Oliver RF. J Embryol Exp Morph. 1966; 15: 331-347
2   Oliver RF. J Embryol Exp Morph. 1967; 18: 43-51
3   Oliver RF. J Embryol Exp Morph. 1970; 23: 219-236
4   Jahoda CAB, Oliver RF. Br J Dermatol. 1981; 105: 623-627
5   Messenger AG. Br J Dermatol. 1984; 110: 685-689
6   Jahoda CAB, Horne KA, Oliver RF. Nature. 1984; 311: 560-562
7   Kobayashi K, Nishimura E. J Invest Dermatol. 1989; 92: 278-282

©1996 Elsevier Science B.V. All rights reserved.
Hair research for the next millenium
D.J.J. Van Neste and V.A. Randall (Eds)

Inflammatory cytokines cascade in the pilosebaceous unit: interleukin-1 as a putative co-actor of androgenetic alopecia ?

Y.F. Mahé, B. Buan, N. Billoni, J.-F. Michelet and B.A. Bernard

L'Oréal, Hair Biology Research Group, 92583 Clichy cedex, France

Introduction

Interleukin (IL)-1α and IL-1β are non-specific mediators of inflammation, active at low concentrations (10^{-15} M), similar to those of endogenous hormones [reviewed in 1]. While both 31kD pro-IL-1α and 17kD IL-1α bind and transduce a signal through the 80kD IL-1R1, the 31kD pro-IL-1β has to be cleaved by an IL-1β converting enzyme (ICE) to generate an active 17kD IL-β. Since keratinocyte lack this activity, in skin, the conversion might occur through the action of extracellular proteases. Several IL-1 responsive genes among which those of chemokines and adhesion molecules have been identified. Thus, the induction of adhesion molecules in the endothelium of the nearest irrigating vessels, combined with a gradient of chemokines might guide the localized extravasation and activation of leukocytes toward the original site of IL-1 production in the skin [reviewed in 2]. Since IL-1 has been reported as an inhibitor of hair follicle growth *in vitro* [3] and *in vivo* in IL-1α trangenic mice [4], we investigated IL-1 transduction potential and designed a rapid routine assay to evaluate IL-1 inflammatory status in human hair follicle.

Materials and methods

mRNA expression
mRNA from 5 plucked hairs was prepared using the QuickPrep® mRNA preparation kit (Pharmacia Biotech S.A.; Brussels, Belgium). Poly-A+ mRNA(s) were then reverse transcribed using the first strand cDNA synthesis kit from Pharmacia and PCR was performed using the Taq polymerase and the 10x buffer commercialized by Amersham (UK). hIL-1α, hIL-1β, hIL-6, hIL-8, hMCAF and hTNFα primers have been previously described in [5]. hIL-1R2 primers (FP:5'-TTCGTGGGAGGCATTACAAGCGGG-3'), (RP:5'-AGGAGGCTT CCTTGACTGTGGTGCG-3') were designed using the PC gene data base program; hIL-1R1 and hGAPDH primers were purchased from Clontech (Palo Alto, CA). 1/15 of the cDNA was used for PCR (1 cycle at 95°C, 4 min followed by 30 cycles (95°C, 25 sec; 57°C, 1 min; 72°C, 1 min) as previously described [5].

Human hair follicle isolation and culture *in vitro*

Individual human hair follicles from facelift surgery were dissected according to [3]. Briefly, 5×10 mm strips of scalp were cut at the dermo-epithelial junction. Anagen follicles with their perifollicular external connective tissue layer were then isolated using fine forceps. They were maintained at 37°C in William's E culture medium supplemented with 2 mM L-glutamine, 10 μg/ml transferrin, 10 ng/ml hydrocortisone and antibiotics.

IL-1α production

Five plucked anagen hairs with an intact outer root sheath were incubated in 1 ml of Williams-E medium supplemented with antibiotics at 37°C during 18 hours. IL-1α in supernatant was evaluated by ELISA using the kit RPN2140 from Amersham.

Results and discussion

Inflammatory cytokines status in normal anagen outer root sheath (ORS)

As shown in Table 1, freshly plucked hair expresses IL-1α and both the transducing (IL1R1) and non-transducing (decoy IL-1R2) IL-1 receptors mRNAs. However, most of the well known IL-1 responsive genes are not expressed in outer root sheath keratinocytes at the time of plucking suggesting that inflammatory signalling is blocked in normal anagen plucked hairs. It is only after triggering by exogenous IL-1 *in vitro* that one could observe the induction of mRNAs coding for the inflammatory cytokines (IL-1β and TNFα and IL-6) and chemokines (IL-8 and MCAF) genes. These results indicate that the IL-1 transduction machinery is functional in normal anagen ORS keratinocytes.

Table 1.
IL-1 signalling in freshly plucked anagen hair follicle (RT/PCR analysis)

	IL-1α	IL-1β	IL-1 R1	IL-1R2	TNFα	IL-6	IL-8	MCAF
T0	+ +	-	+ +	+ +	-	-	-	-
Medium 6 hrs	+ +	-	+ +	+ +	±	-	±	±
IL-1α 6 hrs	+ + +	+ +	+ +	+ + +	+	+	+	+

Inhibitory effect of IL-1 on growth and survival of human hair follicle *in vitro*

As shown in Fig. 1, IL-1β (20 ng/ml) slightly inhibits (20% inhibition) the growth rate of human hair follicles *in vitro*. The most dramatical effect of IL-1 was in fact to rapidly decrease the number of growing follicles since from day 8 of culture, none of the 12 follicles were growing anylonger in the IL-1-treated sample (half life = 5.4 days) while in the control experiment (half life = 7.6 days), 5 out of 12 follicles (40%) continued their growth at a normal rate. This inhibitory effect was not restricted to IL-1β since in a separate experiment, IL-1α (25 ng/ml) was also found to inhibit the growth of human hair follicles *in vitro* (data not shown). These results are comparable to those reported in [3] and confirm that IL-1 is a negative signal for human hair follicle growth *in vitro*. In addition, Kupper and Groves have recently shown that trangenic mice which overexpress IL-1α in basal keratinocytes develop baldness [4]. These observations indicate that IL-1 might be an aggravating factor of androgenetic alopecia *in vivo*.

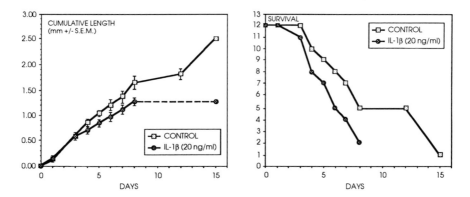

Figure 1. Inhibitory effect of IL-1α on human hair follicle growth and survival in vitro

IL-1α production in supernatants of freshly plucked anagen hair follicles

In order to correlate human hair follicle IL-1 production *in vitro* and a precise clinical stage of alopecia, we evaluated the potential of freshly plucked hairs to produce IL-1α in the supernatant of an overnight *in vitro* culture. As shown in Table 2, we surprisingly found that among a population of 85 volunteers, while 21.2% were found non-producers (< 0.3 pg/ml), 43.5% showed low levels of production (< 5.0 pg/ml), 21.2% were high producers (5-10 pg/ml) and 14% could be considered as heavy producers (> 10 pg/ml).

Table 2.
Classification of volunteers according to their rate of IL-1α production

	non-producers <0.3 pg/ml	low < 5.0 pg/ml	high 5-10 pg/ml	heavy >10 pg/ml
General population (n = 85)	18	37	18	12
Alopecic population (n = 65)	16	28	12	9
Non-alopecic population (n = 20)	2	9	6	3

Conclusions and perspectives

Altogether, our data suggest that monitoring of hair follicle inflammatory cytokine status combined with adapted anti-IL-1 strategies might be of therapeutical relevance for alopecic patients with high IL-1 production rates. In addition, an induction of DHT synthesis by IL-1 has been reported in fibroblasts [6] suggesting that a cross-talk might exist between IL-1 and androgen metabolism. Thus IL-1 status can no longer be ignored when considering therapeutical strategies against androgenetic alopecia. Whether this cross-talk occurs in the hair follicle as well as whether hair follicle inflammatory status monitored *in vitro* correlates or not with a precise stage of alopecia remains to be established.

References

1 Mahé YF, Oppenheim JJ. In Roit IM, Delves PJ, eds. Encyclopedia of Immunology. London. Academic Press. 1992; 2: 897-901
2 Kupper TS, Groves RW. J Invest Dermatol. 1995; 105: 62S-66S
3 Harmon CS, Nevins TD. Lymphokine and Cytokine Res. 1993; 12: 197-202
4 Kupper TS, Groves RW. J Invest Dermatol. 1994; 103: 422
5 Mahé YF, Hirose K, Clausse B, Chouaib S, *et al*. Biochem Biophys Res Comm. 1992; 1: 121-126
6 Kasasa SC, Soory M. Inflammation Res. 1995; 44: S291

IL-1 and IL-1-RA expression in cultured dermal papilla cells is regulated by cytokines

R. Hoffmann, A. König, E. Wenzel and R. Happle

Department of Dermatology, Philipp University, Deutschhausstraße 9, 35033 Marburg, Germany

Introduction

In alopecia areata (AA), the cascade of immunological events is not lethal for crucial elements of the hair follicle, which is why AA is usually reversible [1]. Cytokines may be responsible for the cessation of the hair cycle, and recently we detected an aberrant lesional expression of IFN-γ, IL-2 and IL-1β in scalp biopsies from patients with active AA [2]. Interestingly, IL-1β appeared to be the most potent inhibitor of hair growth *in vitro* [3]. Following this line of thought, we have hypothesized that IL-1β might be a crucial mediator of hair loss [4].

The induction and periodic elicitation of an allergic contact dermatitis is at present the most effective approach to treat AA [5]. If it is true that the hair loss in AA results from lesional IL-1β overexpression, the immunologic mechanisms induced by the contact dermatitis should interfere with the IL-1 bioactivity *in vivo*. Indeed we were able to show that, despite an augmented inflammation after DCP-treatment, the IL-1β mRNA levels were significantly reduced, whereas cytokines such as IL-10, IL-8, TNFα and TGFβ1 were markedly overexpressed within treated scalp [2]. The cytokines of the contact dermatitis may have a variety of effects on the AA specific infiltrate. They may induce proteins that neutralize IL-1 bioactivity. In this regard IL-10 has been shown to be a potent inducer of the IL-1-RA (receptor antagonist) gene [6].

Because dermal papilla cells (DPC) are likely target cells in AA and only little is known about their likely immune functions, we decided to investigate expression levels and search for inducers for IL-1β and IL-1-RA in DPC and to elucidate whether typical cytokines of an allergic contact dermatitis are able to modulate the IL-1 expression, possibly by inducing the IL-1-RA. In this way we wanted to clarify crucial pathways involved in the induction of hair regrowth in AA after treatment with contact allergens.

Materials and methods

Chemicals

The chemicals were purchased from Sigma (Deisenhofen, Germany), whereas the cytokines were bought from Laboserv (Gießen, Germany). A human anti IL-1β antibody was bought from genzyme (USA). ELISA-assays came from RD-Biosystems (USA).

Isolation of human hair follicles and cultivation of dermal papilla cells

Intact, viable anagen hair follicles and DPC were dissected as described [7]. DPC were only used in their third passage and incubated for 16 hours with various mediators [IL-1β (100 ng/ml), IL-2 (500 U/ml), IL-4 (100 ng/ml), IL-6 (250 ng/ml), IL-8 (200 ng/ml), IL-10 (100 ng/ml), IL-13 (250 ng/ml), TNFα (100 ng/ml), IFNγ (50 ng/ml), TGFβ1 (20 ng/ml), PGE_2 (1 μM), diclofenac (10 mg/ml) and PMA (1 μM)]. For PMA-incubation a time-kinetic of IL-1β and IL-1-RA expression was established. In some experiments (PMA, IL-1β and TNFα treatment) a neutralizing human anti IL-1β-antibody (10 μg/ml) was added.

ELISA analysis

After stimulation, supernatants and cell lysates were harvested. ELISA-analysis for IL-1β and IL-1-RA (RD-Biosystems) were performed as described by the supplier. Supernatants and lysate volumes were equal. ELISA results were expressed per mg protein.

Results

Time-dependent induction of IL-1β and IL-1RA proteins by phorbolester

Our approach allowed the detection of IL-1β and IL-1-RA proteins only in cell lysates of DPC. Incubation with phorbolester (PMA, 1 μM) led to a time-dependent increase of both proteins. IL-1β expression reached its peak expression level after 8 hours, whereas IL-1-RA expression was maximal after 12 hours PMA treatment (data not shown).

Effect of various mediators on the accumulation of IL-1β and IL-1RA protein

PMA, IL-1β and TNFα appeared to be inducers for IL-1β and IL-1-RA. Treatment with IL-4, IL-8, IL-10, IL-13, IFNγ and TGFβ1 had no effect with regard to constitutive or TNFα or IL-1β-elicited IL-1β or IL-1-RA expression. Induction of IL-1RA by PMA was completely abrogated by co-incubation with actinomycin D or cycloheximide, whereas IL-1β induction was abrogated by actinomycin D treatment only. The induction of IL-1β and IL-1RA by IL-1β was completely, and for TNFα incompletely, abrogated by addition of neutralizing human anti IL-1β-antibodies.

pg Cytokine in Cytosol per mg Total Cellular Protein

	Interleukin-1β	Interleukin-1 Receptor Antagonist
None	31 ± 9	389 ± 37
PMA	788 ± 81	6700 ± 620
PMA+ Aktinomycin	28 ± 8	320 ± 32
PMA+ Cyclohex.	771 ± 75	331 ± 35
TNFα	3726 ± 430	1200 ± 154
TNFα+ Anti-IL-1	1005 ± 320	340 ± 28
TNFα+ IFNγ	5050 ± 632	650 ± 53
TNFα+ IL-10	4950 ± 420	2400 ± 210
TNFα+ TGFβ1	3600 ± 320	1050 ± 110
IL-1β	4200 ± 395	1300 ± 125
IL-1β+ Anti-IL-1	200 ± 20	370 ± 42
IL-1β+ IFNγ	5550 ± 532	985 ± 101
IL-4	40 ± 7	420 ± 43
IL-8	42 ± 6	280 ± 35
IL-10	35 ± 11	295 ± 34
IL-13	38 ± 12	429 ± 5
TGFβ1	32 ± 9	276 ± 26
IFNγ	35 ± 8	299 ± 32

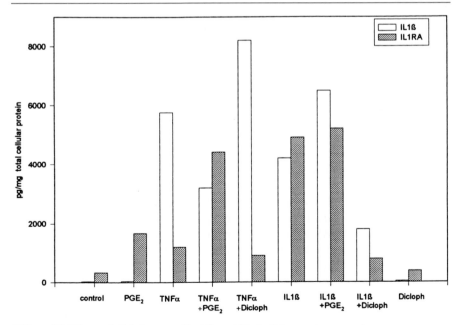

Effect of PGE$_2$ and diclofenac on IL-1β and IL-1-RA protein expression

Effect of PGE$_2$ and diclofenac on IL-1β and IL-1-RA protein expression

PGE$_2$ appeared to be a strong inducer of IL-1-RA, whereas IL-1β expression was not affected. TNFα–elicited IL-1β expression was inhibited, whereas IL-1β-elicited IL-1β expression was augmented by PGE$_2$. PGE$_2$ augmented the TNFα and IL-1β-elicited IL-1-RA expression. The cyclooxygenase inhibitor diclofenac in combination with TNFα or IL-1β had an adverse effect. Diclofenac was ineffective on basal IL-1β or IL-1-RA expression (Fig. 1).

Discussion

Several observations favor the hypothesis that IL-1 is a potent inhibitor of hair growth and constitutes an effector cytokine in AA leading to hair growth arrest and subsequent hair loss. If this hypothesis holds true, any treatment for AA should neutralize harmful lesional IL-1 levels. A possible pathway is the induction of proteins that modulate the IL-1 response. Those endogenous inhibitors should be able to down-regulate the IL-1 bioactivity thus promoting hair regrowth. In this regard the IL-1RA appears to be a likely candidate, because IL-1RA has been found in several cell types of the skin and is very effective in modulating an IL-1 response [8].

We have evidence that human DPC express IL-1β and IL-1-RA constitutively and after stimulation with several mediators *in vitro*. DPC are able to induce IL-1β *via* an autocrine pathway and neutralizing anti IL-1β-antibodies antagonize the effect of IL-1β or TNFα. In acute AA we have found aberrant mRNA levels for IFNγ, IL-1β and IL-2 in scalp biopsies. The cells which synthesize these cytokines are unknown. *in vitro*, DPC fail to secrete IL-1β after stimulation with IFNγ as it has been shown for keratinocytes [9] and we can therefore conclude that DPC are unlikely the source of IL-1β during the immune response present in early AA. Hair matrix keratinocytes or outer root sheath keratinocytes may be more important in this regard.

The elicitation of a contact dermatitis involves a cascade of events leading to a highly coordinated up- and down-regulation of several mediators. IL-1β, TNFα and prostanoids have been found during the inflammatory response. With regard to the IL-1-RA the role of prostanoids has been so far underestimated and to our knowledge we report herein for the first time that PGE$_2$ is a strong inducer of IL-1-RA, at least in DPC. Remarkably, TNFα and PGE$_2$ co-stimulation led to an inhibition of IL-1β induction but augmented the IL-1-RA induction in DPC. In successfully treated AA we found in scalp biopsies decreased mRNA levels for IL-1β as compared to untreated AA, but increased levels for TNFα [2].

In summary, within the rather sheltered microenvironment of the dermal papilla, DPC can now be regarded to be immunologically active cells. The cytokines IL-4, IL-8, IL-10, IL-13, IFNγ and TGFβ1 had no effect with regard to constitutive or TNFα or IL-1β-elicited IL-1β or IL-1-RA expression. PGE$_2$ is a strong inducer of IL-1-RA in DPC and the presence of IL-1-RA may be important to maintain a physiologic homeostasis during IL-1 induction and release. In the late phase of the therapeutic allergic contact dermatitis the combination of PGE_2 and TNFα may be responsible for the therapeutic effect in AA.

Acknowledgements

This work was supported by a grant from the Deutsche Forschungsgemeinschaft (Ho 1598/1- 2), Bonn, Germany.

References

1 Perret CM, Happle R. Treatment of alopecia areata. In: Orfanos CE, Happle R. (eds.) Hair and hair diseases. Springer-Verlag, Berlin, Germany. 1990; 571-587
2 Hoffmann R, Wenzel E, Huth A, Steen P, Schäufele M, Henninger HP, Happle R. Cytokine mRNA-levels in alopecia areata before and after treatment with the contact allergen diphenylcyclopropenone. J Invest Dermatol. 1994; 103: 530-533
3 Harmon CS, Nevis TD. IL-1α inhibits human hair follicle growth and hair fiber production in whole-organ cultures. Lymphokine Cytokine Res. 1993; 12: 197-203
4 Steen PHM van der, Boezeman JBM, Happle R. Topical immunotherapy for alopecia areata: Re-evaluation of 139 cases after an additional follow-up period of 19 months. Dermatology. 1992; 184: 198-201
5 Hoffmann R, Happle R. Does interleukin-1 induce hair loss? Dermatology. 1995; 191: 273-275
6 Cassatella MA, Meda L, Gasperini S, Calzetti, Bonora S. Interleukin-10 upregulates IL-1 receptor antagonist production from lipopolysaccharide-stimulated human polymor-phonuclear leucocytes by delaying mRNA degradation. J Exp Med. 1994; 179: 1695-1699
7 Messenger AG. The culture of dermal papilla cells from human hair follicles. Br J Dermatol. 1984; 110: 685-689
8 Chan LS, Hammerberg C, Kang K, Sabb P, Tavakkol A, Cooper KD. Human dermal fibroblast interleukin-1 receptor antagonist and interleukin-1β mRNA and protein are co-stimulated by phorbol ester: Implication for a homeostatic mechanism. J Invest Dermatol. 1992; 99: 315-322
9 Gueniche A, Schmitt D. Effect of γ-interferon on IL-α, β and receptor antagonist production by normal human keratinocytes. Exp Dermatol. 1994; 3: 113-118

K$^+_{ATP}$ channel openers inhibit the bradykinin-induced increase of intracellular calcium in hair follicle outer root sheath keratinocytes

F. Pruche, N. Boyera and B.A. Bernard

L'OREAL, Hair Biology Research Group, C. Zviak Research Center
92583 Clichy cedex, France

Introduction

The increase in cytosolic concentration of free calcium $[Ca^{++}]_i$ is a crucial mechanism of signal transduction in keratinocytes [1]. The increase could be due either to calcium release from internal stores or Ca^{++} influx from extracellular space or both [2, 3]. In this study we have compared bradykinin (BK) induced $[Ca^{++}]_i$ increase in outer root sheath (ORS) keratinocyte primary culture and epidermal growth factor (EGF) induced $[Ca^{++}]_i$ increase in A 431 cells, an epidermoid cell line with a greatly increased number of EGF receptors [4]. In addition, the effects of K$^+_{ATP}$ channels openers (minoxidil and minoxidil sulfate) pre-treatment were evaluated in this assay.

Materials and methods

Hair follicle ORS keratinocytes were grown from scalp skin removed during plastic surgery procedure. The scalp biopsy was incubated for 20 h at 4°C in phosphate buffered saline containing 2.4 U/ml dispase. The ORS keratinocytes were removed and incubated with trypsin 0.125% 30 mn at 37°C. Cells were cultured during 6 days in G. Rheinwald and H. Green medium [5] and then passed in KGM medium before seeding onto cover-slips. A 431 cells were grown in DMEM medium with 10% calf serum. For intracellular calcium studies, cells were washed with Hepes buffer (10 mM Na-Hepes pH 7.4, 5 mM KCl, 140 mM NaCl, 10 mM Glucose, 1 mM $MgCl_2$, 2 mM $CaCl_2$) and loaded with the calcium sensitive dye FURA-2 acetoxymethyl ester (Molecular Probes, Oregon USA) at a concentration of 5 µM for 60 min at 37°C. They were rinsed with Hepes buffer. Measurement of emitted fluorescence was made using a dual excitation system. The excitation wavelengths were 340 nm (bound) and 380 nm (free) and the emission wavelength 510 nm. $[Ca^{++}]_i$ is expressed as ratio units calculated from measured fluorescence at the two excitation wavelengths.

464

Results

BK provokes a transient rise of $[Ca^{++}]_i$ in ORS keratinocytes and this effect is inhibited by minoxidil sulfate and to a lesser extent by minoxidil (Fig. 1).

The $[Ca^{++}]_i$ peak duration after EGF addition is longer than after BK treatment and could be attributed to a calcium influx from extracellular space. This effect was confirmed by inhibition of this influx by calcium chelation with EGTA (data not shown) (Fig. 2).

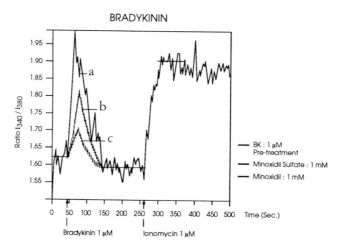

Figure 1. {Ca^{++}}, response of ORS keratinocytes after (a) addition of 1 μM BK, followed by the addition of 1 μM Ionomycin; (b) 1 mM minoxidil pre-treatment and (c) 1 mM minoxidil sulfate pre-treatment.

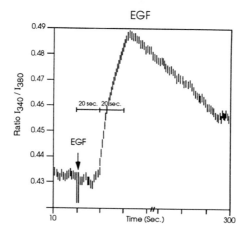

Figure 2. {Ca^{++}}, response of A 431 keratinocytes after addition of 100 ng/ml EGF.

Minoxidil sulfate is more efficient than Minoxidil and shows a dose dependent response curve from 50 μM to 1 mM, with an IC50 = 100 μM and > 1 mM, respectively (Fig. 3).

The results obtained with the reference compounds P1075, diazoxide, pinacidil and minoxidil underline the relationship between inhibition of inward calcium flux and stimulation of hair growth (Fig. 4).

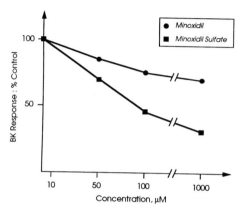

Figure 3. Inhibitory effect of minoxidil and minoxidil sulfate on BK-response. The cells (ORS keratinocytes primary culture) were treated with the compound for 120s just before BK treatment (1 μM). The results represent the mean of two independent experiments.

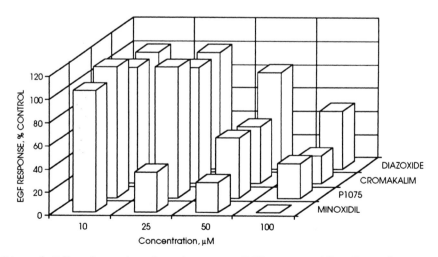

Figure 4. Effect of potassium channel openers on EGF- response. The cells (A 431) were treated with the compound for 120s and EGF (100 ng/ml) was injected. Values represent the mean of two independent experiments.

Discussion

In normal human keratinocytes or A 431 epidermoid cells, BK and EGF trigger $[Ca^{++}]_i$ increase by internal stores mobilization and Ca^{++} influx stimulation, respectively. Minoxidil inhibits both of these effects. By contrast minoxidil sulfate was found to only inhibit BK-induced calcium release from internal stores (ORS keratinocytes) and to have no effect on EGF-induced influx (A 431). Hair follicle keratinocyte proliferation and differentiation could be regulated by modulation of various signal transduction pathways including activation of a G-protein-coupled receptor and by stimulation of phosphatidylinositol hydrolysis. Thus sulfatation might be crucial not only for minoxidil biodisponibility but also for the targets of its action (i.e. calcium intracellular stores mobilization versus calcium influx).

References

1 Sharpe GR, Fisher C, Gillespie JI, Greenwell JR. Arch Dermatol Res. 1993; 284: 445-450
2 Rosenbach T, Liesegang C, Binting S, Czarnettzki BM. Arch Dermatol Res. 1993; 285: 393-396
3 Aoyama Y, Seishima M, Mori S, Kitajima Y, Okano Y, Nozawa Y. J Dermatol Science. 1995; 9: 111-116
4 Peppelenbosch MP, Tertoolen LGJ, de Laat SW. J Biol Chem. 1991; 266: 19938-19944
5 Rheinwald G, Green H. Cell. 1975; 6: 317-330, 331-344

Minoxidil potentiates the mitogenic properties of growth factors *in vitro* in the absence of streptomycin

D.A. Sanders[1], I. Fiddes[2], D.M. Thompson[1], M.P. Philpott[1], G.E. Westgate[3] and T. Kealey[1]

[1]Department of Clinical Biochemistry, Cambridge University, Addenbrooke's Hospital, Hills Road, Cambridge CB2 2QR, UK
[2]Department of Biological Sciences, Anglia Polytechnic University, East Road, Cambridge CB1 1PT, UK
[3]Unilever Research, Colworth House, Sharnbrook, Bedford, MK44 1LQ, UK

Introduction

It has long been recognized that minoxidil and other K$^+$ channel agonists will stimulate hair growth *in vivo* [1, 2]. Their mode of action has, however, remained obscure, but there is strong circumstantial evidence in the cell biology literature to indicate that K$^+$ channel agonists should be mitogens.

First, the *in vitro* addition of a range of K$^+$ channel blockers will block mitogen-induced cell proliferation in a range of cell types including T lymphocytes, melanoma cells and Schwann cells [3, 4]. Second, a range of mitogens will increase the K$^+$ conductance *in vitro* of a range of cell types including T lymphocytes, melanoma cells and neuroblastoma cells [3, 4]. Third, Ca^{2+}-activated K$^+$ channel activity is induced in 3T3 fibroblasts by the Ras/Raf signal transduction pathway and this channel activity can also be induced by the addition of EGF and PDGF [5].

Paradoxically, however, the addition of K$^+$ channel openers to a range of cell types *in vitro* has not unequivocally stimulated mitogenesis; *in vitro* studies looking at the effect of minoxidil on cell proliferation have shown either no effect or an inhibition of growth of fibroblasts [6-8], keratinocytes [9, 10] and endothelial cells [11]. Some reports have indicated that minoxidil will stimulate cell proliferation of keratinocytes *in vitro* [12, 13], but only in the presence of very high concentrations of minoxidil (three orders of magnitude higher than those seen in the blood *in vivo*). Other reports [14, 15] also suggest that minoxidil stimulates keratinocytes and hair follicles *in vitro*, but these results are based only on ^{3}H-thymidine uptake studies and may be an artefact of thymidine metabolism as no actual stimulation of keratinocyte or hair follicle growth was shown.

However, these *in vitro* studies appear to have been carried out in the presence of streptomycin. The aminoglycoside antibiotics, which include streptomycin, have been reported to inhibit K$^+$ channel activity [16-18] which might account for the *in vitro* paradoxes. To investigate this, we have employed

NIH 3T3 fibroblasts as a model for mitogenesis.

Materials and methods

Cell culture

NIH 3T3 fibroblasts were plated out at 10^4 cells per well in 24 well multi-well plates in Dulbecco's modified Eagle's medium (MEM) at 37°C in 5% CO_2/95% air, supplemented with 2 mM L-glutamine. For specific experiments, this was further supplemented with 5% or 10% fetal calf serum (FCS) or on occasion with 0.05 mM minoxidil, 1 mM or 5 mM Tolbutamide, 2 mM Tetramethylammonium (TEA), 1 mM Glibenclamide, 10 nM Apamin, 100 units ml^{-1} penicillin, 100 mg ml^{-1} streptomycin, 5% Controlled Process Serum Replacement-2 (CPSR-2) or growth factors as described below. Some pharmacological agents were dissolved in DMSO or ethanol, but those experiments were controlled with equal volumes of vehicle. Cells were counted in a haemocytometer, in triplicate.

Results

When NIH 3T3 fibroblasts were grown in medium supplemented with 5% FCS, 100 units ml^{-1} penicillin and 100 mg ml^{-1} streptomycin, cell numbers increased over five fold to $57,077 \pm 4232$ cells per well; n = 5 (mean ± SEM). The addition of 10 mg/ml minoxidil led to a marked, statistically significant stimulation of growth ($84,938 \pm 4,596$ cells per well; n = 5; p<0.001). But in the presence of streptomycin (100 mg/ml) minoxidil had no effect on cell numbers.

When cells were grown with 10% FCS ($119,401 \pm 7,959$ cells per well; n = 5), addition of 10 mg/ml minoxidil also led to a slight, but statistically significant stimulation of growth ($134,564 \pm 5,254$ cells per well; n = 5; p<0.05).

The K$^+$ channel blocker tolbutamide (5 mM), or combinations of the blockers tolbutamide (1 mM)/tetraethylammonium (2 mM) or glibenclamide (1 mM)/apamin (10 nM) completely blocked the minoxidil induced stimulation of growth, whilst having no effect on growth in the absence of minoxidil.

Fibroblasts maintained in 5% CPSR-2 also increased their cell numbers ($41,533 \pm 3,556$ cells per well; n = 5; p<0.001) over 7 days, although this was less than with 5% FCS. Minoxidil (10 μg/ml), which potentiated the growth of fibroblasts in 5% FCS, had no effect on fibroblasts maintained with 5% CPSR-2, which confirms that minoxidil is not a mitogen per se, but potentiates the effects of mitogens (CPSR-2 is growth factor-depleted FCS).

Addition of 10 ng/ml IGF-1 to wells containing 5% CPSR-2 resulted in a significant stimulation of cell growth ($92,667 \pm 7,306$ cells per well; n = 5; p<0.001). This IGF-1 stimulated growth was further potentiated by 10 μg/ml minoxidil ($137,400 \pm 8,681$ cells per well; n = 5; p<0.001). PDGF (10ng/ml) also stimulated the growth of fibroblasts maintained in 5% CPSR-2 (74,833 ± 13,534; n = 4; p<0.001). Moreover, this stimulation of growth by PDGF was also potentiated by minoxidil (99,958 ± 14,503 cells per well; n = 4; p<0.001).

Discussion

These findings indicate that the earlier reports that minoxidil, *in vitro*, inhibited mitogenesis, or only stimulated it at very high concentrations, were artefactual and attributable to the presence of streptomycin. It now appears that minoxidil *in vitro* will potentiate the mitogenic effects of FCS, IGF-1 and PDGF, using NIH 3T3 fibroblasts as a model. It remains to be established which K^+ channels minoxidil is activating in the 3T3 fibroblast, and whether those are to be found in the hair follicle, but our earlier findings that IGF-1 is a major hair follicle mitogen [19] would indicate that the NIH 3T3 is a good model for IGF-1 mitogenesis in the hair follicles. It will now be of interest to use the NIH 3T3 model to test the effects of other agonists of K^+ channels, and to use it as a screen for developing new hair follicle stimulants.

The mechanism by which the opening of K^+ channels potentiates mitogenesis is obscure, but such an opening would render the intracellular potential more negative. Since the influx of extracellular Ca^{2+} is a major mitogenic signal, it might be expected that its electrochemical gradient would be augmented by minoxidil. However, its proportional augmentation would be small, and it is possible that minoxidil is triggering a voltage-mediated cascade.

References

1   Dargie HJ, Dollery CT, Daniel J. Lancet. 1977; ii 515-518
2   Headington JT, Novak E. Curr Ther Res Clin Exp. 1984; 36: 1098-1106
3   Dubois J-M, Rouzaire-Dubois B. Prog Biophys Mol Biol. 1993; 59: 1-21
4   Nilus B, Droogmans G. NIPS. 1994; 9: 105-110
5   Huang Y, Rane SG. J Biol Chem. 1994; 269: 31183-31189
6   Katsuoka K, Schell H, Wessel B, Horstein OP. Arch Dermatol Res. 1987; 279: 247-250
7   Murad S, Pinnell S R. J Biol Chem. 1987; 262: 11973-11978
8   Priestley GC, Lord R, Stavropoulos P. B. J Dermatol. 1991; 125: 217-221
9   Bernd A, Breuer M, Dold K, Holzmann H. Arnzneim-Forch Drug Res. 1990; 40: 413-416
10 O'Keefe E, Payne RE. J Invest Dermatol. 1991; 97: 534-536
11 Norris WD, Johnson G, Donald GS. Cell Biol Int Rep. 1989; 13: 555- 562
12 Baden HP, Kubilus J. J Invest Dermatol. 1983; 81: 558-560
13 Tanigaki-Obana N, Ito M. Arch Dermatol Res. 1992; 284: 290-296
14 Cohen R L, Alves M E, Weiss VC, West DP, Chambers DA. J Invest Dermatol. 1984; 82: 90-93
15 Harmon CS, Lutz D, Ducote J. Skin Pharmacol. 1993; 6: 170-178
16 Oosawa Y, Sokabe M. Am J Physiol. 1986; 250: C361-C364
17 Nomura K, Naruse K, Watanabe K, Sokabe M. J Membrane Biol. 1990; 115: 241-251
18 Takeuchi S, Wangemann P. Hearing Research. 1993; 67: 13-19
19 Philpott M P, Sanders D A, Kealey T. J Invest Dermatol. 1994; 102: 857-861

1996 Elsevier Science B.V.
Hair research for the next millenium
D.J.J. Van Neste and V.A. Randall (Eds)

Minoxidil sulfate effect on internal calcium of the cells in epidermis and epidermal appendages

M. Ohtsuyama and M. Morohashi

Department of Dermatology, Faculty of Medicine, Toyama Medical and Pharmaceutical Univ., Toyama, Japan

Introduction

Although minoxidil sulfate (MXDS) has been used as a therapeutic agent to stimulate hair growth, the mechanism of action of MXDS on hair growth has only been poorly understood. Recently we found that MXDS opened Cl channels and decreased cytosolic calcium in dissociated rhesus eccrine clear cells [1]. These data can however hardly be translated into hair growth function. Therefore, we investigated the effect of MXDS and testosterone, as an androgen, on cytosolic calcium in keratinocytes using a fluorescent spectrophotometer. The different effect of MXDS and androgen on cytosolic calcium may support the hypothesis that MXDS induces hair re-growth by triggering passage from telogen into anagen.

Materials and methods

Second-passage normal human epidermal keratinocytes (NHEK) were purchased from Kurabo Co. (Tokyo Japan). Keratinocytes were incubated in KGM which consisted of KBM (modified MCDB 153 media with 0.15 mM calcium) supplemented with 140µg/ml bovine pituitary extract (BPE), 0.1 ng/ml EGF, 0.5µg/ml hydrocortisone, 5µg/ml insulin and antibiotics (gentamycin and amphotericin B) for 24 hours under an atmosphere of 95% air and 5% CO_2 at 37°C. Then the cells were trypsinized and maintained in KGM. Finally, after the cells were supplemented with 10% DMSO and 10% FBS, they were frozen at-80°C for later use.

Keratinocytes were loaded with Fura 2-AM (5µM) for 1 hour at 37°C. After cells were washed by Krebs Ringer Bicarbonates (KRB), 2 ml of cell suspension in KRB were placed in a chamber kept at 37°C which was set in a fluorescent spectrophotometer (Shimazu RF-5000). The excitation wavelength was switched 340 nm to 380 nm alternatively. The emission wavelength was fixed at 500 nm. The ratio 340 nm/380 nm of the fluorescence was calculated and printed out. Drugs dissolved in KRB were added into the chamber for the stimulation.

472

Results

1) MXDS (0.5 mM, 1 mM) moderately, and with a time lag, decreased cytosolic calcium in a transient manner (Figs. 1a and 1b). MXDS (1 mM)-induced a more pronounced cytosolic calcium decrease as compared with MXDS (0.5 mM).

2) Minoxidil (MXD; 0.5 mM, 1 mM) also decreased cytosolic calcium although less than MXDS (Figs. 2a and 2b).

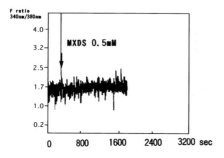

Figure 1a. MXDS (0.5mM) decreases {Ca}, transiently

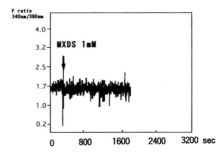

Figure 1b. MXDS (1mM) decreases {Ca}, transiently

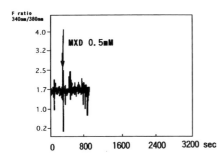

Figure 2a. MXD (0.5mM) decreases {Ca}, transiently

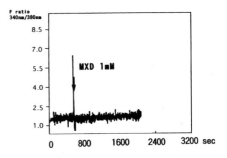

Figure 2b. MXD (1mM) decreases {Ca}, transiently

3) Testosterone (1 μM, 3 μM, 10 μM) increased cytosolic calcium dramatically in a dose dependent manner (Figs. 3a, 3b and 3c). There was about 1-min time lag after stimulation to increase cytosolic calcium, the level remaining constant during stimulation with testosterone.

4) Calcium ionophore, ionomycin (10 μM) as a control drug, increased cytosolic calcium immediately (Fig. 4).

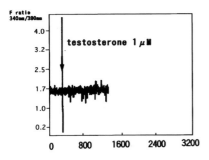

Figure 3a. Testosterone (1mM) does not increases {Ca}

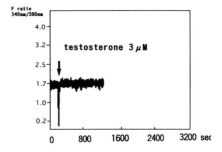

Figure 3b. Testosterone increases {Ca}

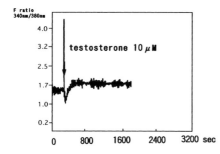

Figure 3c. Testosterone increases {Ca}

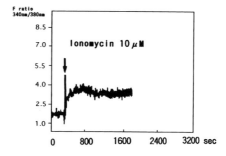

Figure 4. Ionomycin increases {Ca}, dramatically

Discussion

Although the mechanism of hair growth has been investigated in various ways, it is not clearly established yet on which region of hair follicle hair growth agents act on. MXDS, an antihypertensive agent, has been reported to stimulate

474

potassium channels in the smooth muscle cells and to increase DNA synthesis in outer root sheath cells (ORSC). Recently we have reported that MXDS decreased cytosolic calcium in dissociated eccrine clear cells [1]. As shown in the results section, MXDS also decreased cytosolic calcium in keratinocytes. On the other hand, testosterone elevated cytosolic calcium although the concentrations of testosterone used to achieve this effect were higher than physiologic levels.

In the light of calcium, EGF which inhibits hair growth increases calcium in the cells [2, 3], but some of potassium channel openers including minoxidil oppose the entry of calcium into the cells and induce hair growth [4]. Thus the MXDS-induced low concentration of cytosolic calcium might play an important role in the regulation of growing hair.

References

1   Ohtsuyama M, Sato F, Toyomoto T, Sato K. J Pharmacol Exp Ther. 1994; 269: 823-831
2   Philpott MP, Kealey T. J Invest Dermatol. 1994; 102: 186-191
3   Peppelenbosch MP, Tertoolen LGJ, De Laat W. S. J Biol Chem. 1991; 266: 19938-19944
4   Buhl AE, Waldon DJ, Conrad SJ, Mulholland MJ, et al. J Invest Dermatol. 1992; 98: 315-319

The motility of cultured dermal cells from human follicles-stimulation by rat papilla cell conditioned medium

A. Ishino[1,2], A.J. Reynolds[1] and C.A.B. Jahoda[1]

[1]Department of Biological Sciences, University of Durham, South Road, Durham, DH1 3LE, U.K.
[2]Shiseido, Pharmaco Science Research Laboratories, Shiseido, 1050 Nippa-cho, Kohokuku, Yokohama-shi, 223, Japan

Introduction

At the beginning of hair follicle development, embryonic dermal cells aggregate to create the cell condensations that are the precursors of the adult hair follicle dermal papilla (DP) [1]. Papilla cells from adult rat vibrissae also display aggregation behavior both *in vitro* and when re-implanted *in vivo* [2]. Little is known of the behavior of DP cells during the hair growth cycle when the DP moves higher in the dermis at catagen and descends again at the start of the next anagen phase, but it is possible that motility plays a role. We have investigated the relative motilities of human DP, dermal sheath (DS) and interfollicular skin fibroblast (SF) cells. In addition, having previously reported that rat DP conditioned medium stimulates rat DP cell motility [3], we have also investigated the effects of rat DP cell conditioned medium on human cell behavior.

Materials and methods

Human hair follicles were dissected from scalp skin biopsies. DP, DS and interfollicular connective tissue were dissected and initiated separately as explant culture to allow cell outgrowth [4, 5]. All cells were initially maintained in Dulbecco's modified Eagle medium (MEM) containing 20% FBS, at 37°C in an atmosphere of 5% CO_2 and 95% air. After 10-14 days, the serum concentration was reduced to 10%. Cell motilities and chemotactic effects of rat dermal papilla conditioned medium (RDPCD) were measured using 48 well modified Boyden chemotactic chamber (Nucleopore). For all experiments, cells were harvested, counted and seeded on polycarbonate (PC) membranes with 12 μm-diameter pores (Nucleopore). Six replicate wells were used for each test medium sample. After 16-h incubation the membranes were removed and the cells were fixed. The cells on the upper surface were removed by scraping with a rubber blade and the remaining migrated cells were stained with Giemsa (SIGMA). Random fields, representing nearly 30% of the total area, were counted and averaged to give the number of nuclei per well as a measure of the chemotactic response. All experiments were carried out using early passage cells (P2 to P4).

Results

Comparison of the motility of DP, DS and SF

To compare the intrinsic motility of the three cell types, DP and DS cells derived from female scalp follicles were plated at 30×10^4 cells per 25 cm^2 dish and SF derived from the same skin were plated at 20×10^4 cells. After 2-weeks incubation, all cells reached confluence, with the DP, DS and SF cells having proliferated to 81.4×10^4, 59.3×10^4 and 127.8×10^4 cells respectively. DP cells were compactly arranged, with groups of cells starting to aggregate. All cells were harvested and seeded on PC membranes at equal densities and their random migrations were assayed against MEM. DP cells showed very poor locomotory ability. SF cells displayed over ten times greater motility than DP cells. DS cell locomotion was intermediate between DP and SF cells (Fig. 1).

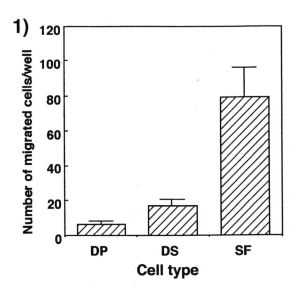

Figure 1. Comparison of intrinsic motility exhibited by DP, DS and SF cell types. Cells derived from female scalp follicles or surrounding connective tissue, were harvested when confluent and seeded at 15×10^3 cells per chamber. Migration assays were performed as described in the Materials and methods. Data are expressed as the mean ± standard error.

Effect of growth state on the motility of human DP.

We have previously reported that rat DP cells in the process of aggregating are many times more motile than aggregated DP cells. We therefore made a comparison between the motility of aggregating and aggregated (density packed) human DP cells. Aggregating phase DP cells and confluent culture of SF cells derived from male scalp were assayed at densities of 9.65×10^5 and 2.14×10^6 cells/25 cm^2 flask respectively. Aggregated or density packed cultures, were assayed when the DP cells had reached a density of 1.51×10^6 while SF cell numbers were at 2.00×10^6 cells/25 cm^2 flask. As SF cell density was relatively constant, the motility of aggregating and aggregated phase DP cells was calcultated as the ratio of DP migration against SF migration at the two phases. The motility of aggregating DP cells was found to be around 20% of SF cells, while the aggregated DP cells showed a depressed level of migration at only 3% of the motility of SF cells tested at this time (Fig. 2).

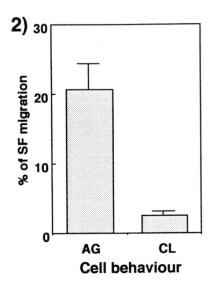

Figure 2. Effect of DP cells state of growth on their motility. Cells derived from male scalp follicles or surrounding connective tissue. The motilities of cells from two phases of DP aggregation were expressed as % of SF migration in corresponding experiments. AG: Aggregating DP and confluent SF cells were harvested and seeded at 13.8×10^3 cells per chamber. CL: Aggregated, or density packed DP cells and confluent SF cells were harvested and seeded at 21.5×10^3 cells par chamber. Data are expressed as the mean ± standard error.

478

Effect of RDPCD on the motility of DP, DS and SF

The effects of RDPCD on the motility of DP, DS and SF were investigated. To prepare conditioned medium, rat DP cells were cultured as previously described. When cells reached the aggregating phase, they were washed three times with MEM, and then incubated in MEM overnight. Conditioned medium was collected, spun at 13000 rpm and then used immediately in assays, or stored frozen. When the RDPCD conditioned medium was tested on human cells, it significantly stimulated the motility of human DP and DS cells, but showed no effect on confluent SF cells' motility (Fig. 3).

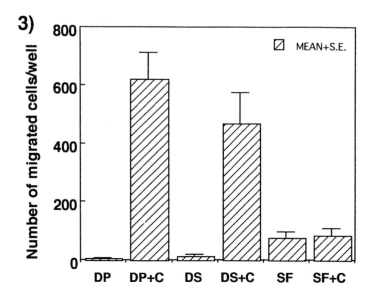

Figure 3. Effect of RDPCD on the motility of DP, DS and SF. This experiment was carried out using the same cells and conditions as in Fig. 1. RDPCD was collected from aggregating rat DP cells. Migration assay was carried out as described in the Materials and methods. Data are expressed as the mean ± standard error. +C: with RDPCD

Discussion

Locomotion, like proliferation, is an important cell behaviour, however up to now few studies have investigated motility in hair follicle cells [6]. We have previously reported that

1) rat DP cells in the process of aggregating are many times more motile than clumped DP cells and

2) conditioned medium collected from aggregating phase rat DP cells stimulates rat DP cell motility. The findings presented here suggest that the intrinsic motility of human DP cells is very low compared with SF cells, and that DS and DP cells are similar in locomotory behaviour. In addition, both human DP and DS cells demonstrated pronounced increases in motility in response to conditioned medium from aggregating rat DP cells.

In relation to the parallels between human DP and DS cells, Taylor *et al.* reported that their synthesis of glycosaminoglycans was similar [7]. Our group has also previously reported that smooth muscle α-actin is expressed at high levels by both DP and DS but not SF cells in culture [8]. It is well known that both extracellular matrix and cytoskeleton are involved in cell movements, so our findings provide a link between the common intrinsic levels of motility demonstrated by DP and DS cells, and their cytoskeletal and extracellular matrix profiles. Exactly how the regulation of DP and DS cell motility might be involved in hair growth is unclear, however cell movement, and the inhibition of cell migration are both important in the hair growth cycle.

Interestingly, human DP cells in our study demonstrated aggregation dependent motility behaviour similar to rat DP cells, with highly confluent cultures having very low motility. This is not unique, as Grotendorst [9] and Soma *et al.* [10] reported that the motility response to growth factors, of both NIH/3T3 and human SF cells, was affected by the density or growth state of the cultures. Confluent human SF cells decreased their migratory potential compared with growing or subconfluent cells [10].

In this preliminary report, RDPCD from aggregating cells was found to specifically stimulate the motility of human DP and DS cells. The mechanism by which RDPCD affects cell migration is currently under investigation, but a number of growth factors are known to affect the motility of cultured fibroblasts. For example PDGF, which is the best known fibroblast mitogen, also has a potent motogenic influence on fibroblast-like cells. PDGF is also produced by smooth muscle cells, with whom papilla cells have features in common [8]. Autocrine motility factors are also not uncommon. Autocrine motility factor (AMF) was purified from melanoma cell conditioned medium and found to stimulate the motility of fibroblast and melanoma cell [11]. Migration stimulating factor (MSF) which is produced by the fibroblasts from fetal skin or cancer patients also stimulates human fibroblast motility [12]. Therefore our working hypothesis is that the RDPCD contains factor(s) which affects DP and DS cell motility.

References

1 Kollar EJ. J Invest Dermatol. 1970; 55: 374-378
2 Jahoda CAB, Oliver RF. J Embryol Exp Morphol. 1984; 79: 211-224
3 Sleeman MA. Thesis, University of Durham. 1995
4 Jahoda CAB, Oliver RF. Br J Dermatol. 1981; 105: 623-627
5 Messenger AG. Br J Dermatol. 1984; 110: 685-689
6 Katsuoka K, Hein R, Schell H, Hornstein OP. Arch Dermatol Res. 1988; 280: 185-186
7 Taylor M, Ashcroft ATT, Westgate GE, Gibson WT, Messenger AG. Br J Dermatol. 1992; 126: 479-484
8 Jahoda CAB, Reynolds AJ, Chaponnier C, Forester JC, Gabbiani G. J Cell Sci. 1991; 99: 627-636
9 Grotendorst GR. Cell. 1984; 36: 279-285
10 Soma Y, Takehara K. Ishibashi Y. Exp Cell Res. 1994; 212: 274-277
11 Liotta LA, Mandler R, Murano G, Katz DA, Gordon KR, Chiang PK, Schiffmann E. Proc Nat Acad Sci, USA. 1986; 83: 3302-3306
12 Grey AM, Schor AM, Rushton G, Ellis I, Schor SL. Proc Natl Acad Sci, USA. 1989; 86: 2438-2442

Beard dermal papilla cells secrete more stem cell factor in culture than non-balding scalp cells or dermal fibroblasts

V.A. Randall[1], A.G. Messenger[2] and N.A. Hibberts[1]

[1]Department of Biomedical Sciences, University of Bradford, Bradford, West Yorkshire, BD7 1DP
[2]Department of Dermatology, Royal Hallamshire Hospital, Sheffield S10 2JF, United Kingdom

Introduction

The extent of the pigmentation of hair follicles is determined by the production of melanin by the hair follicular melanocytes and its subsequent transfer into the precortical hair matrix keratinocytes. Although the structural and morphological events involved in the various stages of follicular morphogenesis have been characterized in some detail, the biochemical regulation of hair pigmentation remains relatively obscure [1-3].

Stem cell factor, otherwise known as SCF, mast cell growth factor, c-kit ligand and Steel factor, and its receptor c-kit, have been shown to be implicated in skin and hair pigmentation [4, 5]. C-kit, a tyrosine kinase receptor, has been mapped to the dominant white spotting (W) locus in mice, whilst the cDNA for stem cell factor has been cloned and mapped to the SL locus. The importance of stem cell factor/c-kit is demonstrated in mice with pigmentary disorders who have defects in these genes [6], and similarly, people with piebaldism, have a mutation in the c-kit gene [7]. In mice, blocking c-kit with specific antibodies caused apoptosis in hair follicular melanocytes, both pre- and post-natally [8, 9]; these results suggest that there is a local source of stem cell factor in the hair follicle.

The hair follicle is a three dimensional tube of epithelial cells which protrudes through the epidermis and dermis containing in its bulb, the mesenchyme-derived dermal papilla. Hair growth is not continuous but cyclic, with a growing anagen phase, a resting telogen phase, and a short transitory catagen phase. The dermal papilla plays an important role in the regulation of the hair cycle and in control of human hair growth e.g. hair diameter [10]. Several reports have shown that the dermal papilla is capable of producing factors which influence the surrounding follicular cells [11,12]. It is, therefore, possible that the dermal papilla will produce factors responsible for controlling melanocyte behaviour and may well be a local source of stem cell factor in the hair follicle.

In humans, the hair follicle is influenced by a variety of hormones including those involved in pregnancy [13] and thyroid hormones [14]. However, androgens are the most important systemic regulators of human hair growth, often involving changes in hair color e.g. darkening of the male beard at puberty [10]. It is believed that androgens act on the hair follicle via the mesenchyme-derived dermal papilla, causing the production of factors which affect the surrounding cells. Itami *et al* [15] have shown that androgens can stimulate the secretion of insulin like growth factor-1 by cultured dermal papilla cells and therefore, it is possible that the production of stem cell factor by dermal papilla cells may also be controlled by androgens.

In order to test the hypothesis that the dermal papilla may be the local source of stem cell factor in the hair follicle, and that androgens may alter the levels produced, this study was designed to investigate the production of stem cell factor by dermal papilla cells. The levels of stem cell factor in conditioned medium produced by dermal papilla cells and dermal fibroblasts derived from androgen-dependent beard, and control, non-balding scalp skin, was measured using an ELISA system. The ability of testosterone to influence the production of stem cell factor by these cells in vitro was also investigated.

Materials and methods

Cell culture

The culture of dermal papilla cells was carried out as described in [16]. Briefly, full depth skin biopsies were obtained from beard skin and non-balding scalp. Using microdissection techniques, the dermal papilla was removed from each hair follicle and 3-5 such dermal papillas were placed in a sterile 35 mm tissue culture dish containing medium E199 + 20% fetal calf serum (FCS). The cultures were passaged into 25 cm² flasks when sufficient cells were present. Corresponding lines of dermal fibroblasts from beard and non-balding scalp skin were also established. Dermal papilla cells and dermal fibroblasts were routinely subcultured in medium E199 containing 10% FCS.

Collection of conditioned medium

Dermal papilla cells and dermal fibroblasts were cultured to confluency in normal growth medium before being washed in 5 ml PBS (x4). The cells were then incubated in serum free medium E199 containing 10 nM testosterone or the ethanol vehicle (0.001%) alone for 15 minutes. This medium was removed and designated «15 minute conditioned medium» . This conditioned medium was used to establish that stem cell factor was actually produced by the cells and not merely residual amounts of serum stem cell factor incompletely removed. The cells were then incubated for 24 hours in serum free medium E199 ± 10 nM testosterone. This medium was then centrifuged (1000 g) to remove cell debris, sterile filtered (0.2 μm) and stored at -20°C until required.

Measurement of stem cell factor

The levels of stem cell factor in conditioned medium and serum free medium were measured using a sandwich ELISA (enzyme linked immunosorbent assay) kit produced by R&D systems Europe, Abingon, U.K. The kit was capable of detecting both natural and recombinant stem cell factor. For each assay, a standard curve of stem cell factor ranging from 0-100 pg/ml was measured. All points were measured in duplicate according to the manufacturers instructions. The minimum detection level of the kit was 3 pg/ml with a sensitivity of 3 pg/ml.

The concentration of stem cell factor in the conditioned medium and serum free medium was calculated from the standard curve. The protein concentration of each medium sample was determined using the standard Bradford [17] protein assay and the stem cell factor content expressed as pg/ml/µg protein. Statistical analysis of the differences in the content of stem cell factor in the various medium was performed using the non- parametric Mann Whitney-U test.

Results

The ELISA system was proved to be very reliable, giving little variation between duplicates and the serial dilution of the pure stem cell factor produced a linear absorbance graph. The serum free medium which had not been conditioned by cells and the «15 minute conditioned medium» contained no detectable stem cell factor.

Medium conditioned for 24 hours by non-balding scalp dermal papilla cells (n=7) contained 3.10 ± 0.55 pg/ml/µg protein [mean ± SEM] of stem cell factor, whilst beard dermal papilla cells (n=6) contained significantly higher (p=0.001) levels of stem cell factor (7.18 ± 1.72 pg/ml/µg protein) (Fig. 1). Dermal

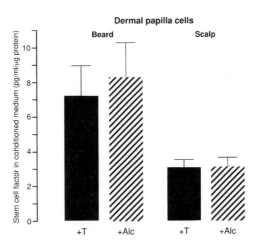

Figure 1. The concentration of stem cell factor in dermal papilla cell conditioned medium

fibroblasts from beard (n=3) and non-balding scalp (n=2) also produced detectable levels of stem cell factor. There were no differences in the amounts produced by beard (1.76 ± 0.79 pg/ml/μg protein) and non-balding scalp fibroblasts (1.42 ± 0.76 pg/ml/μg protein), but the levels were significantly lower (p=0.004) than that produced by beard dermal papilla cells. Testosterone in vitro had no effect on the amounts of stem cell factor produced by any cell type.

Discussion

Dermal papilla cells and dermal fibroblasts derived from beard and non-balding scalp skin were shown to be capable of producing stem cell factor in culture. No stem cell factor was detected in the «15 minute conditioned medium», thereby indicating that the stem cell factor was actually secreted by the cells in the 24 hour period, and not present in the flasks as a residual contamination from previous incubation conditions.

There were no differences in the production of stem cell factor by dermal fibroblasts or any testosterone stimulation. However, androgen-dependent beard dermal papilla cells secreted significantly higher levels of stem cell factor than non-balding scalp dermal papilla cells or dermal fibroblasts. In vivo, beard hairs are generally highly pigmented under androgenic stimulation which could account for these differences. The lack of testosterone in vitro stimulation could possibly be explained by a slow response to testosterone by the stem cell factor genes, or more likely, the genes are triggered by events prior to, or in early anagen, whereas dermal papilla cells used in this study were taken from later in the hair cycle.

The results of this study indicate that the dermal papilla could act as a local source of stem cell factor in the hair follicle and may be important in the regulation of hair follicle pigmentation. Androgens may be capable of altering the production of stem cell factor by the dermal papilla only at specific times in the hair cycle. Cultured dermal papilla cells do contain androgen receptors [18] and can respond to androgens in vitro in culture by secreting additional mitogenic factors [15, 19], thereby showing the validity studying these cells.

References

1   Slominski A, Paus R, Plonka P, Chakraborty A, Maurer M, Pruski D, Lukiewicz S. J Invest Dermatol. 1994; 102: 862-869
2   Slominski A, Paus R. J Invest Dermatol. 1993; 101: 90S-97S
3   Chase HB. Adv Skin Biol. 1966; 8: 503-507
4   Ortonne JP, Prota G. J Invest Dermatol. 1993; 101: 82S-89S
5   Williams DE, DeVries P, Namen AE, Widmer M, Lyman SD. Dev Biol. 1992; 151: 368-378
6   Zsebo KM, Williams DA, Geissler EN, Broudy VC, Martin FH, Atkins HL, Hsu R-Y, Birkett NC, Okino KH, Murdock DC, Jacobsen FW, Langley KE, Smith KA, Cattanach BM, Galli SJ, Suggs SV. Cell. 1990; 63: 213-224

7 Fleischman RA, Saltman DL, Stasyny V, Zneimer S. Proc Natl Acad Sci USA. 1991; 10: 885-889
8 Nishikawa S, Kusakabe M, Yoshinaga K, Ogawa M, Hayshi S-I, Kurisada T, Eva T, Sakakura T, Nishikawa SI. EMBO J. 1991; 10: 2111-2118
9 Okura M, Maeda H, Nishikawa S, Mizoguchi M. J Invest Dermatol. 1995; 105: 322-328
10 Randall VA. Clin Endocrinol. 1994; 40: 439-457
11 Itami S, Kurata S, Sonoda T, Takayasu S. J Invest Dermatol 1991; 96: 57-60
12 Randall VA Thornton MJ, Hamada K, Redfern CPF, Nutbrown M, Ebling FJ, Messenger AG. Ann NY Acad Sci. 1991; 642: 355-375.
13 Lynfield YL. J Invest Dermatol. 1960; 35: 323-327
14 Jackson D, Church RE, Ebling FJ. Br J Dermatol. 1972; 87: 361- 367
15 Itami S, Kurata S, Sonoda T, Takayasu S. Br J Dermatol. 1995; 132: 527-532
16 Messenger AG. Br J Dermatol. 1984; 110: 685-689
17 Bradford MM. Biochemistry. 1976; 72: 248-254
18 Randall VA, Thornton MJ, Messenger AG. J Endocrinol. 1992; 133: 141-147
19 Hibberts NA, Quick JR, Messenger AG, Randall VA. Br J Dermatol. 1994; 131(suppl): 427

Author index

Subject index

496

Colour plates

Generalized congenital hypotrichosis and male pseudohermaphroditism

J.-J. Stene *et al.*

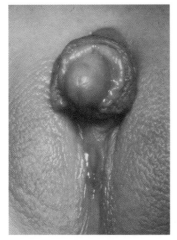

Figure 1. Sexual ambiguity

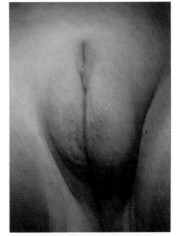

Figure 2. After surgical correction

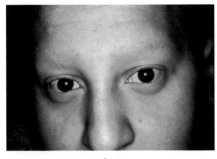

Figure 3. Hypotrichosis

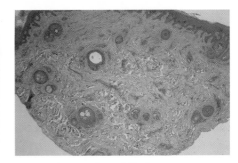

Figure 4. Rare hair follicles

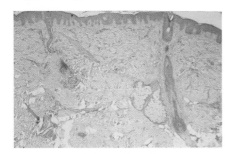

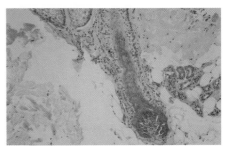

Figures 5 and 6. Trichomalacia and apoptosis

Histological changes in rat vibrissal follicles after electrolysis and the optimum length of time to apply the current

K. Tezuka *et al.*

page 127

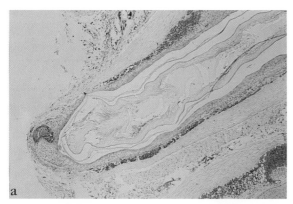

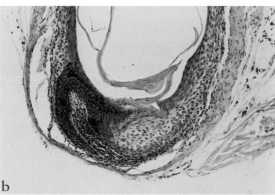

Figure 1 (a-b) Vibrissal follicles at 10 weeks after the 4-sec thermolysis which shows successful electrolysis

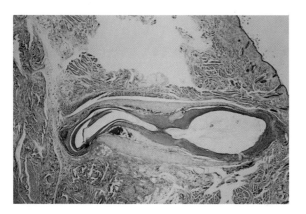

Figure 2. Vibrissal follicles at 10 weeks after the 40 sec blend which shows over treatment

What is new in scalp cosmetic surgery ?

P. Pouteaux and D. Van Neste

page 131

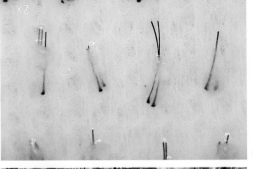

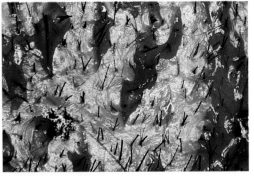

a

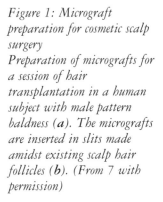

Figure 1: Micrograft preparation for cosmetic scalp surgery
*Preparation of micrografts for a session of hair transplantation in a human subject with male pattern baldness (**a**). The micrografts are inserted in slits made amidst existing scalp hair follicles (**b**). (From 7 with permission)*

b

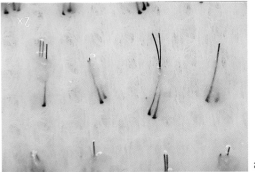

a

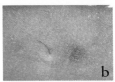

b

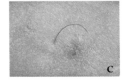

c

Figure 2: Cosmetic surgery techniques applied in the research laboratory (modified after [6])
*Specimen preparation, skin incision and micrograft implantation has been performed onto nude mice in a similar way as shown in figure. 1. This results in «hairy islands» producing 1 up to 3 human hairs in the nude mouse skin (tattoos serve as site markers). This serial photography, performed 3 months after grafting onto nude mice, illustrates a single hair growing from a micrograft placed just between the two tattoos: (**a**) immediately after clipping, (**b**) 4 days later and (**c**) 15 days later. When hair follicles were horizontally sectionned, there was always less hair growth (lower two thirds of the follicle) or no growth at all when the lower third of the follicle was engrafted (Caroline Tételin personal communication).*

Recognition of cellular differentiation in the human hair follicle at the light microscope level using SACPIC staining

M. Nutbrown and V.A. Randall

page 161

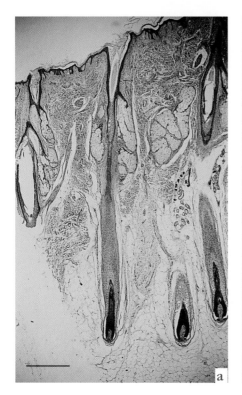
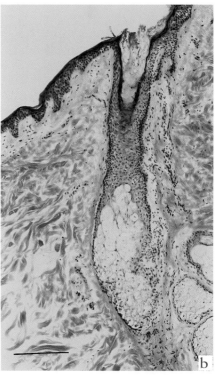

Figure 1a. Human scalp skin in wax stained with SACPIC
Keratinized parts of hair fibres (yellow) are easily distinguished. Collagen and the outer root sheath clearly stain a different blue from non-keratinizing epithelial cells of sebaceous glands and hair fibre. Scale bar: 600 μm

Figure 1b. Section of frozen human scalp skin stained with SACPIC
Collagen is stained an intense blue. Dark blue/black nuclei surrounded by purple cytoplasm are seen in the non-keratinizing portions of the epithelial tissues. Keratinized epithelium shows strong red staining. Scale bar: 200 μm

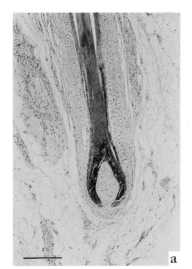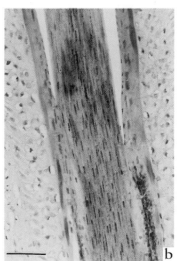

Figure 2a. Human anagen hair follicle; wax section stained with SACPIC
The individual layers of Henle, Huxley and the cuticle of the inner root sheath (all shades of red) are easily discerned. Differentiation of these layers is also distinguished by the changes in staining intensity and hue. Non-keratinizing epithelial cells all display dark blue nuclei with a purple/dark pink cytoplasm. Scale bar: 200 μm

Figure 2b. High power view of anagen follicle; wax section stained with SACPIC
This view shows the Henle and Huxley layers and inner root sheath at about three times dermal papilla height. Keratinizing cells of Henle's layer can be distinguished from non-keratinizing cells by the increased intensity of staining. Trichohyalin granules (orange/brown) can be seen in Huxley's layer in the lower part of the micrograph. Several changes can be seen in the staining pattern of the hair fibre, from the lower region of pre-keratinization (pink/blue) to higher portions of the fibre (yellow) which are fully keratinized. Scale bar: 50 μm

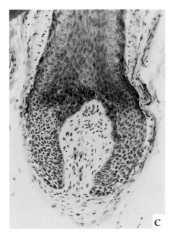

Figure 2c. Bulb of anagen hair follicle from frozen section of human scalp skin (SACPIC)
The extracellular matrix of the dermal papilla stains pale blue whereas the dermal papilla cells themselves are an intense blue with darker nuclei. The epithelial cells of the germinative layers and undifferentiated matrix have blue/purple nuclei with paler cytoplasm which contrasts with the brown/black deposits of melanin in the cells of the adjacent presumptive cortical region. Scale bar: 60 μm

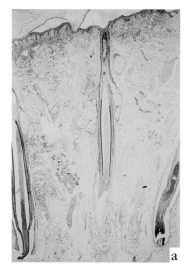
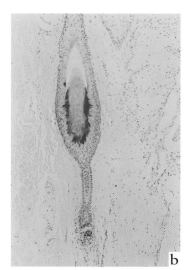

Figure 3a. Wax section of hair follicle at the end of catagen or in early telogen (SACPIC)
The keratinized hair fibre is stained mostly yellow with red tinges at the brush end of the club hair. The collapsing sac of the connective tissue sheath (pale blue) extends below the end of the hair fibre. Scale bar: 500 μm

Figure 3b. Late catagen/telogen follicle, oblique wax section (SACPIC)
The epithelial tissue including the epithelial stalk with the ball of the dermal papilla at its end are stained blue. Differential staining of the keratinized (yellow) and partly keratinized (red) hair fibres is evident. Scale bar: 120 μm

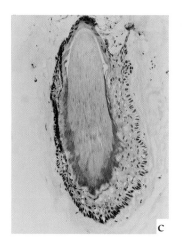

Figure 3c. Detail of brush end of hair fibre in telogen follicle from a frozen section of human scalp skin (SACPIC)
Distinction can easily be made between the fully keratinized hair fibre (yellow) and the brush border (red) of the end of the club hair. The non-keratinizing epithelial cells (blue) are clearly distinguished from the pale blue of the connective tissue sheath. Scale bar: 60 μ

Regeneration of the human scalp hair follicle after horizontal sectioning : implications for pluripotent stem cells and melanocyte reservoir

J.C. Kim *et al.*   page 135

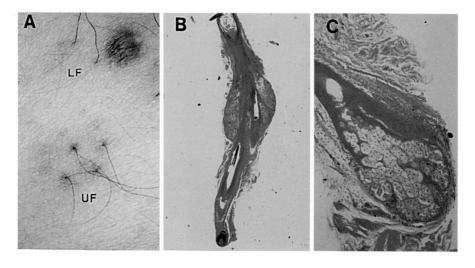

Figure 1. **A** *: Surface view of the leg, 8 months after grafting upper and lower 1/2 grafts.*
UF : regrown hairs from upper 1/2 grafts ; LF : regrown hairs from lower 1/2 grafts.
B *: Longitudinal section of a regenerated follicle from an upper 1/2 graft, 2 years after grafting (magnification x10).*
C *: Light micrograph of the sebaceous gland regenerated from a lower 1/2 graft, 2 years after grafting (magnification x100)*

©1996 Elsevier Science B.V. All rights reserved.
Hair research for the next millenium
D.J.J. Van Neste and V.A. Randall (Eds)

Reconstitution of hair follicles by rotation culture

A. Takeda *et al.*   page 191

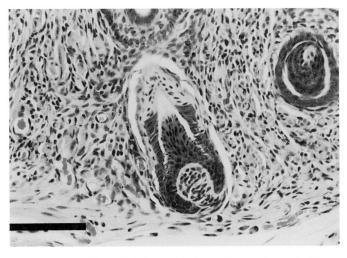

Figure 1. Reconstruction of hair follicles at 10 days after grafting of cell aggregates produced by rotation and flotation culture (H&E stains). Scale bar=100 μm

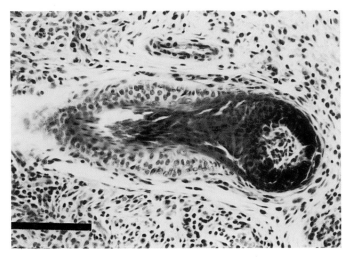

Figure 2. Reconstruction of hair follicles at 10 days after grafting of cell aggregates produced by rotation culture only (H&E stains). Scale bar=100 μm